ACE THE BOARDS:
DERMATOPATHOLOGY

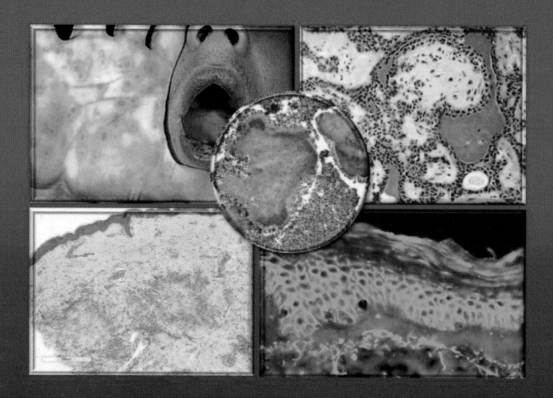

RAJENDRA SINGH, MD

ASHLEY ELSENSOHN, MD
CHRISTINE AHN, MD
AKANKSHA GUPTA, MD

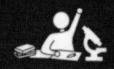

ACE MY PATH
PathPresenter

First Edition

ISBN: 9798882959660
Copyright ©2024: Akanksha Gupta, MD
Follow us on Twitter @AceMyPath
Email: acemypath@gmail.com
Website: www.acemypath.com

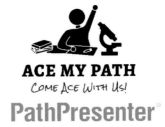

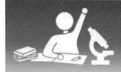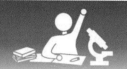
It is with immense pleasure that I commend Raj Singh and his team for this remarkable contribution to the field of dermatopathology education – "Ace the Boards: Dermatopathology."

Raj's dedication to teaching and knowledge sharing is truly inspiring. Through his innovative online platform, Path Presenter, he has empowered countless learners with access to exceptional educational resources. His tireless efforts extend beyond the virtual realm, with the organization of engaging in-person and online events that foster a vibrant community of dermatology and pathology professionals.

Raj's expertise extends far beyond his deep understanding of dermatopathology. He possesses a unique talent for collaborating with skilled technologists, ensuring the seamless development and delivery of these invaluable resources. Driven by a genuine passion for education, Raj has consistently invested both his time and personal resources into these endeavors, recognizing the profound impact they have on learners worldwide.

Ace the Boards: Dermatopathology represents the culmination of Raj's vision and commitment. This groundbreaking book offers a comprehensive and accessible learning experience, featuring over 400 QR codes linking to virtual slides, a wealth of high-quality clinical and microscopic images, and a clear, concise presentation perfectly tailored for board preparation.

I have no doubt that Ace the Boards: Dermatopathology will achieve the same level of success as Raj's renowned platform. This exceptional resource is poised to become an indispensable tool for students, residents, and dermatopathologists seeking to excel in their field.

RONALD P. RAPINI, M.D.
Marvin E. Chernosky, M.D. Endowed Distinguished Chair
Department of Dermatology
Professor of Pathology
University of Texas Medical School and MD Anderson Cancer Center
Houston, TX

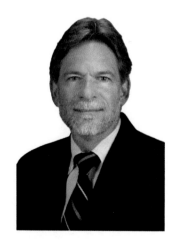

Dr. Rapini is the Distinguished Chernosky Professor and chair of the Department of Dermatology at McGovern Medical School. Dr. Rapini also serves as chair of the Department of Dermatology at The University of Texas MD Anderson Cancer Center, and professor of Pathology at both institutions. He has served as the president of the American Board of Dermatology, the American Society of Dermatopathology, the American Society for Mohs Surgery, the Houston Dermatological Society, and the Texas Dermatological Society. Several society awards have recognized his work, such as the Walter Nickel Award from the American Society of Dermatopathology for excellence in teaching in 2005. He also received the Founder's Award from American Society of Dermatopathology in 2012, and the Robert G. Freeman Mentoring and Leadership award from the Texas Dermatological Society in 2013.

He is the sole author of the textbook, Practical Dermatopathology (2005, Mosby), which is widely used around the world, and the former lead co-editor of the two-volume text Dermatology (2nd. ed 2007, Mosby). He has published over 152 peer-reviewed articles and has been a speaker at 473 meetings in the US and throughout the world. He has also authored 65 textbook chapters.

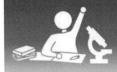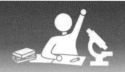
For generations, pathology knowledge has been transferred by our dedicated teachers on multiheaded microscopes diligently pointing out features on the slide that help formulate a differential diagnosis and approach to pathologic classification. However, this pedagogical method is limited to a small number of local students that can sit around a microscope. The purpose of authoring another book on dermatopathology was to simulate this method of learning for readers who do not have the benefit of having spectacular teachers patiently doing the same.

The book is unique, as it not only straight away presents the most characteristic clinical and histological features for every diagnosis, it also allows the readers to scan QR codes that link to whole slide annotated images. In the current technologically advanced world, mobile devices are ubiquitous and work even in remote locations. This technology bridges the educational divide and allows readers worldwide to directly open and interact with the whole slide images as if they are sitting across from an esteemed faculty at the multiheaded microscope.

The book would not be possible without the leadership of two esteemed colleagues-Ashley Elsensohn and Christine Ahn who have dedicated innumerable hours putting the material together and ensuring that the content is updated and accurate Ashley's organizational skills and Christine's attention to detail are par excellence, and their dedication and passion kept the entire team motivated and on track during the marathon schedule of 12 months to complete the book.

The chapter authors Jesús Alberto Cárdenas de la Garza, Lorena Maia Campos Costa, George Mukosera, Terrance J Lynn, Snehal Sonawane, Pooja Srivastava, Angela Jiang, Franchesca Choi, Daniel Gonzalez, Aayushma Regmi, Chelsea Huang, Nathan Bowers, Cassy Drew, Chiara Tognaccini, Michael Greas, Marina Ibraheim, and Michael Lee dedicated numerous hours and attention to complete this book. Having the opportunity to work with so many talented individuals from various places and stages in their careers was a true joy.

Above all, this would not have been possible without the vision and hard work of Akanksha Gupta. She has been the visionary who brought the concepts of Ace My Path books to life and works with great passion to ensure the books are of the highest quality and presented in a way that is very reader focused. We had previously collaborated to write "Surgical Pathology Reimagined" and the immense love and feedback received from all around the globe encouraged us to author this book.

The purpose of these books has not only been to be a great resource, but to ensure it feels and functions like a 21st century book that uses modern technology to enhance the reader's experience. We have tried our best to ensure that it becomes a useful and handy resource for pathology and dermatology trainees as well as practicing pathologists, especially those that have not gone through a dermatopathology fellowship. Recent updates from literature have been included to ensure it is also useful for practicing dermatopathologists.

Finally, this book would not have been possible without the unwavering support of my wife, Manisha, and my children, Satyen and Kritika who have been the selfless anchors of my life. I will always stay indebted to them as well as my numerous mentors and colleagues who have guided me at every step of my life.

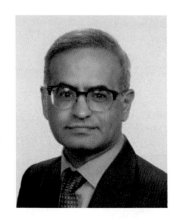

RAJENDRA SINGH, MD
Director of Dermatopathology
Director, Digital Pathology
Summit Health, New Jersey, NJ

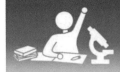 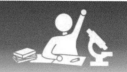
"A Game-Changer in Dermatopathology: A Must-Have Reference
This groundbreaking dermatopathology book modernizes the way we approach skin pathology - a true game-changer in the field. One of the standout features of this book is its innovative use of annotated whole slide images (WSI), easily accessible through QR codes. This unique approach allows readers to delve into the microscopic details of excellent histological images and in addition of 448 WSI, tremendously enhancing the learning experience and providing an outstanding visual aid. Each diagnosis is accompanied by up-to-date information, reflecting the latest advancements in the field and with a special focus is put on the differential diagnostic aspects. The information is presented in a concise and organized manner. Authored by experts in skin pathology, this book seamlessly integrates comprehensive information on most common inflammatory and neoplastic skin diseases, making it an indispensable resource for both dermpath and non-dermpath pathologists and fellows in preparation for the board exams. The emphasis on keeping content to the point enhances the book's practicality, allowing dermpathologists and general pathologists to efficiently navigate and make informed decisions while signing out cases. This dermatopathology book with its integration of annotated WSI and comprehensive coverage of common diagnoses is a milestone. I recommend it to anyone involved in dermatopathology."

WERNER KEMPF, MD
Professor of Dermatology
Consultant Dermatopathologist at the Dept of Dermatology
University Hospital Zürich, Zürich, Switzerland

"I am honored to endorse Professor Rajendra Singh's superb dermatopathology text, "Ace My Path, Ace the Boards: Dermatopathology" Dr Singh and colleagues share a comprehensive set of clinical and pathologic descriptions and images across the spectrum of dermatopathology. Each entity is presented with color photos of the clinical presentation and histology, and bullet points in text on key features including differential diagnosis. The pages link by 2D barcode to PathPresenter images easily accessible by cellphone or hyperlink from the digital format.

This book is relevant to all students of dermatopathology- as a board review resource for residents and fellows, and also as a convenient reference for those of us later in our profession, sitting continuing proficiency exams. "

MICHAEL HITCHCOCK MBCHB, MBA
Clinical Lead Pathologist
Anatomic Pathology Services
Auckland District Health Board, Auckland, New Zealand

"In Ace My Path: Dermatopathology, Dr Rajendra Singh and his colleagues introduce a ground-breaking educational resource for learning and mastering skin pathology, preparing for board and certification examinations, and to serve as an essential reference for both pathologists and dermatopathologists alike. This authoritative yet compact atlas provides succinct descriptions of all the essential entities encountered in routine work. An unprecedented benefit is direct access to 440 digitized whole slide histopathological images in Path Presenter online. This work is supplemented by some 2000 additional images detailing gross and microscopic features, immunohistochemistry, and other ancillary information."

RAYMOND BARNHILL, MD
Professor of Pathology
Co-Director, Dermatopathology
David Geffen School of Medicine at UCLA, Los Angeles, CA

"As a hematopathologist with a passion for medical education, I am thoroughly impressed by this comprehensive dermatopathology textbook Its accessibility and practicality stand out, making it an invaluable resource not just for those specializing in dermatopathology but for pathologists across various subspecialties. The innovative integration of annotated whole slide images via QR codes transforms this

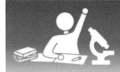 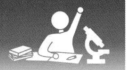

book into an interactive learning tool, bridging the gap between traditional textbooks and digital pathology. The concise yet comprehensive coverage of common diagnoses, combined with the latest updates in the field, ensures that this book is not only a reference but a cornerstone for real-time diagnostic decision-making Its clarity and to-the-point information make it an essential companion for both seasoned and novice pathologists. I wholeheartedly endorse this book for its remarkable contribution to the field of pathology and medical education."

KAMRAN M MIRZA, MD PHD
Professor of Hematopathology
Department of Pathology
University of Michigan Health, Ann Arbor, MI

"I am delighted to endorse this Ace the Boards: Dermatopathology textbook edited by Dr Raj Singh. This book is unique because, in partnership with PathPresenter, it provides the reader with easy access to over 440 carefully selected and annotated whole slide images Besides this innovative attribute, the book is perfectly designed for those who want to quickly master dermatopathology. The text is concise, perfectly highlights key points, and contains countless stunning photos."

LIRON PATANOWITZ, MD
Professor and Chair of Pathology
Director of Pathology Informatics Fellowship
University of Pittsburg Medical Center, Pittsburg, PA

"This is certainly a resource that will enable one to ace their dermatopathology boards! It combines beautiful histologic and clinical images with easy-to-read bulleted text. In addition, each case has a link to an excellent, illustrative digital slide. I would have loved to have this resource when I was studying for my board examination. Furthermore, I think this text will be a valuable reference for practicing dermatopathologists for the efficient way it presents critical information."

STEVEN BILLINGS, MD
Professor of Dermatopathology
Co-director of the Dermatopathology section
Cleveland Clinic, Cleveland, OH

"Raj has been a leader in creating online educational resources for dermatopathology. This book serves as a wonderful introduction to dermatopathology for beginners and as an excellent reference for those in practice. The quality of both path and clinical images is excellent Well done Raj!

DIRK M ELSTON, MD
Professor and Chair
Department of Dermatology and Dermatologic Surgery
Medical University of South Carolina, Charleston, SC

"This book sets the new standard of conveying knowledge in the field of pathology with a concise text accompanied by multiple illustrations; including easy-to-access high quality whole slide images."

DR ARNAUD DE LA FOUCHARDIÈRE, MD, PhD
Département de Biopathologie
Centre Léon Bérard, 28, rue Laennec, Lyon, France

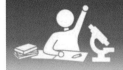 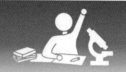

"To my wife, Manisha, daughter Kritika and son, Satyen who have selflessly sacrificed a lot and allowed me to follow my passions. To all my friends, mentors and colleagues who have been supportive and encouraging every step of the way."

- RAJENDRA SINGH, MD

"I would like to thank my family, friends, and mentors over the years-- I have been blessed with love and support! Also thank you to my colleagues and trainees at Loma Linda University, who make me better both professionally and personally."

- ASHLEY ELSENSOHN, MD

"To my mentors, colleagues, and co-authors, for all of their hard work on this team effort, and to all of the budding dermatologists and dermatopathologists who may benefit from this book."

- CHRISTINE AHN, MD

"To God, for instilling a "purpose of life" in me. To my passionate mentors, for instilling in me the passion for Pathology. To my parents, Maya Gupta and Jugalkishore Gupta, for instilling my values and my character and for living a life that I can take inspiration from. To my loving husband, Ashish Gupta, for demonstrating going after one's ambition, encouraging me to fulfill my dreams and pushing me every day to become my best self. And lastly, to my son and best friend, Siddharth Gupta, for reminding me every day that I matter!"

- AKANKSHA GUPTA, MD

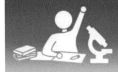
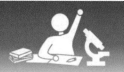
MAIN EDITOR / AUTHOR

RAJENDRA SINGH, MD
Director of Dermatopathology
Director, Digital Pathology
Summit Health, New Jersey, NJ

ASSOCIATE EDITORS / AUTHORS

AKANKSHA GUPTA, MD
Founder and CEO, Ace My Path, LLC
Medical Director, Pathology Laboratory
McLaren Central Michigan, Mt Pleasant, MI
Hematopathologist and Surgical Pathologist
Integrated Pathology Associates, MI

ASHLEY ELSENSOHN, MD, MPH
Assistant Professor of Dermatology and Pathology
Loma Linda University
Loma Linda, CA

CHRISTINE AHN, MD
Assistant Professor of Dermatology and Pathology
Wake Forest University School of Medicine
Winston-Salem, NC

AUTHORS

ANGELA JIANG, MD
Assistant Professor of Dermatology
Oregon Health and Sciences University
Portland, OR

DANIEL GONZALEZ, MD
Dermatopathologist
Compass Dermatopathology
San Diego, CA

MICHAEL GREAS, MD
Assistant Professor
Dermatopathologist, Hematopathologist
Loma Linda University
Loma Linda, CA

NATHAN BOWERS, MD, PhD
Dermatologist & Dermatopathologist
Knoxville Institute of Dermatology
Knoxville, TN

SNEHAL SONAWANE, MD
Assistant Professor
University of Illinois at Chicago
Chicago, IL

JESUS ALBERTO CARDENAS-DE LA GARZA, MD
Assistant Professor & Dermatologist
Universidad Autónoma de Nuevo León
Monterrey, Mexico

POOJA SRIVASTAVA, MD
Dermatopathologist
Marshfield Clinic
Marshfield, WI

TERRANCE LYNN, MD, MS, MHCI
Molecular Genetic Pathology Fellow
University of Nebraska
Omaha, NE

MARINA KRISTY IBRAHEIM, MD
Dermatology Resident
Loma Linda University
Loma Linda, CA

MICHAEL LEE, MD
Dermatology Resident
Loma Linda University
Loma Linda, CA

AAYUSHMA REGMI, MBBS
Pathology Resident
Loyola University Medical Center
Chicago, IL

CHELSEA HUANG, MD
Pathology Resident
Loma Linda University
Loma Linda, CA

LORENA MAIA CAMPOS COSTA, MD
Pathology Resident
Wake Forest University
Winston-Salem, NC

FRANCHESCA CHOI, MD RPh
Dermatology Resident
University of Wisconsin, Madison, WI

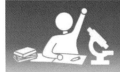
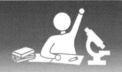

CASSANDRA DREW PROEBSTLE, MD
Family Medicine Resident
Kaiser Permanente Fontana
Fontana, CA

GEORGE TINOTENDA MUKOSERA, PhD
Medical Student
Loma Linda University
Loma Linda, CA

CHIARA TOGNACCINI
Medical Student
California University of Science and Medicine
Colton, CA

REVIEWERS

NEHA SETH, MD
Hematopathology fellow 2024-25
Donald and Barbara Zucker School of Medicine
at Hofstra/Northwell, Greenvale, NY
Former Practicing Hematopathologist
CMC Vellore, TN India
Sehgal Path Lab, Mumbai, India

ZARINE KAMALUDDIN, MD
Assistant Professor
UPMC Shadyside, PA

AAKASH BHATIA, MBBS, MD
Hematopathology and Surgical Pathology
University of Texas MD Anderson Cancer Center, TX

PRIH ROHRA, MD
Cytopathology fellowship
Surgical Pathology fellowship
MD Anderson Cancer Center, Houston, TX
Practicing Pathologist
Midvalley Pathology, Weslaco, TX

ABHILASHA NITIN BORKAR, MD
Cytopathology fellowship
Loyola University Medical Center
Chicago, IL
Resident Physician
UTHSC, Memphis, TN

RADHIKA SEKHRI, MD
Surgical Pathology Fellow (PGY4)
Vanderbilt University
Nashville, TN

HARINI VENKATRAMAN RAVISANKAR, MD
Post Doc fellow, Dept of Hematopathology
Indiana University

HARSHITA MEHROTRA, MD
Fellow, Oncologic Surgical Pathology
Department of Pathology and Laboratory Medicine
Memorial Sloan Kettering Cancer Center

MANASA MORISETTI, MD
Resident Physician
Anatomic and Clinical Pathology Department,
LSU Health Shreveport

BHANUPRIYA KAKARALA, MD
Resident Physician
Anatomic and Clinical Pathology
Boston Medical Centre

KOMAL LAKHANI MD
Resident Physician
Anatomic and Clinical Pathology
Cooperman Barnabas Medical Center/ Rutgers Health

TEHMINA HASHIM, MD
Research Assistant, Dept of Pathology
University of Illinois at Chicago

T RAMA DEVI, MD
Assistant professor of pathology
Present **DM** Oncopathology resident
Gujarat Cancer Research Institute (GCRI)
Ahmedabad, India

ABHINAV GROVER, MD
Resident Physician
Pathology and Laboratory Medicine
Medical College of Wisconsin

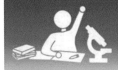 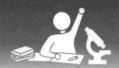

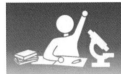
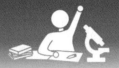

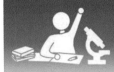
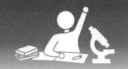

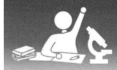
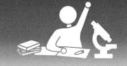

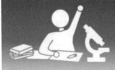
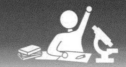

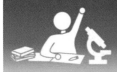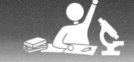

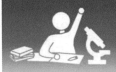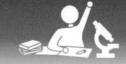

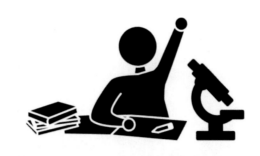

ACE MY PATH

Come Ace With Us!

SECTION 1: NEOPLASTIC
DERMATOPATHOLOGY

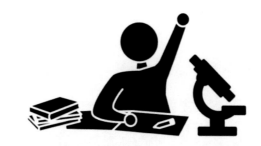

ACE MY PATH
Come Ace With Us!

CHAPTER 1: CYSTS

ASHLEY ELSENSOHN, MD

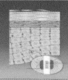

CHAPTER 1: CYSTS

CYSTS

Dermal cyst with loose keratin contents

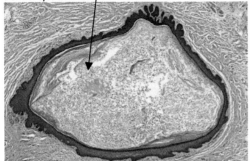

Loose, lamellar keratin contents

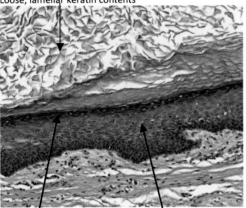

Granular layer   Squamous epithelium

Path Presenter

EPIDERMOID CYST

CLINICAL FEATURES
- Firm skin colored subcutaneous nodule with central punctum and **cheesy contents** with a **pungent odor**
- Typical locations are the trunk, face, neck, and scalp
- Clinical Differential Diagnosis: Dermoid Cyst, Calcinosis Cutis, Branchial cleft Cyst, Dilated Pore of Winer, Lipoma, Dermatofibroma

HISTOLOGIC FEATURES
- Cyst lined by squamous epithelium with **granular layer**
- Contains **lamellated keratin**

OTHER HIGH YIELD POINTS
- Differentiates towards the follicular infundibulum, also called an **Infundibular cyst**
- "Epidermal inclusion cyst" is somewhat a misnomer since most are not associated with inclusions or prior trauma
- Small epidermoid cysts are known as milia

DIFFERENTIAL DIAGNOSIS
- PILAR CYST - compact eosinophilic keratin and an absent granular layer
- FOLLICULAR HYBRID CYST - elements of epidermoid cyst in addition to other areas reminiscent of other follicular cysts such as a pilar cyst
- VERRUCOUS CYST - acanthotic, papillated cyst wall with hypergranulation, prominent keratohyalin granules, and koilocytes

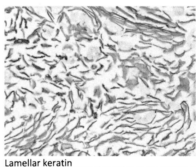

Lamellar keratin   Subcutaneous nodule with central punctum

Papillated squamous epithelium

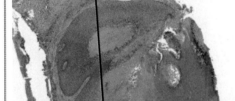

Compact eosinophilic keratin

VERRUCOUS CYST

CLINICAL FEATURES
- Firm skin colored subcutaneous nodule often with central pore
- Clinical Differential Diagnosis: Dermoid Cyst, Calcinosis Cutis, Branchial cleft Cyst, Dilated Pore of Winer, Lipoma, Cellular Dermatofibroma

HISTOLOGIC FEATURES
- **Epidermal cyst** lined by papillated epithelium with **hypergranulosis** and irregular **keratohyalin granules**
- Vacuolated keratinocytes resembling **koilocytes** may be seen

OTHER HIGH YIELD POINTS
- Pathogenesis: Type of epidermal inclusion cyst with papillomatous cyst wall associated with infection by the **human papilloma virus (HPV)**
- It resembles an **epidermoid cyst with viral changes** and acanthotic and/or papillomatous epithelium

DIFFERENTIAL DIAGNOSIS
- EPIDERMOID CYST - absent koilocytes and papillation (no viral changes present). Loose lamellar keratin
- PILAR CYST - absent granular layer without koilocytes or papillation (no viral changes present)

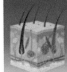
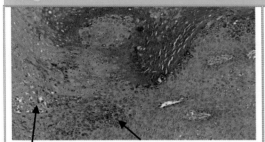

Koilocytes   Hypergranulosis

Path Presenter

- PROLIFERATING PILAR CYST - Rolls and scrolls appearance on low power
  Absent koilocytes and papillation (no viral changes present)

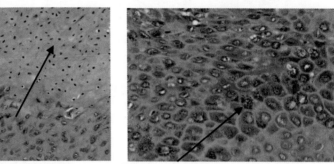

Rounded parakeratosis   Hypergranulosis and prominent keratohyalin granules

Dermal cyst (often on scalp skin)

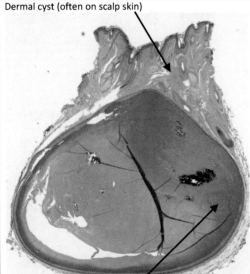

Compact eosinophilic keratin
Trichilemmal keratinization—no granular layer

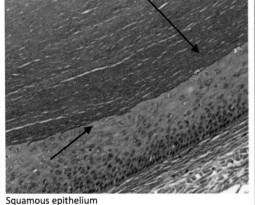

Squamous epithelium

Path Presenter

PILAR CYST

CLINICAL FEATURES

- Firm skin colored nodule without a central punctum
- Most pilar cysts are located on the **scalp** but can be seen at other locations. May be inherited as an autosomal dominant trait
- Clinical Differential Diagnosis: Epidermoid cyst, Lipoma, Proliferating Pilar cyst

HISTOLOGIC FEATURES

- Cyst wall lined by **squamous epithelium** with abrupt keratinization, **absent granular layer**
- **Compact**, deeply eosinophilic homogenized **keratin**
- Focal calcification of contents or cholesterol cleft in middle can be seen

OTHER HIGH YIELD POINTS

- Differentiates towards the follicular isthmus. Derived from outer root sheath/ trichilemma – no granular layer (aka **trichilemmal keratinization**)

DIFFERENTIAL DIAGNOSIS

- EPIDERMOID CYST - granular layer present, loose lamellar keratin
- FOLLICULAR HYBRID CYST - elements of epidermoid cyst in addition to other areas reminiscent of other follicular cysts such as a pilar cyst
- PROLIFERATING PILAR CYST - rolls and scrolls appearance on low power

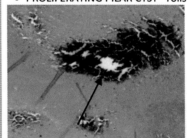
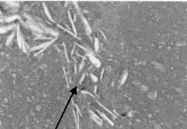

Focal calcification   Cholesterol clefts

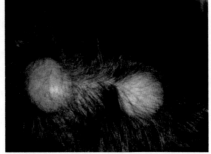

Subcutaneous, firm nodule(s) on the scalp

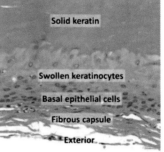

Solid keratin

Swollen keratinocytes

Basal epithelial cells

Fibrous capsule

Exterior

Image by Mikael Häggström, MD

Rolls and scrolls appearance (multilobular)

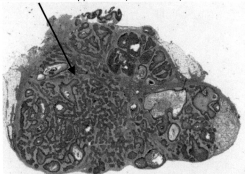

Squamous epithelium

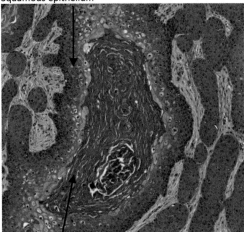

Abrupt trichilemmal keratinization

Path Presenter

PROLIFERATING PILAR CYST

CLINICAL FEATURES

- Firm subcutaneous nodule, may be ulcerated, often on **scalp of older woman**, often **large >6cm**, rarely locally destructive or malignant behavior
- Clinical Differential Diagnosis: Pilar Cyst, Epidermoid Cyst, Adnexal Neoplasm, Dermoid Cyst, Basal Cell Carcinoma, Angiosarcoma, Cylindroma, Lipoma

HISTOLOGIC FEATURES

- **Multilobulated** tumor composed of lobules of **squamous epithelium** showing abrupt **trichilemmal keratinization**
- Also-called "**rolls and scrolls**" appearance
- Peripheral palisading and thickened basement membrane may be noted
- Focal keratinization with squamous eddies. **Focal atypia, no infiltration**
- Sometimes **cholesterol clefting** seen

OTHER HIGH YIELD POINTS

- Also called a proliferating pilar "tumor." Some consider this to be a **low-grade squamous cell carcinoma**, needs to be **re-excised**
- Suspect trichilemmal carcinoma if not on scalp, recent rapid growth, significant atypical, or mitotic activity

DIFFERENTIAL DIAGNOSIS

- SQUAMOUS CELL CARCINOMA - infiltrative growth, cytologic dysplasia
- TRICHILEMMAL CARCINOMA - infiltrative growth pattern, cytologic dysplasia
- PILOMATRICOMA - presence of ghost cells, blue matrical areas

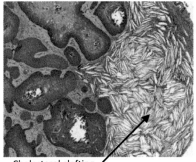 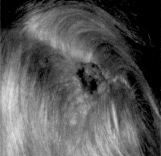

Cholesterol clefting | Large, ulcerated nodule on the scalp

Dermal cyst, debris filled cyst

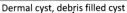

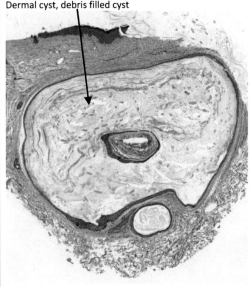

VELLUS HAIR CYST

CLINICAL FEATURES

- Typically **multiple** skin colored to pigmented, soft 1-5mm dome shaped papules on the **chest,** with an onset before young adulthood
- Typically parasternal but can be more generalized
- Clinical Differential Diagnosis: Acne Vulgaris, Eruptive Syringoma, Keratosis Pilaris, Trichostasis Spinulosa

HISTOLOGIC FEATURES

- **Debris-filled cyst** lined by pseudostratified columnar epithelium. May have admixed mucin secreting cells
- Many small **"football shaped" vellus hairs** within the cyst-- more keratin in cyst than in steatocystoma
- In general, represents epidermoid cyst with loose keratin and many small vellus hairs within cyst
- A small hair follicle may be seen at the base of the cyst

OTHER HIGH YIELD POINTS

- Associated with Lowe syndrome and **renal failure**
- Occasionally associated with **pachyonychia congenita 2 (keratin 17 mutation)**, as is steatocystoma multiplex

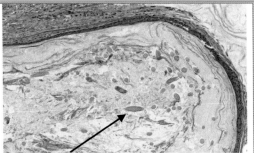
Numerous small, "football-shaped" vellus hairs

Path Presenter

DIFFERENTIAL DIAGNOSIS
- STEATOCYSTOMA - sebaceous glands in cyst wall, wavy "shark tooth" bright red cuticle
- EPIDERMOID CYST - absence of vellus hairs, only keratin present within cyst
- PILAR CYST - absence of vellus hairs, only compact eosinophilic keratin present within cyst

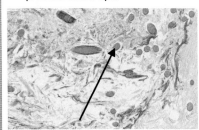

Vellus hairs within cyst | Multiple, soft dome-shaped papules on chest wall

STEATOCYSTOMA
CLINICAL FEATURES
- Yellowish cystic papule containing a **yellowish oily fluid** on the face, trunk, or extremities. Often **multiple** appear in **early adulthood**
- Clinical Differential Diagnosis: Acne Vulgaris, Epidermoid Cyst, Dermoid Cyst, Vellus Hair Cysts

HISTOLOGIC FEATURES
- Intradermal cyst lined by thin squamous epithelium. Center often "empty"
- Cyst lining has characteristic **wavy eosinophilic "shark tooth" cuticle**
- Compressed small **sebaceous glands** within or close to the **cyst wall**

OTHER HIGH YIELD POINTS
- Can be inherited as **autosomal dominant** trait (**Keratin 17** gene)

DIFFERENTIAL DIAGNOSIS
- EPIDERMOID CYST - loose keratin, absence of sebaceous glands in wall
- DERMOID CYST - adnexal structures (to include hair follicles) in wall
- MILIUM - loose keratin, absence of sebaceous glands in wall

Sebaceous glands within cyst wall

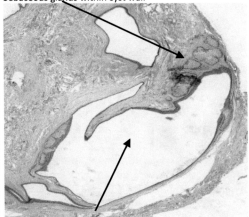

Often "empty" cyst contents

Sebaceous glands within cyst wall

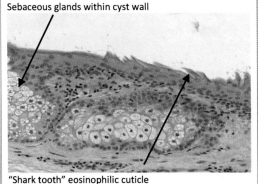

"Shark tooth" eosinophilic cuticle

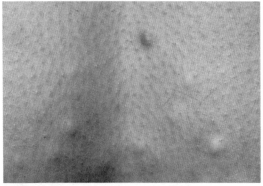
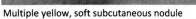

Multiple yellow, soft subcutaneous nodule | Path Presenter

Simple, unilocular cyst on eyelid skin

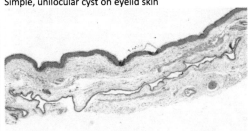

HIDROCYSTOMA
CLINICAL FEATURES
- Solitary, small **clear to bluish** cystic lesion located near the **eyelid** margin
- Sensitive to temperature changes - increases with heat and decreases with cold temperatures
- Multiple hidrocystomas are a feature of **ectodermal dysplasia** and focal dermal hypoplasia (**Goltz syndrome**)

Unilocular, empty cyst

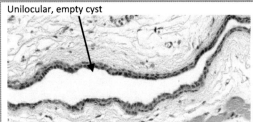

Two layers of cuboidal epithelial cells

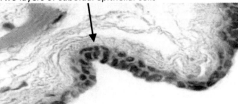

Path Presenter

- Clinical Differential Diagnosis: Epidermoid Cyst, Venous Lake, Chalazion, Basal Cell Carcinoma, Sebaceous Carcinoma

HISTOLOGIC FEATURES

- **Unilocular** cystic cavity lined by **two layers** of **cuboidal epithelial cells**
- Cyst appears **empty or contains clear fluid**
- Apocrine hidrocystomas tend to be multilocular compared to unilocular in eccrine hidrocystoma

OTHER HIGH YIELD POINTS

- May have **eccrine or apocrine** cells, with either merocrine or decapitation secretion
- Apocrine differentiation may have characteristic luminal, frond-like protrusions

DIFFERENTIAL DIAGNOSIS

- EPIDERMOID CYST – filled with loose lamellar keratin

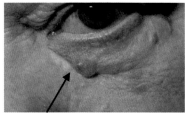
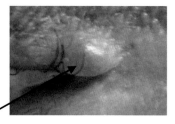

Clear to blue cystic nodule on the eyelid

Unilocular cyst

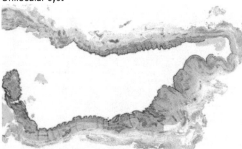

Psuedostratified columnar epithelium

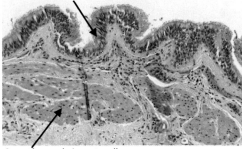

Smooth muscle in cyst wall

Path Presenter

BRONCHOGENIC CYST

CLINICAL FEATURES

- Developmental cyst at **suprasternal notch.** May be on anterior neck or chin
- **Solitary, present at birth, >50% asymptomatic**
- May present with **respiratory distress**, chest or back pain, **dysphagia**
- Complications include compression of vital structures (airway), ulcers/fistulas
- Rarely adenocarcinoma and rhabdomyosarcoma have been described
- Clinical Differential Diagnosis: Thyroglossal Duct Cyst, Goiter, Squamous Cell Carcinoma

HISTOLOGIC FEATURES

- **Unilocular** cyst lined by ciliated **pseudostratified columnar epithelium** with or without goblet cells containing bluish mucoid cytoplasm
- **Smooth muscle common** in wall. Occasional lymphoid follicles and cartilage

OTHER HIGH YIELD POINTS

- Most common cyst of middle mediastinum. Result of anomalous development of the ventral foregut and lung budding during first trimester
- **Goblet cells** can be present but not a prominent feature – **50%**
- **Circumferential smooth muscle** around cyst and cartilage are clues!

DIFFERENTIAL DIAGNOSIS

- BRANCHIAL CLEFT CYST - less circumferential smooth muscle, no cartilage
- THYMIC CYST - thymic tissue present
- EPIDERMOID CYST - filled with keratin, no goblet cells, squamous epithelium

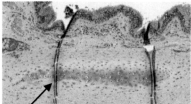
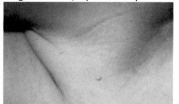

Cartilage

Skin colored nodule at suprasternal notch

Path Presenter

Dermal cyst with debris-filled contents

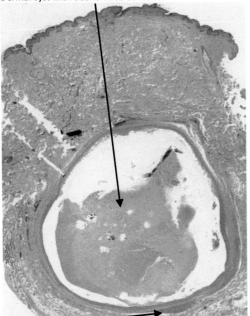

Lymphoid follicle along epithelial lining

Unilocular cyst

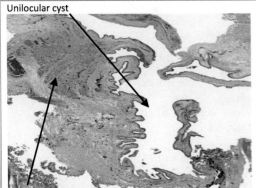

Thyroid follicles

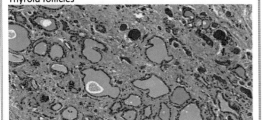

Path Presenter

BRANCHIAL CLEFT CYST

CLINICAL FEATURES

- Developmental cyst or sinus along the anterior border of the sternocleidomastoid muscle **(lateral neck)**. Can be **bilateral in 2-3%**
- The cyst can become inflamed and develop abscesses/draining sinus if ruptures. Swallowing or breathing difficulties if local impingement
- Clinical Differential Diagnosis: Cystic Hygroma, Epidermoid Cyst, Hemangioma, Goiter, Squamous Cell Carcinoma of Head and Neck

HISTOLOGIC FEATURES

- Cyst with lining of either **pseudostratified columnar epithelium** with or without cilia **or squamous epithelium** with granular layer
- **Lymphoid follicles** usually present. Abundant smooth muscle NOT present

OTHER HIGH YIELD POINTS

- Develops due to failure of obliteration of the **second branchial cleft** in embryonic development

DIFFERENTIAL DIAGNOSIS

- BRONCHOGENIC CYST - abundant smooth muscle present, typically midline
- THYMIC CYST - thymic tissue present at least focally in cyst wall
- EPIDERMOID CYST - absence of lymphoid follicles, squamous epithelium

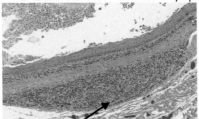
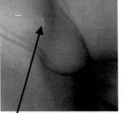

Lymphoid follicle

Cyst along anterior border of the neck

THYROGLOSSAL DUCT CYST

CLINICAL FEATURES

- Developmental cyst on the **midline anterior neck near the hyoid bone**
- Clinical Differential Diagnosis: Cutaneous Ciliated Cyst, Bronchogenic Cyst, Branchial Cleft Cyst, Dermoid Cyst, Epidermoid Cyst, Lipoma, Thyroid

HISTOLOGIC FEATURES

- **Unilocular** cyst with pseudostratified squamous or cuboidal ciliated epithelial lining. **Typically lined by respiratory type epithelium**
- **Surrounding thyroid follicles**
- May have goblet cells or lymphoid aggregates

OTHER HIGH YIELD POINTS

- Midline of neck **moves with swallowing**, unlike bronchogenic cyst

DIFFERENTIAL DIAGNOSIS

- BRONCHOGENIC CYST, BRANCHIAL CLEFT CYST, THYMIC CYST - Absence of thyroid follicles in all entities

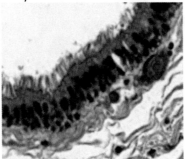
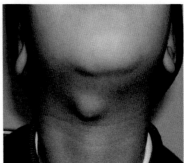

Respiratory epithelium

Midline subcutaneous mass

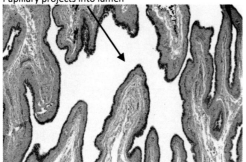
Papillary projects into lumen

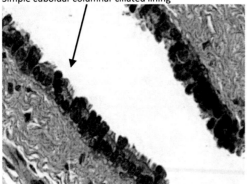
Simple cuboidal-columnar ciliated lining

CUTANEOUS CILIATED CYST

CLINICAL FEATURES
- **Solitary** cyst most common on the **upper legs of females**
- Can also occur on the abdomen and vulva
- Clinical Differential Diagnosis: Epidermoid cyst, Lipoma

HISTOLOGIC FEATURES
- Unilocular or multilocular cyst, **simple cuboidal-columnar ciliated** epithelium
- Cyst epithelium may form papillary projections into the lumen
- No mucous cells
- Non-circumferential smooth muscle

OTHER HIGH YIELD POINTS
- Paramesonephric **(mullerian) duct origin**
- Ciliated columnar epithelium resembles that of **Fallopian tube**

DIFFERENTIAL DIAGNOSIS
- MEDIAN RAPHE CYST - more smooth muscle bundles, clinically on ventral surface of male genitalia
- BRONCHOGENIC CYST - circumferential smooth muscle, cartilage may be present, clinically on or near neck
- BRANCHIAL CLEFT CYST - lymphoid follicles, common location- on or near neck
- APOCRINE HYDROCYSTOMA - not ciliated, common location - eyelids

Path Presenter

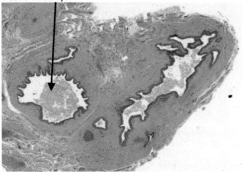
Debris-filled cyst

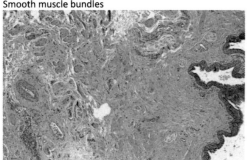
Smooth muscle bundles

Path Presenter

MEDIAN RAPHE CYST

CLINICAL FEATURES
- Developmental cyst on the **ventral aspect of penis/scrotum/perineum** in young males. Usually **solitary.** Can occur from meatus to anus
- Clinical Differential Diagnosis: Apocrine Hidrocystoma, Dermoid Cyst, Epidermal Inclusion Cyst, Glomus Tumor, Hidradenoma Papilliferum

HISTOLOGIC FEATURES
- **Debris-filled** cyst lined by **pseudostratified columnar** epithelium. May have admixed mucin secreting cells
- Variable lining (ciliated, cuboidal, decapitation secretion)
- **Nerve and smooth muscle bundles**

OTHER HIGH YIELD POINTS
- Surrounding skin with characteristics of **genital skin**, with **random smooth muscle**, not circumferential
- Develops from aberrant urethral epithelium without connection to the urethra

DIFFERENTIAL DIAGNOSIS
- CUTANEOUS CILIATED CYST - fewer smooth muscles, on thigh of females
- EPIDERMOID CYST - filled with lamellar keratin, squamous epithelial lining
- PILAR CYST - filled with compact keratin, absence of granular layer, scalp

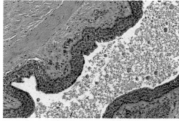
Pseudostratified columnar lining

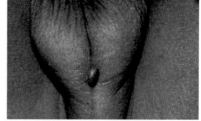
Cyst on ventral aspect of scrotum

Keratin-filled cyst

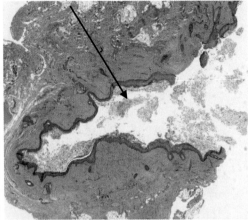

Adnexal structures in cyst wall

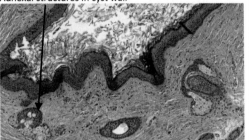

Shark tooth cuticle lining

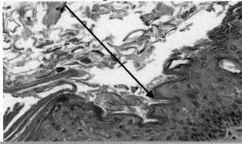

DERMOID CYST

CLINICAL FEATURES
- Firm nodule, **noted in the first year of life** at the embryonic closure zones
- Typically present at birth and located on the **lateral eyebrow**
- Other locations: midline neck, nasal root, forehead, mastoid area, scalp
- Clinical Differential Diagnosis: Epidermoid Cyst, Hemangioma

HISTOLOGIC FEATURES
- Cyst lining with stratified **squamous epithelium** and a **granular layer**
- Cyst with **adnexal structures in the wall**— hair, sebaceous lobules, eccrine/apocrine glands, and/or smooth muscle
- Bright red shaggy **shark tooth cuticle** on lining

OTHER HIGH YIELD POINTS
- Wall commonly **resembles epidermoid cyst, however adnexal structures** present within cyst wall. If occurs midline imaging to look for a dura connection

DIFFERENTIAL DIAGNOSIS
- EPIDERMOID CYST - absence of adnexal structures in cyst wall
- STEATOCYSTOMA - sebaceous glands but not hair follicles within cyst wall
- VELLUS HAIR CYST - numerous vellus hairs present, no adnexal wall structures

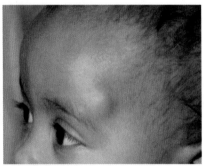

Subcutaneous nodule lateral eyebrow

Path Presenter

Cystic cavity with abundant inflammation

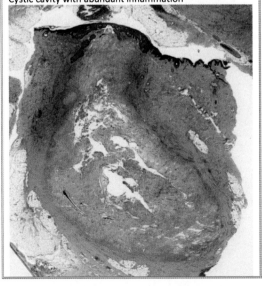

PILONIDAL CYST

CLINICAL FEATURES
- Most commonly presents as a **surface pit** in the **upper gluteal cleft** or sacrococcygeal area of **young males**
- Can be painful, swollen and inflamed
- Clinical Differential Diagnosis: Crohn's Disease, Dermoid Cyst, Epidermoid Cyst, Hidradenitis Suppurativa

HISTOLOGIC FEATURES
- **Numerous naked hair shafts** with **dermal inflammation**
- Acute and chronic inflammation around sinus tracts or cystic cavity lined by squamous epithelium
- Admixed broken hair shafts and keratin debris

OTHER HIGH YIELD POINTS
- Base of spine, thought to result from patients own hair penetrating the skin
- Part of **follicular occlusion tetrad** with hidradenitis suppurativa, dissecting cellulitis of the scalp, and acne conglobate
- Also called a **pilonidal "sinus"** which is likely more accurate, given these often do not have true cyst linings

Numerous hair shafts

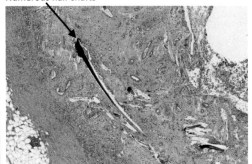

Path Presenter

DIFFERENTIAL DIAGNOSIS
- CROHN'S DISEASE - granulomas present, lack of numerous hair shafts
- HIDRADENITIS SUPPURATIVA - lack of numerous hair shafts, apocrine gland involvement
- RUPTURED EPIDERMOID CYST - squamous epithelial lining, only keratin debris, lack of hair shafts

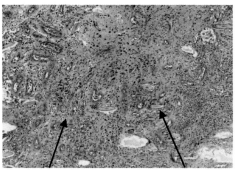 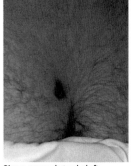

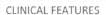

Abundant granulation tissue with admixed hair shafts | Sinus near gluteal cleft

Localized deposit of mucin

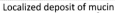

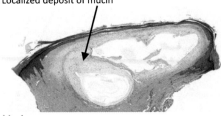

Mucin

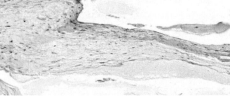

Translucent solitary nodule dorsal distal finger

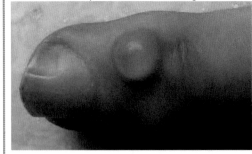

DIGITAL MUCOUS CYST
CLINICAL FEATURES
- This typically is a **translucent or flesh colored**, **solitary** lesion on the **dorsal distal finger** that can drain a **clear viscous fluid**
- When present on the proximal nail fold a characteristic **nail plate groove** can occur
- Can have connection to the underlying or adjacent joint
- Clinical Differential Diagnosis: Acquired Digital Fibrokeratoma, Giant Cell Tumor of the Tendon Sheath, Infantile Digital Fibromatosis

HISTOLOGIC FEATURES
- Localized deposit of **mucin** (acid mucopolysaccharides) in a cystic space of the dermis
- Absence of true epithelial lining
- Mucin can be confirmed by **Alcian blue** or **colloidal iron**

OTHER HIGH YIELD POINTS
- "Cyst" is somewhat of a misnomer as there is no epithelial lining in a digital mucous cyst

DIFFERENTIAL DIAGNOSIS
- FOCAL CUTANEOUS MUCINOSIS - histologically similar, clinical location is key
- SUPERFICIAL ANGIOMYXOMA - vascularity and neutrophils present in addition to large mucin deposits
- METAPLASTIC SYNOVIAL CYST - lined by polygonal cells and villous structures

Path Presenter

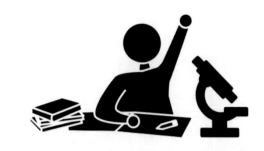

ACE MY PATH

Come Ace With Us!

CHAPTER 2: BENIGN EPIDERMAL LESIONS

MARINA IBRAHEIM, MD

BENIGN EPIDERMAL LESIONS

Pseudohorn cysts in an acanthotic SK

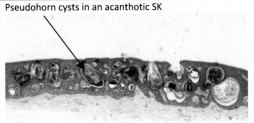

Hyperkeratotic SK

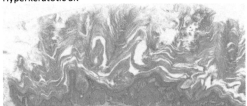

Reticulated SK

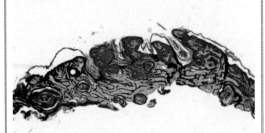

Irritated and inflamed SK

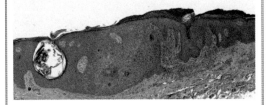

Path Presenter

SEBORRHEIC KERATOSIS (SK)
CLINICAL FEATURES
- **"Stuck-on"** brown-to-black **warty, waxy plaques** on **sun-exposed areas** such as the head, neck, and trunk
- Commonly seen in adults

HISTOLOGIC FEATURES
- Highly varied morphology histologically: lesions may appear **acanthotic, hyperkeratotic, reticulated, irritated, inflamed**
- Melanoacanthoma and **clonal** seborrheic keratoses have also been described
- Epidermal acanthosis
- Papillomatosis with overlying hyperkeratosis
- Small to medium size basaloid cells with squamoid differentiation separated by **pseudohorn cysts**
- Squamous eddies common in irritated seborrheic keratosis

OTHER HIGH YIELD POINTS
- String sign: lesions extending to a uniform depth within the epidermis create an invisible line that is parallel to the surface of the epidermis
- Multiple SK's in patients with internal malignancy-Leser Trelat sign

DIFFERENTIAL DIAGNOSIS

EPIDERMAL NEVUS
- Hyperkeratosis, acanthosis, and papillated epidermal hyperplasia

VERRUCA VULGARIS
- **Exophytic, papillomatous epidermal proliferation**
- **Compact hyperkeratosis** with **vertical columns of round parakeratosis**; hemorrhagic crust at the peaks
- Infolding of elongated rete ridges toward base of lesion

SQUAMOUS CELL CARCINOMA
- Well-differentiated with foci of keratinization, **mild cellular atypia, preservation of basement membrane**

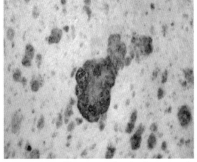 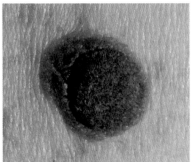

Brown, warty, stuck-on annular plaque on sun-exposed areas

Band-like lichenoid infiltrate at dermal-epidermal junction

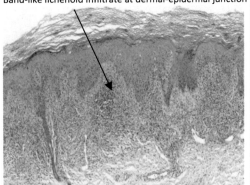

LICHEN PLANUS-LIKE KERATOSIS (BENIGN LICHENOID KERATOSIS)
CLINICAL FEATURES
- **Solitary papule or plaque** varying in color (flesh-colored, pink, brown, or erythematous) commonly **presenting on the trunk, extremities, or the face**
- Pruritus may be present, though **typically asymptomatic**
- **May manifest adjacent to solar lentigo**
- More common in women, Caucasians

HISTOLOGIC FEATURES
- Extensive **band-like lichenoid inflammation at the dermal-epidermal junction (DEJ) with interface change**
- **Orthokeratosis** accompanied by **parakeratosis**
- Variable epidermal acanthosis and **civatte bodies(dyskeratosis)**

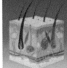
Interface change

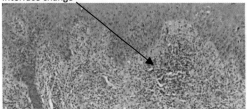

Orthokeratosis

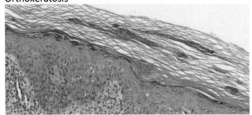

Civatte body

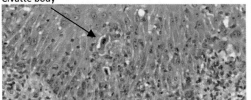

Path Presenter

- Features of a seborrheic keratosis or solar lentigo may be seen at the specimen's periphery
- Melanin pigment incontinence and plasma cells may be observed
- **Eosinophils rarely observed**

OTHER HIGH YIELD POINTS
- Clinical differential diagnosis may include basal cell carcinoma, lentigo maligna, lichen planus, solar lentigo, prompting biopsy
- Diagnosis made histopathologically

DIFFERENTIAL DIAGNOSIS

LICHEN PLANUS
- Compact hyperkeratosis, wedge shaped hypergranulosis
- Parakeratosis typically absent
- **Lichenoid inflammation at DEJ**
- **Eosinophils typically absent**

LICHENOID ACTINIC KERATOSIS
- **Atypia in lower layers of epidermis** associated with **a lichenoid infiltrate**
- Parakeratosis

LICHENOID DRUG ERUPTION
- Compact hyperkeratosis, wedge shaped hypergranulosis with or without parakeratosis
- **Lichenoid inflammation at DEJ**
- **Admixed eosinophils**

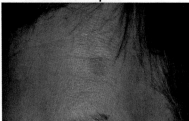
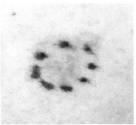

Pink-to-brown patch on forehead   Pink pearlescent papule

Papillomatous structure

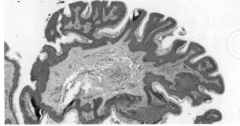

Acanthosis

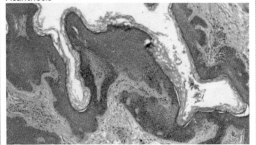

Path Presenter

ACROCHORDON

CLINICAL FEATURES
- **Soft, skin colored or brown pedunculated papule** commonly found on the neck, axillae, or inguinal folds (areas of friction)
- Associated with **obesity, diabetes, and pregnancy**

HISTOLOGIC FEATURES
- **Papillomatous structure** (finger-like projections) demonstrating exophytic growth; variable acanthosis
- Contains **fibrovascular core and adipose tissue; adnexal structures not present**

OTHER HIGH YIELD POINTS
- Clinical differential diagnosis include verruca vulgaris, intradermal nevus, and seborrheic keratosis

DIFFERENTIAL DIAGNOSIS

NEUROFIBROMA
- Variably circumscribed, **unencapsulated lesion. Proliferation of spindle cells with wavy nuclei** enmeshed in loose myxoid stroma
- Scattered mast cells may be observed

NEVUS LIPOMATOSIS
- **Nevoid lesion with mature fat within dermis;** adipocytes present as individual cells or small aggregates

INTRADERMAL NEVUS
- **Symmetric, well-circumscribed melanocytic proliferation**
- Melanocytic nests within superficial dermis demonstrating maturation

Fibrovascular core

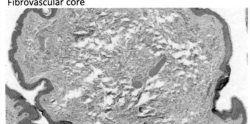

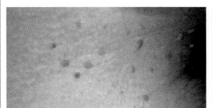

Numerous pedunculated brown papules

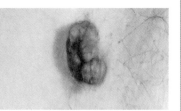

Pink pedunculated papule

Endophytic proliferation

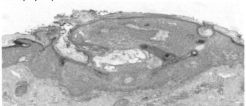

Squamous eddies throughout

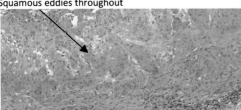

Brown papule on left cheek

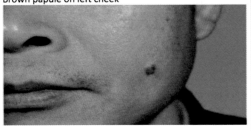

Path Presenter

INVERTED FOLLICULAR KERATOSIS
CLINICAL FEATURES
- **Lesions are typically nonspecific morphologically**
- May appear as solitary white, pink, or tan papule on an adult's face

HISTOLOGIC FEATURES
- **Endophytic proliferation** of squamous epithelium and basaloid cells
- **Papillomatous projections** extending into the **dermis**
- Lymphohistiocytic infiltrate in dermis
- **Squamous eddies** present at base of lesion

OTHER HIGH YIELD POINTS
- Clinical differential diagnosis may include actinic keratosis and squamous cell carcinoma in situ

DIFFERENTIAL DIAGNOSIS
SEBORRHEIC KERATOSIS, IRRITATED
- Epidermal acanthosis with squamous eddies
- Papillomatosis with overlying hyperkeratosis
- Small to medium size basaloid cells with squamoid differentiation separated by **pseudohorn cysts**

SQUAMOUS CELL CARCINOMA
- Well-differentiated with foci of keratinization, **mild cellular atypia, preservation of basement membrane**

TRICHILEMMOMA
- **Endophytic proliferation of clear squamoid cells** arranged in a lobule **with peripheral palisade**
- Basement membrane appears thick, glassy, and eosinophilic
- Overlying focal hypergranulosis and hyperkeratosis

Low power: Acanthosis, hyperkeratosis, papillomatosis

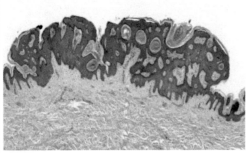

Path Presenter

EPIDERMAL NEVUS
CLINICAL FEATURES
- Linear, warty plaque **present since birth or childhood**
- Typically found on the extremities or trunk

HISTOLOGIC FEATURES
- **Congenital hamartoma; not melanocytic** in origin
- **Acanthosis**
- **Hyperkeratosis**
- Papillomatosis

OTHER HIGH YIELD POINTS
- May follow lines of Blaschko
- Histopathologically looks almost identical to seborrheic keratosis

DIFFERENTIAL DIAGNOSIS
SEBORRHEIC KERATOSIS
- Develops in adults in third decade of life or beyond
- Epidermal acanthosis

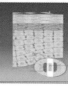

Acanthosis

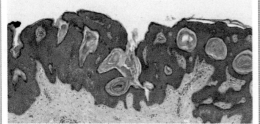

Hyperkeratosis

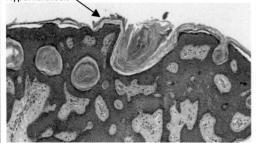

- Papillomatosis with overlying hyperkeratosis
- Small to medium size basaloid cells with squamoid differentiation separated by **pseudohorn cysts**

LICHEN STRIATUS

- Not present at birth; resolves spontaneously
- Lichenoid inflammation with spongiosis and dyskeratosis

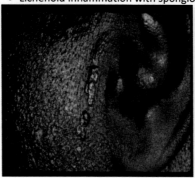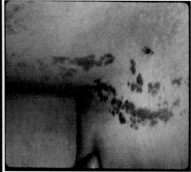

Warty brown plaques in blashchoid distribution

At low power: notably, foci of acantholysis observed

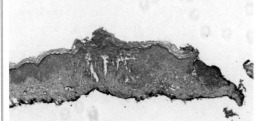

Focal acantholytic dyskeratosis

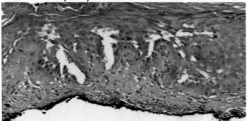

Parakeratosis overlying acantholysis

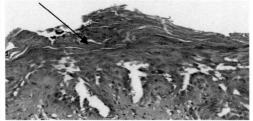

Path Presenter

GROVER'S DISEASE (TRANSIENT ACANTHOLYTIC DYSKERATOSIS)

CLINICAL FEATURES

- **Papulovesicular eruption** affecting the **chest or back**
- May follow after heat exposure, prolonged bed rest; **areas under occlusion**
- Affects **middle-aged men** more commonly

HISTOLOGIC FEATURES

- A number of variants have been described, including spongiotic, superficial pemphigus-like, pemphigus-like, Dariers-like, and Hailey-Hailey-like
- **Focal acantholytic dyskeratosis**
- Overlying parakeratosis; scale, crust

OTHER HIGH YIELD POINTS

- **Direct immunofluorescence testing is negative**

DIFFERENTIAL DIAGNOSIS

DARIER'S DISEASE

- **Abnormal adhesion between keratinocytes** with deranged epidermal keratinization
- Features include acanthosis, hyperkeratosis, and acanthosis
- Suprabasal acantholysis and dyskeratosis are classic findings and appear as **corps ronds** (pyknotic nuclei with clear perinuclear halo) and **grains** (flat parakeratotic cells that appear like rice grains)
- **Direct immunofluorescence testing is negative**
- Electron microscopy demonstrates loss of desmosomes, desmosome/keratin intermediate filament disturbances, and aggregates of keratin intermediate filaments

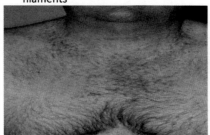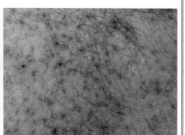

Papulovesicular eruption scattered across the chest

Endophytic proliferation

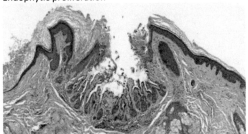

Finger-like projections

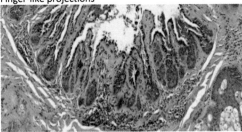

Acantholytic dyskeratosis

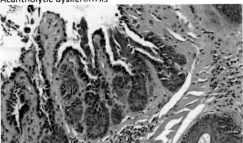

Corps Rond   Grains

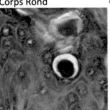 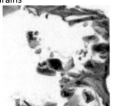

Path Presenter

WARTY DYSKERATOMA

CLINICAL FEATURES

- Solitary, umbilicated papule with **keratotic plug** in the center
- Commonly found on the head, neck

HISTOLOGIC FEATURES

- **Endophytic (invaginated) proliferation with fingerlike projections** within the proliferation
- Overlying parakeratosis and hyperkeratosis
- **Acantholytic dyskeratosis** with corps ronds and grains within the endophytic proliferation

OTHER HIGH YIELD POINTS

- Diagnosis determined by histopathology

DIFFERENTIAL DIAGNOSIS

DARIER'S DISEASE

- **Abnormal adhesion between keratinocytes** with deranged epidermal keratinization
- Features include acanthosis, hyperkeratosis, and acanthosis
- Suprabasal acantholysis and dyskeratosis are classic findings and appear as **corps ronds** (pyknotic nuclei with clear perinuclear halo) and **grains** (flat parakeratotic cells that appear like rice grains)
- **Direct immunofluorescence testing is negative**
- Electron microscopy demonstrates loss of desmosomes, desmosome/keratin intermediate filament disturbances, and aggregates of keratin intermediate filaments

GROVER'S DISEASE

- A number of variants have been described, including spongiotic, superficial pemphigus-like, pemphigus-like, Dariers-like, and Hailey-Hailey-like
- **Focal acantholytic dyskeratosis**
- Overlying parakeratosis; scale, crust

ACANTHOLYTIC ACANTHOMA

- Composed of **benign-appearing keratinocytes**
- Acanthosis, acantholysis, and hyperkeratosis may be observed
- Resembles **"dilapidated brick wall"** seen with Hailey-Hailey Disease

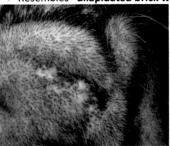 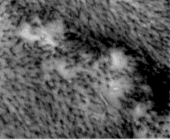

Umbilicated papules in the scalp   Keratotic plug in the center

Compact hyperkeratosis

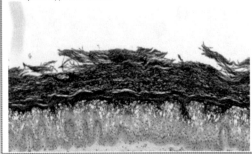

EPIDERMOLYTIC HYPERKERATOSIS (BULLOUS ICHTHYOSIFORM ERYTHRODERMA OR EPIDERMOLYTIC ICHTHYOSIS)

CLINICAL FEATURES

- A type of **congenital ichthyosis** inherited in **an autosomal dominant manner**
- Generalized erythematous, vesiculobullous, and scaly eruption present at birth or early childhood
- Red-brown, scaly skin with furrowing may be observed
- Clinical features exist on a spectrum

HISTOLOGIC FEATURES

- **Compact hyperkeratosis with orthokeratosis**
- **Consumption of the granular layer** appearing as **vacuolar degeneration,**

Orthokeratosis

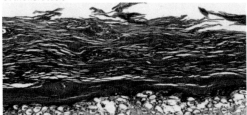

Vacuolar degeneration

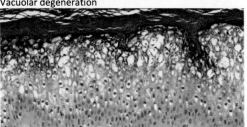

Path Presenter

keratohyalin granules, and lack of or the absence of the granular layer

OTHER HIGH YIELD POINTS

- Occurs due to mutations in keratin genes 1 and 10
- Patients with linear epidermal nevi and this pattern histologically may have offspring who will develop this condition; finding may indicate mosaicism in the parent

DIFFERENTIAL DIAGNOSIS

ICHTHYOSIS BULLOSA OF SIEMENS

- Due to mutation in **keratin 2 gene**
- Mild hyperkeratosis
- **Epidermolysis typically confined to granular layer**

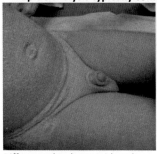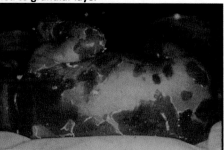

Diffuse erythroderma with scale   Erosions due to eruptions of bullae

---

Acanthosis

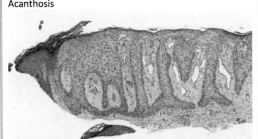

Clear cells with clear demarcation between affeced and unaffected cells

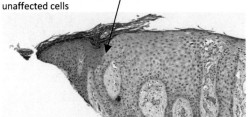

Microbascesses due to neutophils in epidermis

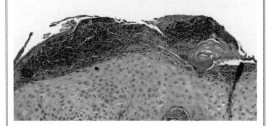

Path Presenter

CLEAR CELL ACANTHOMA (PALE CELL ACANTHOMA)

CLINICAL FEATURES

- **Solitary**, well-circumscribed, **shiny red-brown plaques** that may have **scaling**
- Commonly manifest on the lower extremity of an adult in the fifth decade

HISTOLOGIC FEATURES

- **Well-demarcated acanthosis** with overlying parakeratosis
- **Clear cells** that stain positive for **PAS**; sharply defined border between clear cells and unaffected cells
- Neutrophils may be scattered throughout epidermis, forming microabscesses

OTHER HIGH YIELD POINTS

- Clinically, scaling may appear "stuck on," in a collarette configuration, or on the periphery of the lesion
- On histopathology, the cells appear clear due to accumulation of **glycogen**

DIFFERENTIAL DIAGNOSIS

PSORIASIS

- **Acanthosis with elongated rete ridges** and diminished granular layer
- Neutrophilic scaly crust

SEBORRHEIC KERATOSIS

- Highly varied morphology histologically
- Epidermal acanthosis
- Papillomatosis with overlying hyperkeratosis
- Small to medium size basaloid cells with squamoid differentiation separated by **pseudohorn cysts**

HIDROACANTHOMA SIMPLEX

- **Discrete nests of small cuboidal cells** within epidermis
- Ductal lumina scattered throughout

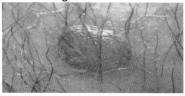

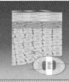

Compact hyperkerkatosis

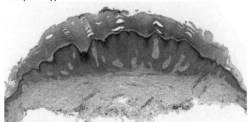

Parakeratosis

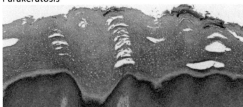

Psoriasiform hyperplasia

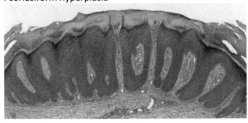

Hypergranulosis and presence of stratum lucidum

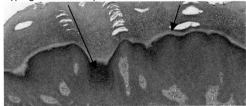

Path Presenter

LICHEN SIMPLEX CHRONICUS/PRURIGO NODULARIS

CLINICAL FEATURES

- Prurigo nodularis: **Multiple pruritic, firm papulonodules** classically affecting the extremities
- Lichen simplex chronicus: **lichenified papules coalescing into plaques with overlying scale** classically affecting the extremities

HISTOLOGIC FEATURES

- Compacted hyperkeratosis with focal parakeratosis and **hypergranulosis**
- **Irregular psoriasiform hyperplasia**
- Focal superficial epidermal necrosis
- Presence of stratum lucidum with hair follicles
- **Vertically oriented dermal collagen**

OTHER HIGH YIELD POINTS

- Focal superficial necrosis may be due to continued excoriation
- Stratum lucidum normally is found only on acral skin; if this layer is noted on a specimen with hair-bearing skin, this may be indicative of repeat excoriation

DIFFERENTIAL DIAGNOSIS

KERATOACANTHOMA

- Type of squamous cell carcinoma that involutes spontaneously
- Histopathologically, lesion appears **crateriform and keratinocytes appear "glassy."** No acanthosis observed
- **Neutrophilic microabscesses**, eosinophils, and elastic trapping may be observed

SQUAMOUS CELL CARCINOMA

- Well-differentiated with foci of keratinization, **mild cellular atypia, preservation of basement membrane**

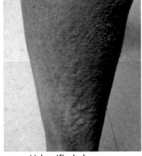 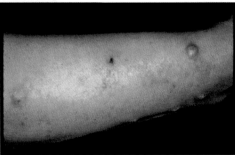

| Lichenified plaque | Multiple pruritic, firm papulonodules |

Horn cysts within rete ridges that resemble antler horns

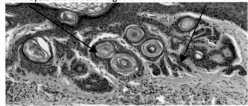

Dangling from cystically dilated hair follicle

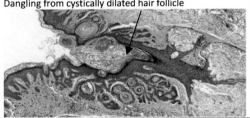

DOWLING- DEGOS DISEASE

CLINICAL FEATURES

- Genetic condition inherited in an **autosomal dominant** fashion
- Hyperpigmented macules coalescing into **reticulated, hyperpigmented patches** affecting the **neck, axillae, and groin**

HISTOLOGIC FEATURES

- Appears **similar to pattern of reticulated seborrheic keratosis** (numerous **horn cysts** in rete ridges that appear almost net-like but **may resemble antler horns**); these appear to **"dangle" from an adjacent hair follicle**
- Hair follicle appears **cystically dilated at level of follicular infundibulum**
- **Hyperpigmentation within rete ridges**

OTHER HIGH YIELD POINTS

- Alternate name for this condition: reticulated pigmented anomaly of the flexures
- Due to defect in **keratin 5**

Hyperpigmentation within rete ridges

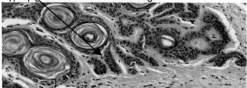

Path Presenter

DIFFERENTIAL DIAGNOSIS

RETICULATED SEBORRHEIC KERATOSIS

- **Reticulated pattern of pseudohorn cysts** in **the absence of dilated follicular infundibula**

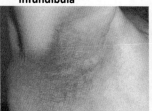 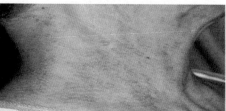

Reticulated, hyperpigmented patches on axilla and neck

Distinct cornoid lamella
Parakeratosis oriented at 45 degree angle

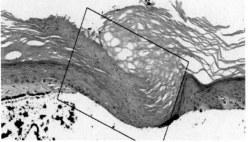

Diminished granular layer beneath cornoid lamella
Dyskeratoic keratinocytes

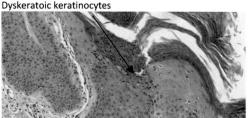

Lichenoid chronic inflammation (patchy)

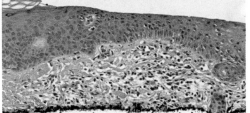

Path Presenter

POROKERATOSIS

CLINICAL FEATURES

- Well-demarcated, **annular, atrophic patch** with **hyperkeratotic rim**
- Lesion may be flesh-colored, pink or brown

HISTOLOGIC FEATURES

- Distinct **cornoid lamella**: **vertical column of parakeratosis at 45 angle** oriented toward center of the lesion. May appear as **"trains"** going in opposite direction
- **Diminished granular layer** and **dyskeratotic keratinocytes**
- Patchy superficial perivascular chronic inflammation that may appear **lichenoid**

OTHER HIGH YIELD POINTS

- Multiple clinical variants have been described, including linear porokeratosis, porokeratosis of Mibelli, plantar porokeratosis, punctate porokeratosis, and disseminated superficial actinic porokeratosis

DIFFERENTIAL DIAGNOSIS

VERRUCA VULGARIS

- Papillomatous exophytic proliferation marked by orthokeratosis and acanthosis, hypergranulosis with keratohyalin-like granules of variable size, and **presence of koilocytes near the granular layer**

POROKERATOTIC ECCRINE OSTIAL AND DERMAL DUCT NEVUS

- Epidermal invagination with overlying porokeratotic cornoid lamella and underlying opening of eccrine duct or hair follicle

HYPERKERATOSIS LENTICULARIS PERSTANS

- Discrete regions of compact hyperkeratosis and focal parakeratosis overlying **atrophic epidermis**
- Band of lichenoid, lymphohistiocytic infiltrate abutting the DEJ

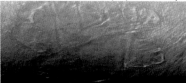 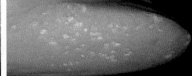

Atrophic patch with rim of scale   Plantar porokeratosis

Psoriasiform Hyperplasia

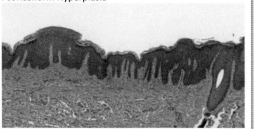

INFLAMMATORY LINEAR VERRUCOUS EPIDERMAL NEVUS (ILVEN)

CLINICAL FEATURES

- Erythematous or brown papules coalescing into plaques in a **blaschkoid distribution**

HISTOLOGIC FEATURES

- **Alternating** regions of **orthokeratosis and parakeratosis**
- **Psoriasiform hyperplasia** and **papillomatosis**
- **Absence of granular layer** underneath regions of parakeratosis

OTHER HIGH YIELD POINTS

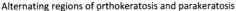
Alternating regions of orthokeratosis and parakeratosis

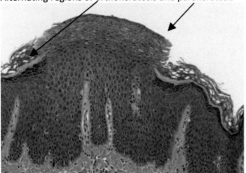

Path Presenter

- Typically manifests in **early childhood**

DIFFERENTIAL DIAGNOSIS

VERRUCA VULGARIS

- **Papillomatous exophytic proliferation** marked by orthokeratosis and acanthosis, hypergranulosis with keratohyalin-like granules of variable size, and presence of **koilocytes** near the granular layer

PSORIASIS

- **Acanthosis** with **elongation of the rete ridges**
- Parakeratosis overlying diminished granular layer
- **Neutrophilic scaly crust** may be observed

SUBACUTE/CHRONIC ECZEMATOUS DERMATITIS

- Acanthosis with overlying parakeratosis and crust, **spongiosis**

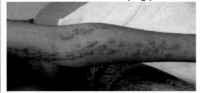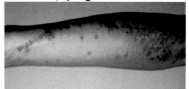

Pink or brown papules coalescing into plaques in a blaschkoid distribution

---

Increased basilar pigmentation

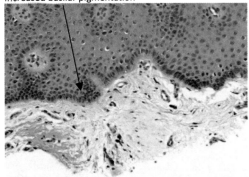

Melanophages in stroma

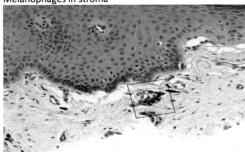

Path Presenter

MELANOTIC MACULE

CLINICAL FEATURES

- **Brown macule** classically found on **mucosal surfaces** such as the mouth or genitalia

HISTOLOGIC FEATURES

- **Increased basilar pigmentation** without increase in melanocytes
- **Melanophages** scattered throughout stroma

OTHER HIGH YIELD POINTS

- If found on genitalia, lesions may appear large, irregular, and darkly pigmented
- Presence of **multiple lesions** may be associated with **genetic conditions** such as LEOPARD Syndrome, Carney Complex, Peutz-Jeger Syndrome, Laugier-Hunziker Syndrome, and Cronkhite-Canada Syndrome

DIFFERENTIAL DIAGNOSIS

POST-INFLAMMATORY PIGMENT ALTERATION

- **Normal number of melanocytes** with **reduced melanin in basal layer** and **pigment incontinence** in dermis

LICHEN PLANUS

- **Compact hyperkeratosis with orthokeratosis, irregular acanthosis with saw-tooth rete ridges; lichenoid, band-like infiltrate** in superficial dermis and vacuolar change; **subepidermal clefting** ("Max Joseph space")

JUNCTIONAL NEVUS

- **No cellular atypia; round to oval melanocytic nests at tips of rete ridges**

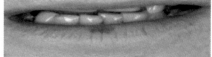

Singular brown macule located on lower vermillion lip

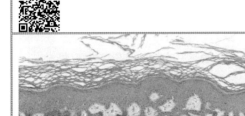

SOLAR LENTIGO

CLINICAL FEATURES

- Discrete **brown macules and patches** found on **sun-exposed areas** such as the **face and dorsal hands**

HISTOLOGIC FEATURES

- **Basal hyperpigmentation of club-shaped rete ridges** that may be described as "dirty socks on a clothes line" or "puppy feet"
- Background of solar elastosis

Basal Hyperpigmentation and club-shaped rete ridges (high-power view)

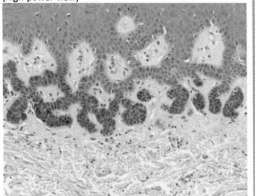

Path Presenter

- Occurs due to **chronic sun exposure**

DIFFERENTIAL DIAGNOSIS

PIGMENTED ACTINIC KERATOSIS
- **Melanin** within **atypical keratinocytes** in lower layers of epidermis
- Dermal melanophages

LARGE CELL ACANTHOMA
- **Acanthosis** with nuclei that are nearly double the size of keratinocytes

LENTIGO SIMPLEX
- Evenly-spaced **dendritic melanocytes in basal layer**

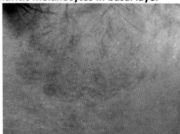

Brown patches found on sun-exposed areas

Papillomatous, exophytic proliferation

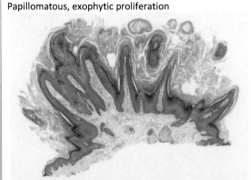

Hypergranulosis

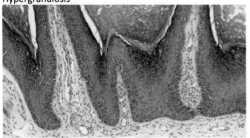

Path Presenter

VERRUCA VULGARIS

CLINICAL FEATURES
- **Filiform** or **hyperkeratotic papules and plaques**
- More commonly seen on the acral skin, including **hands and feet**; can be seen on the knees. Children more commonly affected than adults

HISTOLOGIC FEATURES
- **Papillomatous, exophytic proliferation of the epidermis**
- **Compact hyperkeratosis, orthokeratosis**, and **mounded parakeratosis**
- **Hypergranulosis** and prominence of **keratohyalin-like granules** within the stratum granulosum
- **Presence of koilocytes,** which appear **raisin-like** or **spoon-like,** typically at or around the granular layer. **Elongation of rete ridges** that appears to slope inward
- Dilation of blood vessels at dermal papillae

OTHER HIGH YIELD POINTS
- If numerous observed, may be due to **immunosuppression**
- **Several variations of verruca vulgaris exist are due to different HPV subtypes** Most common type is due to HPV 2.
- Plantar wart: HPV 1, Myrmecia: HPV 1, Verruca plana: HPV 3, Condyloma acuminatum: HPV 6, 11, 16, 18, Epidermodysplasia verruciformis: HPV 5, 8, Bowenoid papulosis: HPV 16, 18, Focal epithelial hyperplasia: HPV 13, 32

DIFFERENTIAL DIAGNOSIS

EPIDERMAL NEVUS
- **Hyperkeratosis, acanthosis**, and papillated epidermal hyperplasia

VERRUCOUS SQUAMOUS CELL CARCINOMA
- Glassy pink keratinocytes, broad lesion with 'bulldozing' into dermis

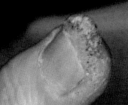

Filiform or hyperkeratotic papules and plaques

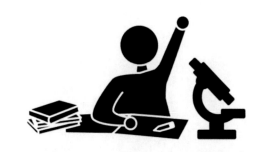

ACE MY PATH
Come Ace With Us!

CHAPTER 3: MALIGNANT
EPIDERMAL LESIONS

MARINA IBRAHEIM, MD

MALIGNANT EPIDERMAL LESIONS

Basaloid islands

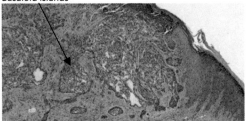

Fibromyxoid stroma surrounding the basaloid islands

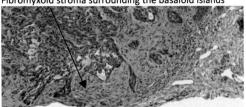

Nodular BCC

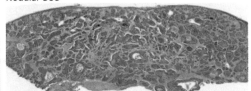

Superficial spreading BCC

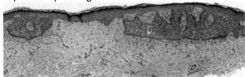

Morpheaform BCC: tadpole-like basaloid islands

Infundibulocystic BCC: pink strands and blue buds

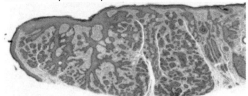

Path Presenter

At low power

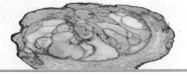

BASAL CELL CARCINOMA (BCC)

CLINICAL FEATURES

- Classically, the nodular variant appears as a **pearly pink to red papule** with **telangiectasias on the head and neck.** Secondary changes such as **ulceration and crusting** may be observed
- Numerous variants have been described; clinically, these may present as pink patches, scars, or may even resemble skin tags

HISTOLOGIC FEATURES

- Multiple variants exist histopathologically, including **nodular**, **superficial**, **infiltrative**, **micronodular**, **morpheaform**, and **infundibulocystic**
- Nodular and superficial types are considered as low risk subtypes based on rate of recurrence. Micronodular, infiltrative and morpheaform considered as high risk subtypes
- **Nodular: collection of nodular, basaloid islands in the dermis** with retraction artifact, peripheral palisading, and fibromyxoid stroma. Basaloid nests show apoptosis and mitosis
- **Superficial:** small buds of basaloid islands extending from the epidermis, retraction artifact, peripheral palisading, and fibromyxoid stroma
- **Infiltrative: spiky basaloid islands with cords extending in the dermis; lacking peripheral palisading or retraction artifact**
- **Micronodular: small nodules of basaloid islands** localized to **reticular dermis** with **fibromyxoid stroma adjacent to the nodules**; small nodules (15 mm in diameter) compose more than 50% of lesion
- **Morpheaform:** thin, **tadpole-like basaloid islands** with **sclerotic stroma** oriented from north to south
- **Infundibulocystic: pink strands of squamous epithelium** with **blue basaloid buds** at the **tips of the strands** that differentiate toward the follicular infundibulum; **central keratinaceous plug**
- **Metatypical:** BCC with focal squamoid differentiation BerEP4 helps in differentiating SCC from BCC. Typically negative in SCC

OTHER HIGH YIELD POINTS

- **Paisley tie differential** (MMEDS): morpheaform BCC, microcystic adnexal carcinoma, desmoplastic trichoepithelioma, syringoma
- **Infundibulocystic BCC** can be associated with **Gorlin-Goltz Syndrome** (nevoid BCC syndrome), an autosomal dominant condition associated with development of **multiple BCCs**

DIFFERENTIAL DIAGNOSIS

TRICHOBLASTOMA

- Basaloid islands in **reticular dermis and subcutis** with peripheral palisading with **fibrous stroma** and **without retraction artifact**

TRICHOEPITHELIOMA

- **Dermal proliferation** with cords and basaloid cells in a **fibrotic stroma**

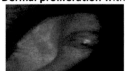

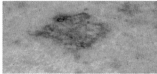

Pink pearly papule with telangiectasia   Pink patch with central scarring

FIBROEPITHELIOMA OF PINKUS

CLINICAL FEATURES

- Flesh-colored or pink **pedunculated papule**
- Most common location: lower back

HISTOLOGIC FEATURES

Pink strands

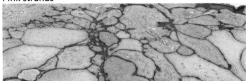

Blue buds

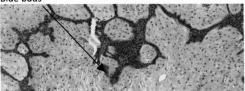

Ducts

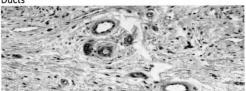

Path Presenter

- Anastomosing epithelium of **pink strands and blue basaloid buds** at the tips
- **Ducts** may be found within the strands
- Embedded in **fibromyxoid stroma**

OTHER HIGH YIELD POINTS

- Considered an **uncommon variant of a BCC**, though some theorize it may be a variant of trichoblastoma
- Ducts present due to its eccrine derivation

DIFFERENTIAL DIAGNOSIS

RETICULATED SEBORRHEIC KERATOSIS

- Epidermal acanthosis, papillomatosis with overlying hyperkeratosis
- Basaloid cells with squamoid differentiation arranged in a reticulated network with **pseudohorn cysts**

ECCRINE SYRINGOFIBROADENOMA

- Reactive proliferation of eccrine ducts with anastomosing strands and ducts

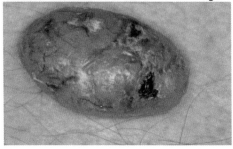

Pink, shiny, pedunculated papule with superficial erosions and crusting

Bowenoid AK

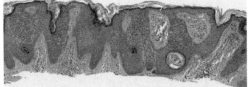

Lichenoid AK with solar elastosis found inferiorly

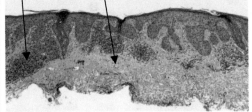

Acantholytic AK   Hypertrophic AK

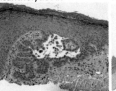 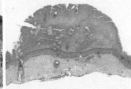

Broad based buds

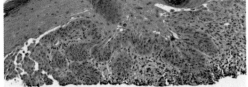

ACTINIC KERATOSIS (AK)

CLINICAL FEATURES

- Pink papule **with scale** typically found on sun-exposed areas

HISTOLOGIC FEATURES

- A number of variants have been described, including Bowenoid, lichenoid, acantholytic, hypertrophic, atrophic, and pigmented
- **Atypical keratinocyte proliferation arising from the basal layer; broad based buds may also extend downward from epidermis**
- Atypical cells surround the follicular infundibulum and form **a shoulder zone** on the periphery of an unaffected follicular structure
- Parakeratosis noted over atypical epidermis; spares intervening hair follicle infundibulum and acrosyringium

OTHER HIGH YIELD POINTS

- **Solar elastoses** may be in background
- May regress or progress to squamous cell carcinoma

DIFFERENTIAL DIAGNOSIS

SQUAMOUS CELL CARCINOMA

- Full thickness atypia of epidermis

LARGE CELL ACANTHOMA

- **Acanthosis** with nuclei that are nearly double the size of keratinocytes

LENTIGO SIMPLEX

- Evenly spaced **dendritic melanocytes in basal layer**

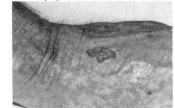 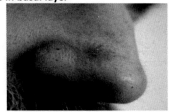

Plaque with overlying yellow-brown scale   Pink papule with overlying scale

Malignant horn and flag sign

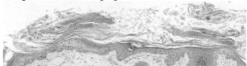

Path Presenter

Hyperkeratosis

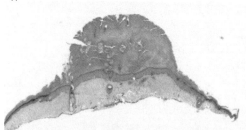

Basilar crowding with cellular atypia

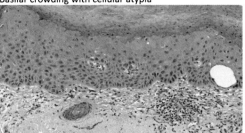

Path Presenter

HYPERTROPHIC ACTINIC KERATOSIS (AK)
CLINICAL FEATURES
- Pink to red papule **with thick scale** that often forms due to repeated rubbing and irritation

HISTOLOGIC FEATURES
- Acanthosis with papillomatosis; **hyperkeratosis**
- **Malignant horn** may be present: **compact eosinophilic stratum corneum** with brick like parakeratosis. These **alternate with pale keratin overlying hair follicle infundibulum** that create the **flag sign**
- **Crowding of the basal layer** with presence of **atypical keratinocytes**. Note the atypia is **not full thickness**

OTHER HIGH YIELD POINTS
- Common site: hand

DIFFERENTIAL DIAGNOSIS

BOWEN'S DISEASE
- Hyperkeratosis with confluent parakeratosis
- **Full thickness atypia; atypical cells in an intraepidermal buckshot or nested pattern**

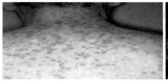 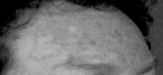

Pink, scaly papules

At low power: hyperkeratosis and parakeratosis

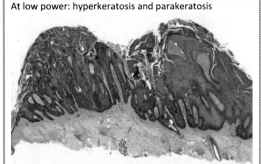

Full thickness atypia with buckshot scatter

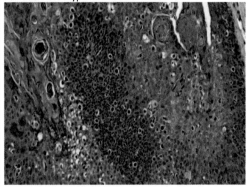

SQUAMOUS CELL CARCINOMA IN-SITU (SCCIS; Bowen's Disease)
CLINICAL FEATURES
- Pink to red **patch or plaque with or without scale**
- May be found on **sun-exposed or photo protected sites** of middle-aged or elderly patients

HISTOLOGIC FEATURES
- **Full thickness atypia** of the epidermis **with loss of normal maturation**: may manifest as a **"wind-blown" pattern**
- Involvement of adnexal epithelium
- Confluent parakeratosis
- **Malignant keratinocytes** advancing throughout **epidermis create a buckshot or nested pattern. Sparing of the basal layer** creates the **"eyeliner sign"**
- **Clear cell change** can be observed: PAS positive, diastase sensitive

OTHER HIGH YIELD POINTS
- Originating from the **follicular epithelium**
- **3-5% progress to invasive SCC**
- **Clear cell change**, if observed, is due to presence of **glycogen** intracellularly

DIFFERENTIAL DIAGNOSIS

BOWENOID PAPULOSIS
- **Acanthosis with full thickness atypia** of keratinocytes

ACTINIC KERATOSIS
- Keratinocyte **atypia restricted to lower layers** of the epidermis: not full thickness

Path Presenter

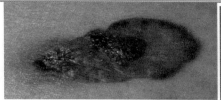
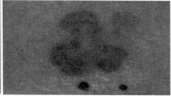

Pink and brown plaque with focal erosion at periphery   Well-demarcated pink plaque

Poorly differentiated SCC

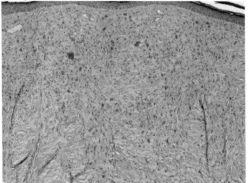

Moderately differentiated SCC

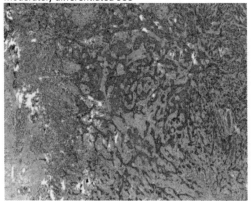

Well differentiated SCC

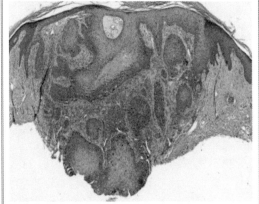

Path Presenter

SQUAMOUS CELL CARCINOMA (SCC)

CLINICAL FEATURES

- **Indurated papule or plaque** with overlying **scale** on skin with a **background of photodamage**

HISTOLOGIC FEATURES

- Infiltration of epithelioid, eosinophilic keratinocytes with atypia
- **Keratin pearls and squamous eddies are common**
- Can be classified as **poorly differentiated, moderately differentiated, and well differentiated**
- **Poorly differentiated: severe cytologic atypia with little squamoid differentiation.** May appear **spindled.** Features associated with keratinization, including keratin pearls are absent
- **Moderately differentiated: prominent** nuclear **atypia,** tumor nests poorly demarcated from surrounding stroma but **features of squamoid differentiation and incomplete keratinization present**
- **Well differentiated: numerous keratin pearls** and **foci of keratinization** indicating **squamous differentiation present;** mild atypia of keratinocytes **with intact basement membrane**

OTHER HIGH YIELD POINTS

- Staging depends on lesion diameter, depth of invasion, degree of differentiation and presence of perineural invasion
- Stains positive for: p63, p40, AE1/AE3
- Does not stain with CK7 or BerEP4
- Acantholytic and Spindle cell variants are considered more aggressive
- **Risk factors** include **photodamage,** prior **radiation, erosive lichen planus, lichen sclerosis,** and **chronic, non-healing wounds**

DIFFERENTIAL DIAGNOSIS

KERATOACANTHOMA

- **Exophytic squamous cell carcinoma** with **full thickness atypia, glassy red keratinocytes,** and **eosinophils, neutrophilic microabscesses**

MICRONODULAR BASAL CELL CARCINOMA

- **Small nodules of basaloid islands** localized to **reticular dermis** with **fibromyxoid stroma adjacent to the nodules**; otherwise, normal dermis present

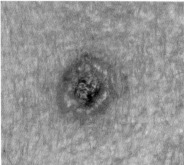
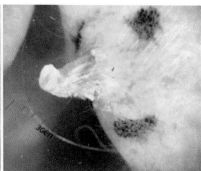

Eroded pink papule   Pink papule with cutaneous horn

At low power: crateriform architecture

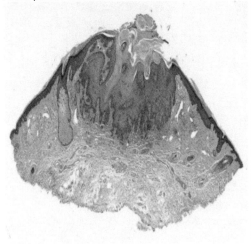

Glassy, red keratinocytes

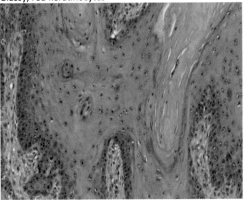

Path Presenter

KERATOACANTHOMA
CLINICAL FEATURES
- Flesh-colored and pink **papule** that **rapidly evolves** into a **dome-shaped nodule** with **keratinaceous center**
- **Spontaneously involutes** after 1-3 months

HISTOLOGIC FEATURES
- May be seen as a type of **well differentiated invasive squamous cell carcinoma** with the capacity to regress
- Squamous cell carcinoma (i.e., full thickness keratinocyte atypia) with **crateriform architecture**
- **Glassy, red keratinocytes, eosinophils,** and **neutrophilic microabscesses** may be seen
- **Elastic fibers** can be **trapped** at periphery of the lesion
- **Hypergranulosis and pseudoepitheliomatous hyperplasia** in hair follicles during early development of the lesion

OTHER HIGH YIELD POINTS
- Rapid growth may be observed after biopsy
- **Acantholysis is never present**
- Multiple KA's can be syndromic-can be seen in Ferguson Smith type and in Generalized eruptive keratoacanthoma of Grzybowski
- Subungual type originates in nailbed and affects toes and fingers. Additional histological findings include presence of dyskeratosis

DIFFERENTIAL DIAGNOSIS
SQUAMOUS CELL CARCINOMA
- Well-differentiated with foci of keratinization, **mild cellular atypia, preservation of basement membrane**

IRRITATED SEBORRHEIC KERATOSIS
- Epidermal acanthosis with **pseudohorn cysts and squamous eddies**

VERRUCA VULGARIS
- **Exophytic, papillomatous epidermal proliferation**
- **Compact hyperkeratosis** with **vertical columns of round parakeratosis;** hemorrhagic crust at the peaks
- Infolding of elongated rete ridges toward base of lesion

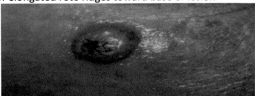

Pink papulonodule with keratinaceous center

At low power

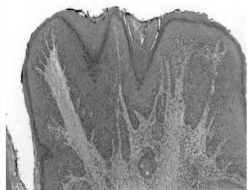

Very little cellular atypia

VERRUCOUS CARCINOMA
CLINICAL FEATURES
- Slow-growing, **white, verrucous papule** found on the **palms, feet,** oral mucosa, or genital **mucosa**

HISTOLOGIC FEATURES
- **Variant of well differentiated SCC**
- **Exo and endophytic squamous proliferation with prominent hyperkeratosis**
- **Endophytic component shows bulbous club like growth pattern and minimal cytological atypia in basal layers**
- Neutrophilic abscesses may be seen
- **Glassy keratinocytes**
- **"Bulldozing" of basal layer** may be observed

OTHER HIGH YIELD POINTS
- Also known as the **Buschke–Lowenstein tumor (if genital), oral florid papillomatosis (if oral),** or **epithelioma caniculatum (palms/feet)**

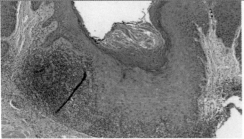

Glassy keratinocytes and basal layer bulldozing

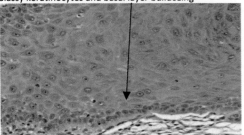

Path Presenter

- Considered a **locally invasive variant of SCC** that **will not metastasize unless if irradiated**
- **Radiation is contraindicated** for this lesion

DIFFERENTIAL DIAGNOSIS

KERATOACANTHOMA

- **Exophytic squamous cell carcinoma** with **full thickness atypia, glassy red keratinocytes**, and **eosinophils, neutrophilic microabscesses**

SQUAMOUS CELL CARCINOMA

- Well-differentiated with foci of keratinization, **mild cellular atypia, preservation of basement membrane**

VERRUCA VULGARIS

- **Exophytic, papillomatous epidermal proliferation**
- **Compact hyperkeratosis** with **vertical columns of round parakeratosis**; hemorrhagic crust at the peaks
- Infolding of elongated rete ridges toward base of lesion

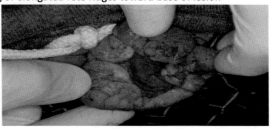

Verrucous nodule with central ulceration and peripheral erosion

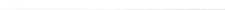

Pagetoid scatter (upward migration of malignant cells)

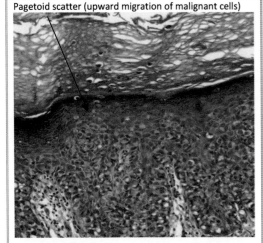

Amphophilic cytoplasm

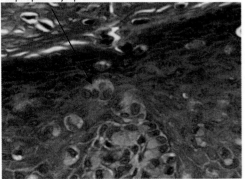

EXTRAMAMMARY PAGET'S DISEASE (EMPD)

CLINICAL FEATURES

- **Pruritic eczematous plaque** found on skin that is rich with **apocrine glands**, including the **vulva, scrotum, and perineum**
- **Intraepidermal proliferation** that arises **from an underlying intraductal carcinoma or de novo**

HISTOLOGIC FEATURES

- Presents with **amphophilic cytoplasm** and **prominent nucleoli**: "Battleship at dusk"
- **Crushed basal layer** may be observed between nests of tumors
- **Tumor cells in nests** in a **buckshot** distribution

OTHER HIGH YIELD POINTS

- Stains negative for: S100, p63
- Positive stains: PAS+, keratin+, CAM 5.2+, CK7+ (cancers from above the diaphragm, lung/breast), CK20+ (CA from below the diaphragm, GI), GATA3+ (breast cancer), CEA+ (gland, polyclonal)

DIFFERENTIAL DIAGNOSIS

BOWEN'S DISEASE

- **Full thickness atypia of keratinocytes within the epidermis**

SUPERFICIAL SPREADING MELANOMA IN SITU

- **Asymmetric proliferation of atypical, epithelioid melanocytes** with abundant cytoplasm, **pleomorphic nuclei**, and **prominent nucleoli**
- **Tumors grow radially**, from one rete to another

SEBACEOUS CARCINOMA

- **Atypical proliferation of sebocytes** (which appear foamy) **comprising >50% of the tumor**
- **Pleomorphic nuclei** and mitotic figures may be observed
- Atypical cells may invade epidermis and demonstrate **pagetoid spread**

Path Presenter

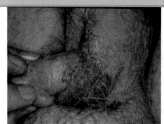
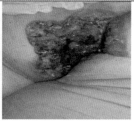

Erythematous plaques with erosions and overlying crust

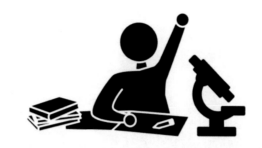

ACE MY PATH
Come Ace With Us!

CHAPTER 4: ADNEXAL NEOPLASMS
WITH FOLLICULAR AND SEBACEOUS
DIFFERENTIATION

DANIEL GONZALEZ, MD

ADNEXAL NEOPLASMS WITH FOLLICULAR AND SEBACEOUS DIFFERENTIATION

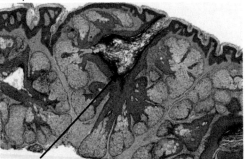

Multiple mature sebaceous lobules

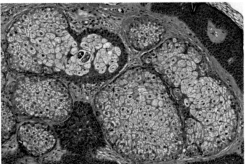

Central dilated follicle

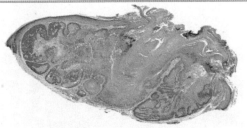

Minimal proliferation of the basal cell layer

Path Presenter

SEBACEOUS HYPERPLASIA

CLINICAL FEATURES

- Asymptomatic **yellowish umbilicated papules**, solitary or multiple, occurring primarily on the forehead and cheeks in adults >40 years old
- Clinically may resemble basal cell carcinoma
- Juxtaclavicular beaded lines variant presents as parallel, closely arranged papules along skin tension lines (Langer's Lines)

HISTOLOGIC FEATURES

- Multiple **mature sebaceous lobules** surrounding a **central dilated follicle**
- No proliferation of the germinative basal cell layer

OTHER HIGH YIELD POINTS

- Typically, fewer fibrous septa and more basal cells compared to normal sebaceous glands
- May be seen in association with an underlying dermatofibroma

DIFFERENTIAL DIAGNOSIS

SEBACEOUS ADENOMA

- Increased proliferation of basaloid cells compared to sebaceous hyperplasia

RHINOPHYMA

- Background inflammatory response (Rosacea)
- Sebaceous lobules are more dispersed and ill-defined

NEVUS SEBACEUS

- Papillomatous and acanthotic epidermis
- Associated eccrine ducts located high in the dermis

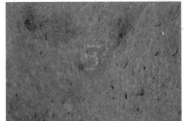
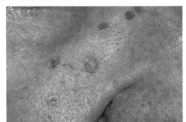

Sebaceous Hyperplasia: Yellow umbilicated papules on the cheeks

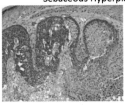
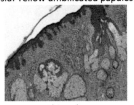
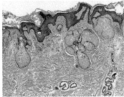

A: Sebaceous Adenoma   B: Rhinophyma   C: Nevus Sebaceus

Lobules of mature sebocytes and basaloid cells

Path Presenter

SEBACEOUS ADENOMA

CLINICAL FEATURES

- **Yellow/pink-colored papule** on the head and neck
- Multiple adenomas may be associated with **Muir-Torre syndrome**

HISTOLOGIC FEATURES

- Multiple well-defined sebaceous lobules separated by thin fibrous septa
- Located in the dermis and may show **multiple epidermal connections**
- Lobules are composed primarily of mature sebocytes and germinative basaloid cells
- **Mature sebocytes outnumber basaloid cells** (>50% of cells)

OTHER HIGH YIELD POINTS

- **Cystic changes** and multiple adenomas may indicate **Muir-Torre syndrome (mutations in MLH1, MSH2, MSH6 genes)**
- EMA(+), CK15(-), BerEp4(-)

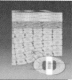

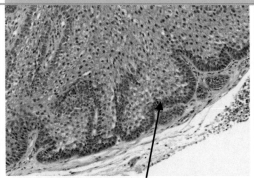

More mature sebocytes than basaloid cells

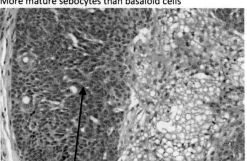

Proliferation of basal cell component

DIFFERENTIAL DIAGNOSIS

SEBACEOMA
- Basaloid cells outnumber mature sebocytes (>50% of cells)

BASAL CELL CARCINOMA WITH SEBACEOUS DIFFERENTIATION
- Increased basal cells
- Fibromyxoid stroma
- Clefting artifact between tumor cells and stroma

SEBACEOUS CARCINOMA
- Cytologic atypia (i.e., mitoses, pleomorphism)
- Infiltrative growth pattern

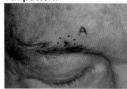

Yellow/pink papule on the head and neck

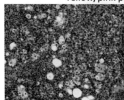 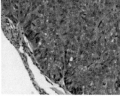 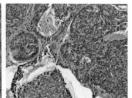

| Sebaceoma | Sebaceous Carcinoma | Basal Cell Carcinoma |

SEBACEOUS EPITHELIOMA/SEBACEOMA

CLINICAL FEATURES
- Yellow to pink papules on the head and neck
- Multiple tumors may be associated with **Muir-Torre syndrome (mutations in MLH1, MSH2, MSH6 genes)**

HISTOLOGIC FEATURES
- Nests or sheets of **basaloid cells** with occasional mature sebocytes
- Located in the upper and mid dermis
- **Basaloid cells outnumber mature sebocytes (>50%)**
- May show **some mitotic activity** and **focal necrosis**

OTHER HIGH YIELD POINTS
- **Cystic changes** and multiple tumors may be associated with **Muir-Torre syndrome (mutations in MLH1, MSH2, MSH6 genes)**
- CK15(+), EMA (-), Ber-Ep4(-)

DIFFERENTIAL DIAGNOSIS

SEBACEOUS ADENOMA
- Mature sebocytes outnumber basaloid cells (>50%)

BASAL CELL CARCINOMA
- Fibromyxoid stroma, clefting artifact between tumor cells and stroma
- Ber-EP4(+), EMA (-), CK15(-)

SEBACEOUS CARCINOMA
- Greater degree of cytologic atypia (i.e., mitoses, pleomorphism) and necrosis
- Infiltrative growth pattern

Proliferation of nests and sheets of basaloid cells
More basaloid cells than mature sebocytes

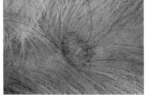

Yellow papule on the head

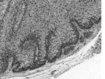 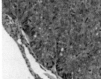 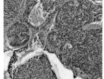

| Sebaceous Adenoma | Sebaceous Carcinoma | Basal Cell Carcinoma |

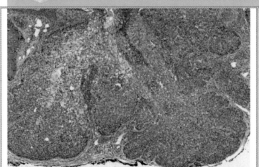
Infiltrative growth of tumor lobules

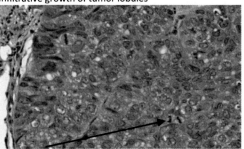
Mitoses are readily identified

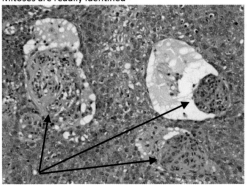
Tumor necrosis

Path Presenter

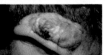
Yellow-red firm nodule

SEBACEOUS CARCINOMA

CLINICAL FEATURES

- Yellow-red firm nodules in older adults
- Most commonly arise in the ocular adnexa and less commonly in the extra-ocular head and neck
- May be associated with Muir-Torre syndrome

HISTOLOGIC FEATURES

- Sheets or lobules of cells separated by thin fibrous stroma
- **Infiltrative and destructive growth pattern** often involving subcutis
- More than half of the lesions also present with pagetoid spread within epidermis, with extension down pre-existing pilosebaceous units in the skin, and pseudoglands of Henle in the conjunctiva
- The cells contain vacuolated or foamy cytoplasm with "scalloping" of the nuclei
- **Pleomorphic nuclei** with prominent nucleoli
- **Mitotic figures** are readily identified
- **Extensive necrosis**

OTHER HIGH YIELD POINTS

- AR (+), Adipophilin(+), EMA(+/-), CEA(-)

DIFFERENTIAL DIAGNOSIS

SEBACEOUS ADENOMA

- Cytologic atypia is absent
- Non-infiltrative growth pattern

SEBACEOMA

- Less cytologic atypia
- Non-infiltrative growth pattern

BASAL CELL CARCINOMA WITH SEBACEOUS DIFFERENTIATION

- Paradoxically shows greater degree of differentiation towards mature sebocytes than sebaceous carcinoma
- EMA (-), Adipophilin(-)
- Both may show Ber-Ep4 expression

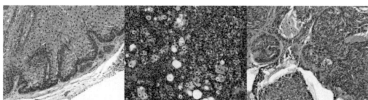
Sebaceous Adenoma   Sebaceoma   Basal Cell Carcinoma

MUIR-TORRE SYNDROME

CLINICAL FEATURES

- Multiple sebaceous tumors in association with internal malignancies (usually gastrointestinal)

HISTOLOGIC FEATURES

- Associated mostly with sebaceous adenoma/sebaceoma and usually not with sebaceous hyperplasia
- **Cystic changes in sebaceous adenomas**

OTHER HIGH YIELD POINTS

- Cystic changes are associated with **microsatellite instability** (MSI-High), a marker of Muir-Torre syndrome
- **Loss of staining for MLH1, MSH2, or MSH6**

DIFFERENTIAL DIAGNOSIS

SEBACEOUS ADENOMA/SEBACEOMA

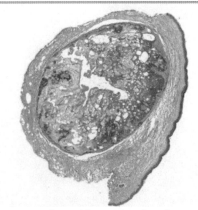
Sebaceous neoplasm with central cystic cavity

Path Presenter

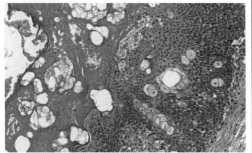

Cystic space (left) lined by neoplastic sebocytes (right)

- Non-syndromic sebaceous adenomas and sebaceomas are difficult to classify on histology alone
- Presence of mutations in MLH1, MSH2, or MSH6 is diagnostic of Muir-Torre syndrome

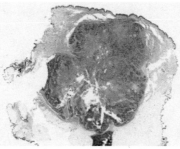

Cystic sebaceous carcinoma, infiltrative

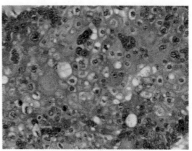

Cytologic atypia and mitoses

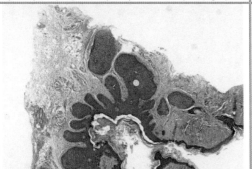

Cystic cavity with surrounding tumor lobules

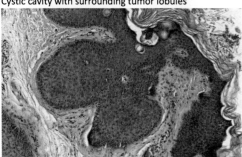

Acanthotic epithelium

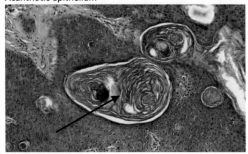

Infundibular keratinization

Path Presenter

PILAR SHEATH ACANTHOMA

CLINICAL FEATURES

- Solitary tan papule with **central depression on the upper lip** of older adults

HISTOLOGIC FEATURES

- Lobules of tumor cells **radiating from a central cystic acanthotic cavity into surrounding dermis**
- Acanthotic epithelium
- **Poorly formed stroma**
- The tumor cells show differentiation toward outer root sheath epithelium and infundibular keratinization

DIFFERENTIAL DIAGNOSIS

DILATED PORE OF WINER

- Central dilated follicle predominates
- No tumor lobules

TRICHOFOLLICULOMA

- Central dilated mother follicle with attached "child" follicles
- Detached tumor lobules are not seen
- Well-formed stroma

FIBROFOLLICULOMA/TRICHODISCOMA

- Anastomosing strands of epithelial cells in a proliferative fibromyxoid stroma
- Lacks a lobular growth pattern

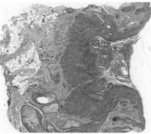

Dilated Pore of Winer

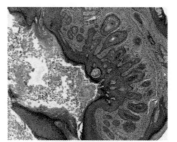

Trichofolliculoma

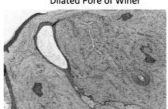

Fibrofolliculoma

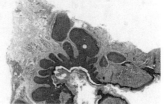

Pilar sheath acanthoma

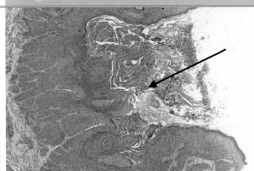
Dilated follicle with central cystic cavity

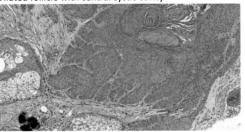
Acanthosis with small papillomatous projections

Path Presenter

DILATED PORE OF WINER

CLINICAL FEATURES

- Small, keratin-filled invagination resembling an **open comedone**
- Most commonly found in adults on the face or trunk

HISTOLOGIC FEATURES

- **Markedly dilated follicle/central cystic cavity** lined by outer root sheath epithelium
- The epithelium shows **acanthosis** and small papillomatous projections into the adjacent dermis
- **Decreased to absent sebaceous glands**

OTHER HIGH YIELD POINTS

- May **contain terminal hairs**

DIFFERENTIAL DIAGNOSIS

PILAR SHEATH ACANTHOMA

- Lobules of tumor cells surround the dilated cavity

TRICHOFOLLICULOMA

- Well-formed dilated follicles radiate from central follicle

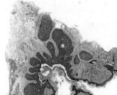
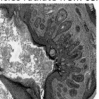

Pilar Sheath Acanthoma   Trichofolliculoma

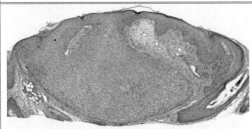
Endophytic lobule of tumor cells

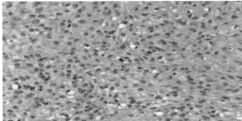
Squamoid to clear cells

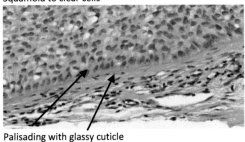
Palisading with glassy cuticle

TRICHILEMMOMA

CLINICAL FEATURES

- Small tan-colored hyperkeratotic papule on the **head and neck**
- Multiple of these are associated with **Cowden syndrome (PTEN gene)**

HISTOLOGIC FEATURES

- Lobules of tumor cells extending from the epidermis into the upper dermis
- Tumor cells are **squamoid to clear** and differentiate towards outer root sheath epithelium
- Thick, glassy **eosinophilic cuticle** composed of basement membrane surrounds the tumor along with **peripheral palisading** of outermost cells
- Desmoplastic trichilemmoma shows nests and strands of epithelial cells with interdigitating hyalinized stroma

OTHER HIGH YIELD POINTS

- Clear cells contain glycogen
- Eosinophilic cuticle is PAS (+) and diastase resistant
- Desmoplastic variant may be mistaken for malignancy
- **CD34(+)**, CK14(+)
- **HRAS mutations**

DIFFERENTIAL DIAGNOSIS

VERRUCA VULGARIS

- Lacks eosinophilic cuticle and pale cells
- Viral cytopathic changes

INVERTED FOLLICULAR KERATOSIS

- Squamous eddies and horn cysts
- Lacks eosinophilic cuticle

SQUAMOUS CELL CARCINOMA

- Lacks eosinophilic cuticle, CD34 (-)
- Often shows more cytologic atypia and infiltrative growth pattern

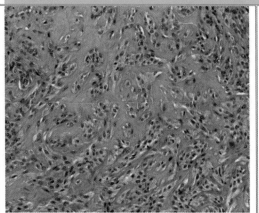

Cords of tumor cells with hyalinized stroma (desmoplastic)

Path Presenter

BASAL CELL CARCINOMA

- Desmoplastic trichilemmoma may closely resemble morpheaform basal cell carcinoma
- Tumor cells in desmoplastic trichilemmoma show thickened eosinophilic basement membrane
- CD34(-)

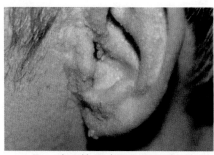

Tan-colored hyperkeratotic papule

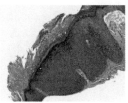 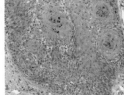 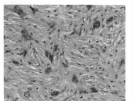

Endophytic verruca   Inverted Follicular Keratosis   Morpheaform BCC

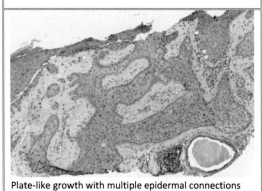

Plate-like growth with multiple epidermal connections

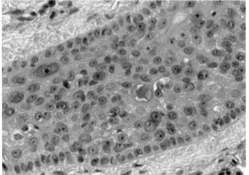

Squamoid cells with peripheral palisade of basal cells

Path Presenter

TUMOR OF THE FOLLICULAR INFUNDIBULUM

CLINICAL FEATURES

- Small keratotic papule on the head and neck
- May occur in association with **Cowden syndrome**, Shopf-Schultz-Passarge syndrome, and nevus sebaceus

HISTOLOGIC FEATURES

- **"Plate-like" growth** of tumor cells with multiple epidermal connections
- The tumor cells are **squamoid to pale**
- Peripheral palisade of basal cells

DIFFERENTIAL DIAGNOSIS

BASAL CELL CARCINOMA

- Cytologic atypia and apoptotic cells
- Fibromyxoid stroma
- Clefting artifact between tumor cells and stroma

TRICHILEMMOMA

- Cytologically similar (outer root sheath epithelium)
- Trichilemmomas show endophytic, lobular architecture as opposed to the "plate-like" growth in tumor of the follicular infundibulum

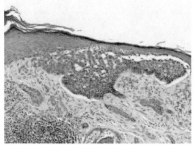 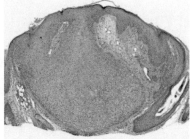

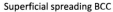

Superficial spreading BCC   Trichilemmoma

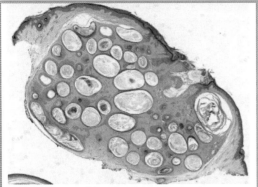
Round cysts resembling doughnuts or swiss cheese

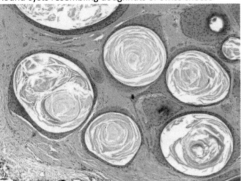
Horn cysts with infundibular keratinization

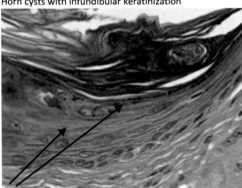
Squamous cells with intact granular layer

Path Presenter

TRICHOADENOMA

CLINICAL FEATURES
- Solitary pale tan papule or nodule on the face and gluteal region in adults

HISTOLOGIC FEATURES
- Dermal proliferation of **multiple round keratin filled cysts** lined by squamous epithelium
- Central large horn cysts with **no hair follicle formation**
- Squamous cells show **infundibular keratinization** with an **intact granular layer**

OTHER HIGH YIELD POINTS
- Tight dermal proliferation of **round cysts resembles "doughnuts" or "Swiss-cheese"**

DIFFERENTIAL DIAGNOSIS

EPIDERMAL INCLUSION CYST
- Large, singular cyst

PILAR SHEATH ACANTHOMA
- Associated with a large central cystic cavity and acanthosis
- Lacks "doughnut" appearance in tumor lobules

SYRINGOMA
- Smaller, tadpole shaped ducts "paisley pattern"
- Ducts are double-layered cuboidal and basaloid cells
- No squamous epithelium, granular layer, or keratinization

DESMOPLASTIC TRICHOEPITHELIOMA
- Desmoplastic stroma
- Tumor cells arranged in small cords and nests
- Granular layer is absent

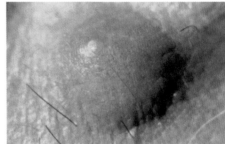
Solitary pale tan nodule

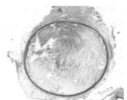 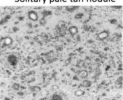 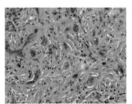

Epidermal inclusion cyst   Syringoma   Desmoplastic Trichoepithelioma

TRICHOFOLLICULOMA

CLINICAL FEATURES
- Pale-tan papule with central tuft of hair on the face of adults

HISTOLOGIC FEATURES
- Large central dilated **"mother" follicle with numerous radiating small "child" follicles**
- Small follicles are seen in various stages of maturation
- Sebaceous Trichofolliculoma will also have proliferation of sebaceous glands

OTHER HIGH YIELD POINTS
- **Child follicles emptying into a mother follicle**

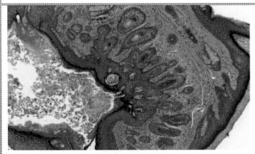
Large central dilated "mother" follicle

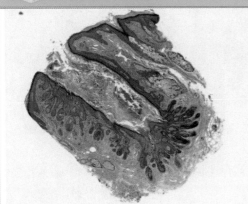

Path Presenter

DIFFERENTIAL DIAGNOSIS
DILATED PORE OF WINER
- Central dilated follicle with acanthosis and without well-formed follicles

TRICHOADENOMA
- No large central dilated follicle
- Composed exclusively of small keratin filled cysts

PILAR SHEATH ACANTHOMA
- Small tumor lobules proliferate beyond the centrally dilated follicle
- No well-formed stroma

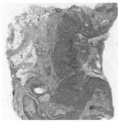 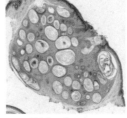 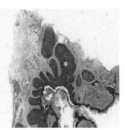

Dilated Pore of Winer   Trichoadenoma   Pilar Sheath Acanthoma

FIBROFOLLICULOMA/TRICHODISCOMA
CLINICAL FEATURES
- Dome shaped, pink, tan colored papule located on the head, neck, and trunk
- Multiple are associated with **Birt-Hogg-Dube**

HISTOLOGIC FEATURES
- Fibrofolliculoma and trichodiscoma are histologic variants of the same entity
- Fibrofolliculoma
    - Central follicle in the dermis with **radiating and anastomosing thin strands of epithelial cells**
    - **Surrounding proliferative fibromucinous stroma**
- Trichodiscoma
    - Well-defined, **loose proliferation of fibromucinous stroma**
    - May see **surrounding follicular epithelium at periphery**
    - Spindle Cell Predominant Trichodiscoma is a variant that shows cellular haphazard proliferation of fibrocytes with abundant mucinous stroma and foci of discrete lipomatous metaplasia

OTHER HIGH YIELD POINTS
- **CD34(+), Factor XIIIa (-) stromal cells**
- **Birt-Hogg-Dube** is an **autosomal dominant** syndrome characterized by mutations in the **FLCN gene** on **chromosome 17p112** encoding **folliculin**
- Recurrent **pneumothorax, lung cysts,** and **chromophobe renal cell carcinoma** are associated with the syndrome

DIFFERENTIAL DIAGNOSIS
NEUROFOLLICULAR HAMARTOMA
- Stromal cells are S100(+) and Factor XIIIa (+) in addition to CD34(+)

TRICHILEMMAL CYST
- Densely packed homogenous keratin

ANGIOFIBROMA
- No associated folliculosebaceous component

NEUROFIBROMA
- S100(+), SOX10(+)
- No associated folliculosebaceous component
- Typically contains mast cells

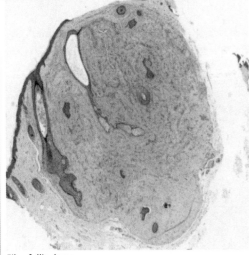

Fibrofolliculoma

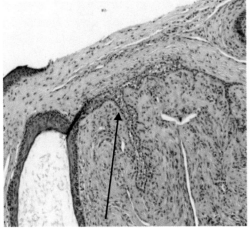

Radiating strands of epithelial cells

Path Presenter

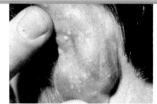

Dome shaped, pink tan colored papule

ORGANOID NEVUS/NEVUS SEBACEUS OF JADASSOHN

CLINICAL FEATURES

- **Multiple grouped yellow/waxy papules or plaque**, usually on the **scalp**

HISTOLOGIC FEATURES

- **Acanthotic and papillomatous** epidermis
- Abnormally formed pilosebaceous structures in the superficial dermis with **hamartomatous** growth pattern
- Vellus hairs predominate in infants/children
- Sebaceous glands are high in the dermis and abnormally distributed; many open directly into the epidermis
- **Ectopic eccrine and apocrine glands with cystic dilation**

OTHER HIGH YIELD POINTS

- Associated with secondary neoplasms: **trichoblastoma, trichilemmoma, syringocystadenoma papilliferum, and basal cell carcinoma**
- Associated with **HRAS and KRAS mutations**

DIFFERENTIAL DIAGNOSIS

EPIDERMAL NEVUS

- Does not have abnormal growth of pilosebaceous units and eccrine glands

ACANTHOSIS NIGRICANS

- Basal keratinocyte hyperpigmentation
- Does not have abnormal growth of pilosebaceous units and eccrine glands

SEBACEOUS ADENOMA/SEBACEOMA

- May present in association with nevus sebaceus
- Lacks papillomatous epidermis and abnormal eccrine glands

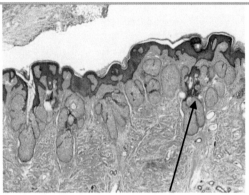

Abnormally formed pilosebaceous structures

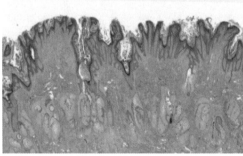

Papillomatous epidermis

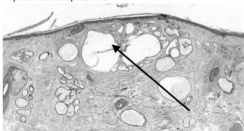

Ectopic eccrine and apocrine glands with cystic dilation

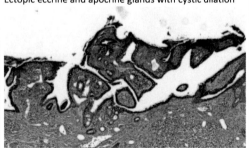

Syringocystadenoma papilliferum

Path Presenter

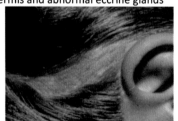

Yellow waxy plaque on the scalp

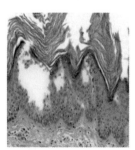

Epidermal Nevus

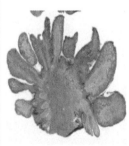

Acanthosis Nigricans

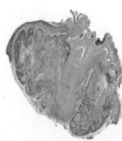

Sebaceous Adenoma

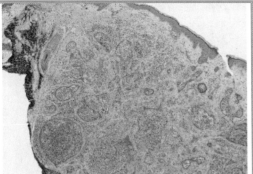

Multiple lobules of tumor cells in the dermis

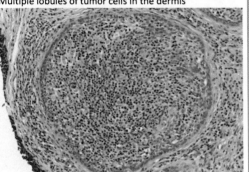

Clear cells with prominent lymphocytic infiltrate

CUTANEOUS LYMPHADENOMA (ADAMANTINOID TRICHOBLASTOMA)

CLINICAL FEATURES
- Solitary dome shaped pale tan nodule on the face, trunk, or legs

HISTOLOGIC FEATURES
- Lobules of **clear cells with peripheral rim of basaloid cells**
- **Prominent lymphocytic infiltrate** within tumor lobules and surrounding stroma
- Associated fibrous stroma

OTHER HIGH YIELD POINTS
- Considered a variant of trichoblastoma, also called adamantinoid trichoblastoma
- CD34(+) spindle cells surrounding tumor lobules

DIFFERENTIAL DIAGNOSIS

BASAL CELL CARCINOMA, ADAMANTINOID VARIANT
- Spindle cells surrounding tumor nests are CD34(-)

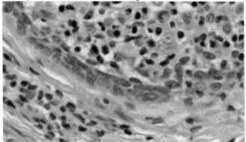

Peripheral palisading of basaloid cells   Path Presenter

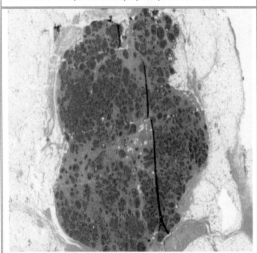

Deep dermal tumor nodule

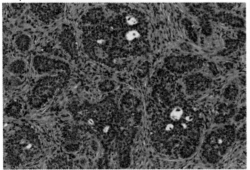

Basaloid cells with surrounding stromal condensation

TRICHOBLASTOMA

CLINICAL FEATURES
- Deep dermal nodule usually greater than 1 cm in size, classically on the scalp

HISTOLOGIC FEATURES
- Large, circumscribed proliferation of **basaloid cells** arranged in nests and lobules
- **Deep dermis** with extension into subcutis
- **No epidermal connection**
- Basaloid cells show differentiation towards the hair germ with formation of primitive hair bulbs
- **Papillary mesenchymal bodies**
- Surrounding fibrous stroma with **no clefting artifact** between tumor cells and stroma
- **Stromal condensation around tumor lobules**

OTHER HIGH YIELD POINTS
- **CK20 highlights scattered Merkel cells** in the tumor nests
- CD34(+) spindle cells surrounding tumor lobules
- Pigment is common

DIFFERENTIAL DIAGNOSIS

BASAL CELL CARCINOMA
- Typically lacks papillary mesenchymal bodies
- Fibromyxoid stroma
- Clefting artifact is seen between tumor cells and stroma, not between collagen bundles
- CK20 does not highlight Merkel cells (absent) in basal cell carcinoma
- Spindle cells surrounding tumor nests are CD34(-)

TRICHOEPITHELIOMA
- Often in the mid to upper dermis
- May show connection with the overlying epidermis

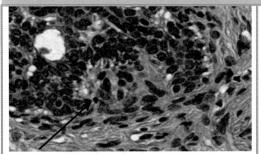

Papillary mesenchymal body

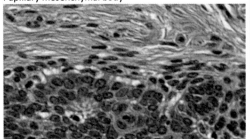

Fibrous stroma with no tumor/stromal clefting

Path Presenter

- Show more features of advanced follicular differentiation such as keratin horn cysts and greater number of papillary mesenchymal bodies

SPIRADENOMA
- Hyalinized basement membrane deposition
- Associated lymphocytes scattered throughout the tumor cells

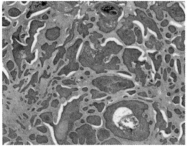

Basal cell carcinoma

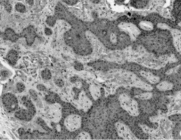

Infundibulocystic Basal Cell Carcinoma

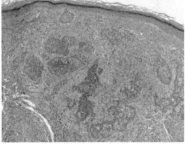

Trichoepithelioma

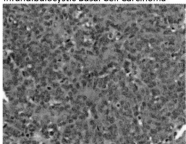

Spiradenoma

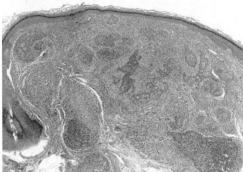

Upper to mid dermal proliferation of basaloid cells

Papillary mesenchymal body

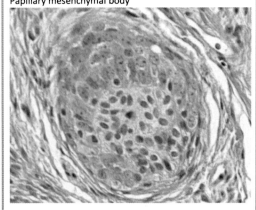

TRICHOEPITHELIOMA

CLINICAL FEATURES
- Pale-tan papule less than 1cm located on the head and neck
- Multiple are associated with **Brooke-Spiegler syndrome** or **Multiple Familial Trichoepithelioma**

HISTOLOGIC FEATURES
- Dermal-based proliferation of basaloid cells arranged in nests and lobules with surrounding fibrous stroma; no apoptosis or mitosis in basaloid nests
- Situated in the **mid to upper dermis**
- Focal **epidermal connection** may be seen
- Fibrous stroma with **clefting artifact present between collagen bundles**
- **Papillary mesenchymal bodies**
- **Desmoplastic trichoepithelioma**
    - Composed of thin cords of tumor cells in a desmoplastic stroma
    - Overlying **central depression/umbilication**
    - Stroma shares characteristics with classic trichoepithelioma (**clefting artifact**)

OTHER HIGH YIELD POINTS
- **CK20** highlights **scattered Merkel cells** in the tumor nests
- CD34(+) spindle cells surrounding tumor lobules

DIFFERENTIAL DIAGNOSIS

BASAL CELL CARCINOMA
- Typically lacks papillary mesenchymal bodies
- Fibromyxoid stroma
- Clefting artifact is seen between tumor cells and stroma, not between collagen bundles
- CK20 does not highlight Merkel cells (absent) in basal cell carcinoma
- Spindle cells surrounding tumor nests are CD34(-)

Fibrous stroma with clefting between collagen bundles

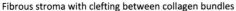

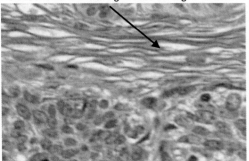

Path Presenter

TRICHOBLASTOMA

- Typically larger and deeper in the dermis and subcutis
- More primitive basaloid appearance
- Lacks epidermal connection

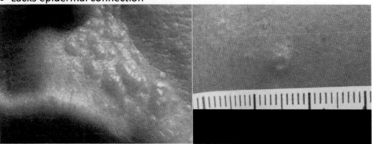

Multiple pale tan papules on the face   Pale tan papule with central depression

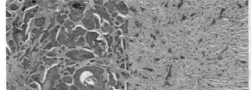
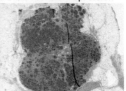

Basal Cell Carcinoma   Morpheaform BCC   Trichoblastoma

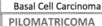

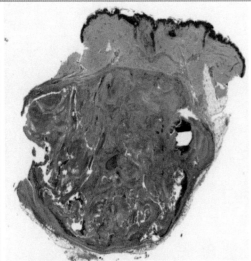

Dermal based nodule

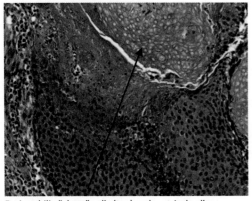

Eosinophilic "ghost" cells (top) and matrical cells (bottom)

PILOMATRICOMA

CLINICAL FEATURES

- Solitary hard, pale-tan nodule on the head, neck, and proximal upper extremities
- "Tent sign" when skin over the tumor is stretched and shows multiple angulations and facets

HISTOLOGIC FEATURES

- Large dermal-based nodule composed of **basaloid "matrical" cells** and **eosinophilic "ghost" or "shadow" cells**
- Eosinophilic cells form from necrotizing basaloid cells
- **Calcifications** are common with admixed foreign body reaction
- **Ossification** may be seen
- Melanin pigment may be seen
- Mitotic figures and atypia can be seen

OTHER HIGH YIELD POINTS

- Mitotic activity and cytologic atypia alone do not constitute malignancy
- Associated with mutations in **CTNNB1** gene encoding **B-catenin**
- **Nuclear and cytoplasmic positivity for B-catenin**
- Aggressive pilomatrixomas are infiltrative but show low degree of cytologic atypia
- May be associated with **Gardner syndrome** (numerous **colorectal polyps** with increased risk of **colorectal cancer**)

DIFFERENTIAL DIAGNOSIS

TRICHILEMMAL (PILAR) CYST
- Contains compact Lacks eosinophilic shadow cells and basaloid cells

PILOMATRIX CARCINOMA
- Infiltrative growth pattern in addition to cytologic atypia, mitoses, and necrosis
- Trichilemmal keratin

BASAL CELL CARCINOMA
- Fibromyxoid stroma
- Clefting artifact is seen between tumor cells and stroma

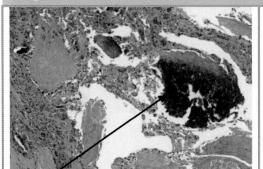

Calcification

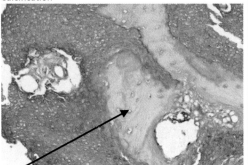

Ossification

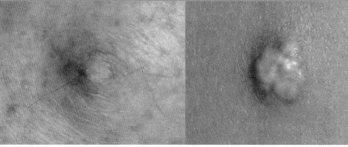

Solitary hard pale nodules   Multiple angulations and facets

Proliferating Pilar Cyst   Pilomatricoma   Basal Cell Carcinoma

Path Presenter

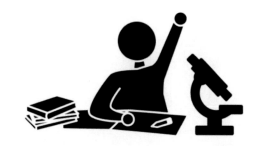

ACE MY PATH
Come Ace With Us!

CHAPTER 5: ADNEXAL NEOPLASMS
WITH ECCRINE AND APOCRINE
DIFFERENTIATION

MICHAEL P LEE, MD

ADNEXAL NEOPLASMS WITH ECCRINE AND APOCRINE DIFFERENTIATION

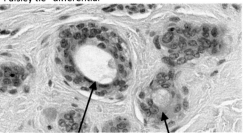

"Paisley tie" differential

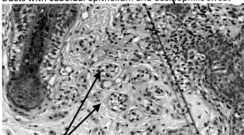

Ducts with cuboidal epithelium and eosinophilic sweat

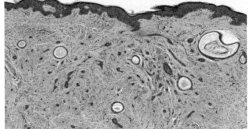

Clear cell variant

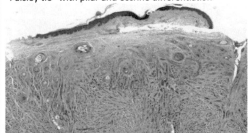

Desmoplastic trichoepithelioma

Path Presenter

SYRINGOMA
CLINICAL FEATURES
- Small yellow to flesh colored papules typically appearing in clusters around the eyelids
- Eruptive type can occur on the chest, back, axillae, and genitals
- **Clear cell variant** associated **with diabetes mellitus**

HISTOLOGIC FEATURES
- **"Paisley tie"** (comma or tadpole shape) islands of basophilic ducts
- Ducts lined by **cuboidal epithelium** and contain **eosinophilic material/sweat**
- Dark red or pink **sclerotic stroma**
- Clear cell changes seen in variant containing abundant glycogen

OTHER HIGH YIELD POINTS
- Syrinx means pipe or duct -> syringoma is an **adenoma** of **acrosyringium** (intraepidermal portion of eccrine sweat duct)
- In Down syndrome, syringomas commonly seen on eyelids

DIFFERENTIAL DIAGNOSIS

DESMOPLASTIC TRICHOEPITHELIOMA
- Cords of basaloid cells and keratin cysts

MORPHEAFORM BASAL CELL CARCINOMA
- Infiltrative basaloid cells with haphazard scar like stroma

MICROCYSTIC ADNEXAL CARCINOMA
- Infiltrative adnexal tumor with biphasic differentiation

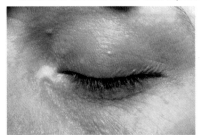
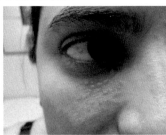

Yellow to flesh colored papules in clusters around eyelids

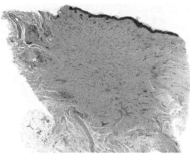

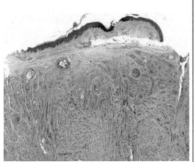

Morpheaform BCC   Microcystic adnexal carcinoma

"Paisley tie" with pilar and eccrine differentiation

MICROCYSTIC ADNEXAL CARCINOMA
CLINICAL FEATURES
- Poorly delineated, skin-colored, indurated plaque or nodule
- Most commonly on the head and neck with a predilection for **perioral area** ("eat a big MAC")
- Slow growing, locally aggressive

HISTOLOGIC FEATURES
- Infiltrative **"paisley tie"** tad pole shaped **eccrine** neoplasm with focal **pilar** differentiation (**biphasic differentiation**)

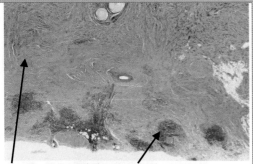
Sclerotic stroma with deep lymphoid aggregates

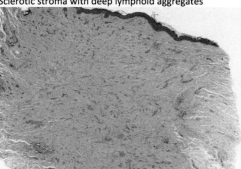
Morpheaform basal cell carcinoma

Path Presenter

- Microcysts or horn cysts in upper portion, bigger basaloid nests in upper part of lesion with smaller nests and single cells at base (zonation)
- Dense pink **sclerotic stroma**
- Frequent **perineural invasion**
- **Usually no cytological atypia-only infiltrative pattern is clue**
- "A syringoma that has gone wild"

OTHER HIGH YIELD POINTS

- Sclerosing sweat duct carcinoma is **monophasic variant** with no pilar component-can show cytologic atypia
- Overlapping features with desmoplastic trichoepithelioma but infiltrative into deep dermis and subcutis and often with perineural extension

DIFFERENTIAL DIAGNOSIS

MORPHEAFORM BASAL CELL CARCINOMA

- Infiltrative basaloid cells with haphazard scar like stroma

DESMOPLASTIC TRICHOEPITHELIOMA

- Cords of basaloid cells and keratin cysts; admixed CK20 positive Merkel cells

SYRINGOMA

- Basophilic ducts with two layered cuboidal epithelium

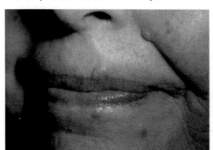
Flesh colored papule of upper lip

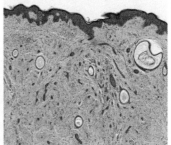
Desmoplastic trichoepithelioma

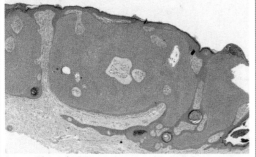
Intraepidermal nests

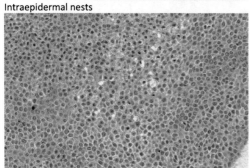
Cuboidal cells within epidermis and ducts

HIDROACANTHOMA SIMPLEX

CLINICAL FEATURES

- Hyperkeratotic plaque on extremities of women

HISTOLOGIC FEATURES

- **Discrete nests** of small cuboidal cells within the epidermis (**intraepidermal**)
- **Cuboidal cells** with ample pink cytoplasm
- Architectural intraepidermal variant of poroma

OTHER HIGH YIELD POINTS

- Can resemble clonal seborrheic keratosis (has **Borst-Jadassohn appearance**), but contains ducts

DIFFERENTIAL DIAGNOSIS

CLONAL SEBORRHEIC KERATOSIS

- Whorled clonal islands of small keratinocytes within epidermis

CLEAR CELL ACANTHOMA

- Acanthotic epidermis with clear cells and distinct transition from surrounding epidermis

SQUAMOUS CELL CARCINOMA

- Full thickness atypia of keratinocytes

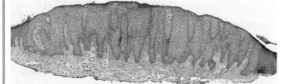
Clear cell acanthoma

Path Presenter

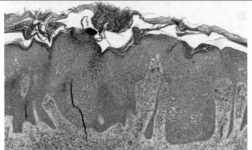
Clonal seborrheic keratosis

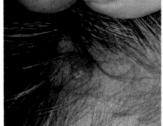
Hyperkeratotic plaque

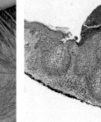
Squamous cell carcinoma in situ

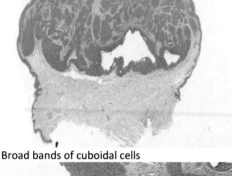
Broad bands of cuboidal cells

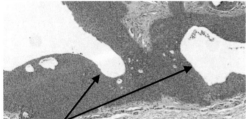
Cuticle lined ducts with ample pink cytoplasm

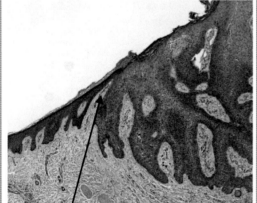
Sharp demarcation from normal epidermis

Path Presenter

POROMA

CLINICAL FEATURES

- Solitary flesh to red colored exophytic nodule commonly on hands or feet; however can be seen at any site

HISTOLOGIC FEATURES

- Acanthotic appearing epidermis with **broad bands of bland cuboidal cells**
- Admixed ducts lined by cuticle, can be highlighted with CEA
- **Sharp demarcation** from normal epidermis
- **Stroma richly vascular** or telangiectatic
- Variants include Hidroacanthoma simplex, which is predominantly intraepidermal; dermal duct tumor is dermal with no connection to epidermis

OTHER HIGH YIELD POINTS

- Can have coagulative necrosis and is an exception to rule that necrosis suggests malignancy

DIFFERENTIAL DIAGNOSIS

SEBORRHEIC KERATOSIS

- Epidermal acanthosis, papillomatosis with overlying hyperkeratosis

NODULAR BASAL CELL CARCINOMA

- Large nodules of basaloid cells with peripheral palisading and clefting

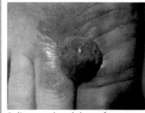
Solitary red nodule on foot

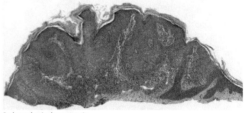
Seborrheic keratosis

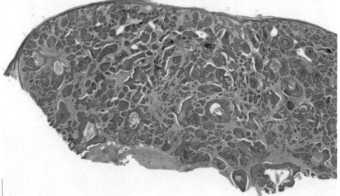
Nodular basal cell carcinoma

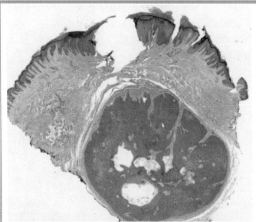

Large dermal nodule

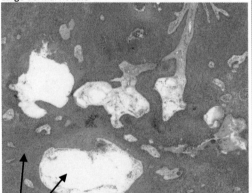

Solid and cystic configurations of cuboidal cells

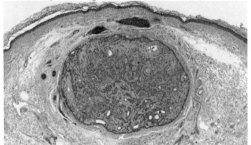

Glomus Tumor

Path Presenter

HIDRADENOMA

CLINICAL FEATURES

- Solitary nodule with predilection for trunks and limbs

HISTOLOGIC FEATURES

- Well circumscribed **large dermal nodule**
- Have **solid** and **cystic configurations** composed of **round polygonal cells with eosinophilic cytoplasm, elsewhere clear cells, mucinous cells and squamoid cells**
- **Admixed ducts**
- **Sclerotic stroma**

OTHER HIGH YIELD POINTS

- Myoepithelial cells are not present in hidradenoma (useful to differentiate in acral site from digital papillary adenocarcinoma)

DIFFERENTIAL DIAGNOSIS

ECCRINE POROMA (DERMAL DUCT TUMOR)

- Acanthosis with broad bands of small cuboidal cells or dermal nodule with poroid cells and admixed ducts

GLOMUS TUMOR

- Dermal nodules composed of small round cells around blood vessels

SQUAMOUS CELL CARCINOMA

- Full thickness atypia

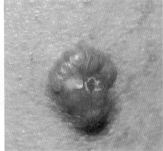

Multilobular reddish nodule

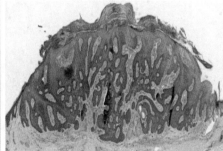

Eccrine poroma

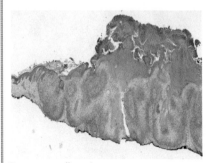

Squamous cell carcinoma

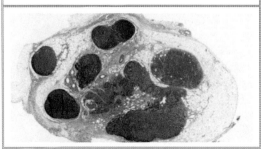

SPIRADENOMA

CLINICAL FEATURES

- Solitary **painful** pink/blue nodule typically on **upper half of body**
- Mostly sporadic, but may present with **cylindromas** and **trichoepitheliomas** in patients with **Brooke-Spiegler**

HISTOLOGIC FEATURES

- **Big blue balls** in the dermis and/or subcutis
- Nodules composed of light (or clear) and dark cells
- **Nodules sprinkled with lymphocytes**

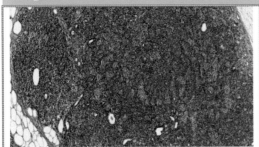
Big blue ball in dermis

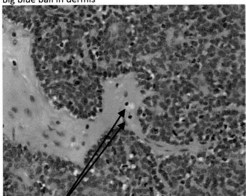
Lymphocytes in nodules

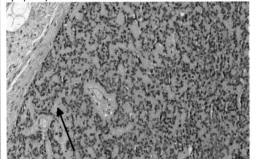
Eosinophylic hyaline droplets and trabeculated network

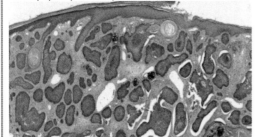
Nodular basal cell carcinoma

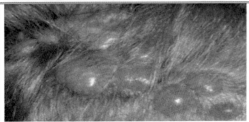
Multiple rubbery nodules on scalp

- Admixed ducts
- Basement membrane material surrounding nodules as well as hyaline deposits admixed with cells in nodules

OTHER HIGH YIELD POINTS

- Overlaps with cylindroma and lesion can have characteristics of both
- May resemble papillary digital carcinoma, although has minimal to no lymphocytes
- BANGLE (painful nodule Differential Diagnosis): Blue rubber bleb nevus, angiolipoma, neuroma/neurilemmoma, glomus, leiomyoma, eccrine spiradenoma

DIFFERENTIAL DIAGNOSIS

CYLINDROMA

- Islands of basaloid nests arranged as a jigsaw puzzle

NODULAR BASAL CELL CARCINOMA

- Large nodules of basaloid cells with peripheral palisading and clefting

PAPILLARY DIGITAL CARCINOMA

- Multinodular tubular and papillary lesion with solid and cystic foci with mitoses and atypia

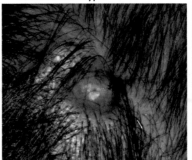
Solitary painful nodule

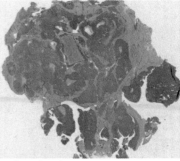
Papillary digital carcinoma

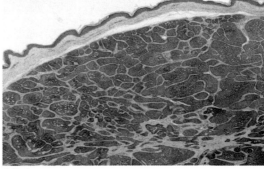
Cylindroma
Path Presenter

CYLINDROMA

CLINICAL FEATURES

- Firm rubbery pink to blue nodule on head and neck
- Can present with multiple nodules, AD inheritance seen in **Brooke-Spiegler**. Results in **turban coverage** of scalp

HISTOLOGIC FEATURES

- **Islands of basaloid nests** with dark blue nuclei and no surrounding cytoplasm (High N:C ratio)
- **"Jigsaw puzzle"**

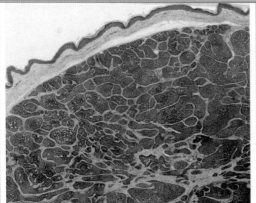
"Jigsaw puzzle" of basaloid nests

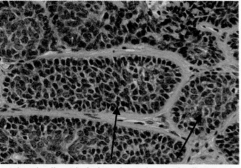
Peripheral cells with dark nuclei and central cells are pale

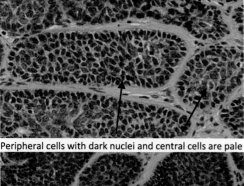
Eosinophilic cuticle and hyaline droplets in nests

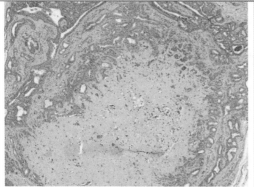
Biphasic tumor with epithelial and mesenchymal features

- Two cell types: **peripheral cells** with **dark nuclei** that palisade and larger **pale grey cells centrally**
- Surrounded by **pink eosinophilic cuticle** representing prominent basement membrane
- **Hyaline droplets** inside nests (more distinct than spiradenoma)

OTHER HIGH YIELD POINTS
- Less lymphocytes than spiradenoma, but can overlap on spectrum

DIFFERENTIAL DIAGNOSIS

SPIRADENOMA
- Big blue ball in the dermis

NODULAR BASAL CELL CARCINOMA
- Large nodules of basaloid cells with peripheral palisading and clefting

HIDRADENOMA
- Nodular proliferation with solid and cystic configuration

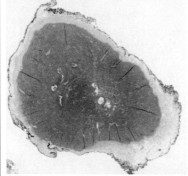
Spiradenoma

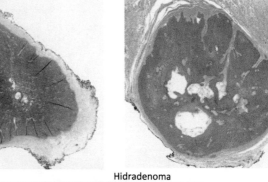
Hidradenoma

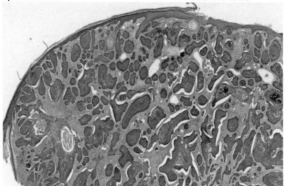
Nodular basal cell carcinoma

Path Presenter

CHONDROID SYRINGOMA/MIXED TUMOR

CLINICAL FEATURES
- Firm solitary subcutaneous nodule on the head or neck of middle-aged patients, but can affect other areas

HISTOLOGIC FEATURES
- Biphasic tumor with **epithelial** and **mesenchymal** components
- **Branching glands** lined by two layers or small ducts lined by single layer of epithelial cells
- Mesenchymal component shows **myxoid/chondroid stroma**
- May see **decapitation secretion** or **keratin cysts**

OTHER HIGH YIELD POINTS
- Chondroitin sulfate stains include **Alcian blue** and **Toluidine blue** ("Blues Brothers")

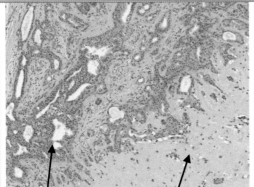

Branching glands and myxoid/chondroid stroma

Chondroma

DIFFERENTIAL DIAGNOSIS

HIDRADENOMA
- Nodular proliferation with solid and cystic configuration

CHONDROMA
- Well circumscribed tumor of chondrocytes; no epithelial component

MALIGNANT MIXED TUMOR
- Poorly circumscribed, lobulated biphasic tumor with atypia and mitoses

Path Presenter

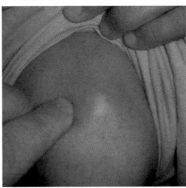

Solitary firm subcutaneous nodule   Hidradenoma

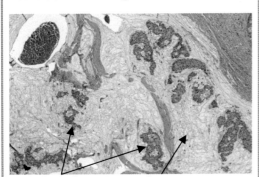

Mucinous stroma extending into subcutis

Basaloid nests floating in a sea of snot

Path Presenter

MUCINOUS CARCINOMA

CLINICAL FEATURES
- Red, painless nodule of head/neck commonly on eyelid
- Can be primary in skin, or metastatic from breast, gastrointestinal, or ovarian

HISTOLOGIC FEATURES
- **Basaloid nests** floating in a sea of snot (**mucinous stroma**)
- Mucinous stroma may extend into subcutis

OTHER HIGH YIELD POINTS
- Primary cutaneous and metastatic mucinous carcinoma appear identical; presence of in situ component (highlighted by myoepithelial markers) favors primary lesions
- Colon adenocarcinoma is CK20+, while breast is not while investigating site

DIFFERENTIAL DIAGNOSIS

BREAST ADENOCARCINOMA
- Dermal neoplasm with ductal differentiation and infiltrative single file pattern

UPPER GI CARCINOMA
- Glandular elements in dermis with atypia

METASTATIC ADNEXAL NEOPLASM
- Focal well-differentiated basophilic neoplasm

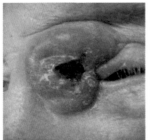

Ulcerated red nodule of eyelid   Breast adenocarcinoma

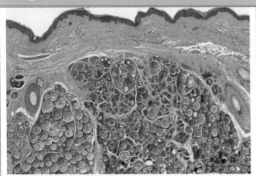
"Swiss chess" or cribiform appearance

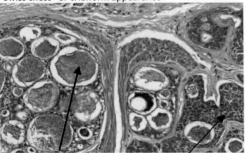
Eosinophilic hyaline like material between basaloid nests

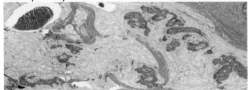
Mucinous carcinoma

Path Presenter

ADENOID CYSTIC CARCINOMA
CLINICAL FEATURES
- Flesh colored papule or nodule of scalp, chest, vulva in elderly
- Can be primary tumor or metastatic from salivary gland carcinoma
- Primary tumors are indolent, but metastatic tumors are aggressive

HISTOLOGIC FEATURES
- **Monomorphic basaloid cells** arranged in tubules, nests, and cords
- "Swiss cheese look" or sieve/colander (cribriform) like appearance
- Admixed small bilayered ducts and pseudocysts
- Prominent eosinophilic hyaline BM-like material between tumor cells, lobules, and luminal surfaces of cystic spaces

OTHER HIGH YIELD POINTS
- Perineural invasion is relatively common
- Lack of fibromyxoid stroma, stromal retraction, and epidermal connection distinguish it from adenoid basal cell carcinoma

DIFFERENTIAL DIAGNOSIS
TRICHOEPITHELIOMA
- Basophilic neoplasm with cribriform pattern

CYLINDROMA
- Islands of basaloid nests arranged as a jigsaw puzzle

MUCINOUS CARCINOMA
- Basaloid nests within mucinous stroma

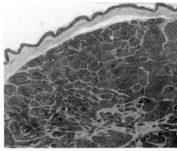
Cylindroma

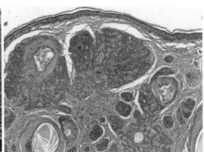
Trichoepithelioma

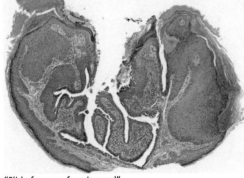
"Slide from surface inward"

Path Presenter

SYRINGOCYSTADENOMA PAPILLIFERUM
CLINICAL FEATURES
- Warty papules or plaques on head/neck
- Most commonly appears at birth or in young children

HISTOLOGIC FEATURES
- Papillary growth composed of fibrovascular cores **opening into surface** ("slide from surface inward")
- **Epidermal hyperplasia** and **papillomatosis** that look like fronds extending upward into clear spaces
- **Numerous plasma cells** in the core of fronds and **decapitation secretion**
- Fibrovascular core surrounded by two layers of cells: inner columnar cells with eosinophilic cytoplasm and outer layer of small cuboidal cells

OTHER HIGH YIELD POINTS
- May ooze serosanguinous fluid (reflects papillae open to epidermal surface)
- One-third arise from **Nevus Sebaceous of Jadassohn**

DIFFERENTIAL DIAGNOSIS
HIDRADENOMA PAPILLIFERUM
- Densely packed glands with papillary projections into cystic lumina (maze-like)

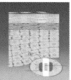

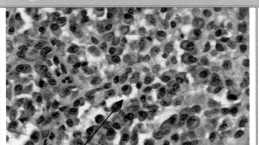

Numerous plasma cells

TUBULAR APOCRINE ADENOMA
- Variably sized well-formed tubules or glands with decapitation secretion

WELL DIFFERENTIATED SQUAMOUS CELL CARCINOMA
- Good squamous differentiation- numerous horn pearls and foci of keratinization

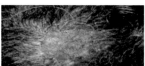

Warty plaque on scalp

HIDRADENOMA PAPILLIFERUM
CLINICAL FEATURES
- Solitary, asymptomatic papule of vulva or perineal area

HISTOLOGIC FEATURES
- Blue dermal nodule with **branching and cystic spaces**
- Papillary projections that are maze like with **no opening to surface or epidermal connection** ("hidden")
- **Decapitation secretion** within lumen, but **no plasma cells**
- Two cell types: columnar layer and underlying myoepithelium

OTHER HIGH YIELD POINTS
- If on acral skin, consider **papillary digital carcinoma**

DIFFERENTIAL DIAGNOSIS
SYRINGOCYSTADENOMA PAPILLIFERUM
- Cystic neoplasm opening onto surface

PAPILLARY ECCRINE ADENOMA
- Duct like structures in dermis with papillary projections

TUBULAR APOCRINE ADENOMA
- Variably sized well formed tubules or glands with decapitation secretion

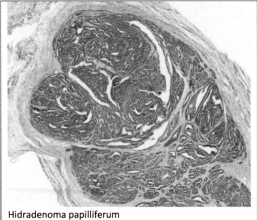

Hidradenoma papilliferum

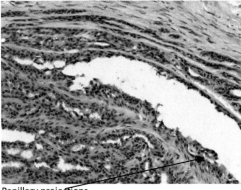

Papillary projections

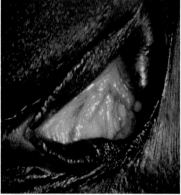

Solitary papule of vulva

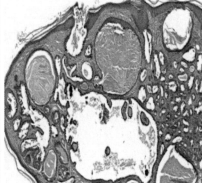

Tubular apocrine adenoma

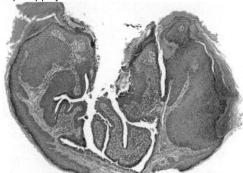

Syringocystadenoma papilliferum

Path Presenter

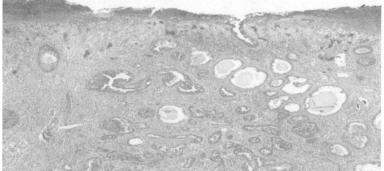

Papillary eccrine adenoma

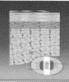
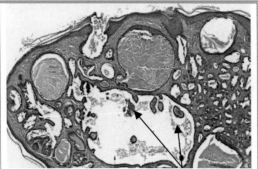
Multiple tubules or glands papillary projections

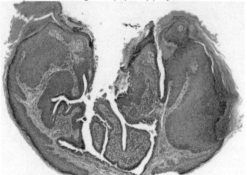
Syringocystadenoma papilliferum

Path Presenter

TUBULAR APOCRINE ADENOMA

CLINICAL FEATURES
- Deep dermal nodule of scalp, axillae, or chest

HISTOLOGIC FEATURES
- Well circumscribed lesion with **tubules or glands**
- Tubules lined by two cell layers filled with **abundant eosinophilic material**

OTHER HIGH YIELD POINTS
- **Decapitation secretion** differentiates from papillary eccrine adenoma
- Can arise from **Nevus Sebaceous of Jadassohn**

DIFFERENTIAL DIAGNOSIS

SYRINGOCYSTADENOMA PAPILLIFERUM
- Cystic neoplasm opening onto surface

PAPILLARY ECCRINE ADENOMA
- Duct like structures in dermis with papillary projections

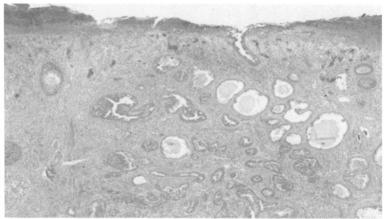
Papillary eccrine adenoma

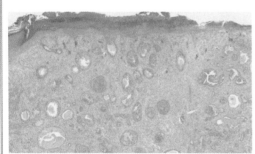
Papillary eccrine adenoma

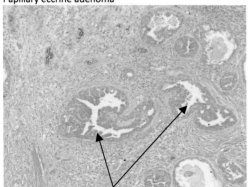
Duct like structures with fronds

PAPILLARY ECCRINE ADENOMA

CLINICAL FEATURES
- Large nodule on the dorsal hand/foot of a child

HISTOLOGIC FEATURES
- Duct like structures with **fronds** in dermis and a surrounding **fibrovascular stroma**
- Lined by two or more layers of polyhedral cells
- Papillary fronds into lumen are variable

OTHER HIGH YIELD POINTS
- Mainly seen in dark skinned patients

DIFFERENTIAL DIAGNOSIS

HIDRADENOMA PAPILLIFERUM
- Densely packed glands with papillary projections into cystic lumina (maze-like)

TUBULAR APOCRINE ADENOMA
- Variably sized well-formed tubules or glands with decapitation secretion

Path Presenter

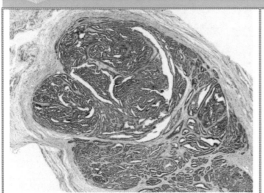
Hidradenoma papilliferum

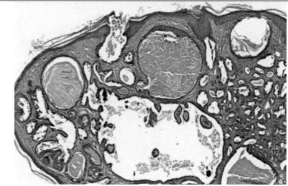
Tubular apocrine adenoma

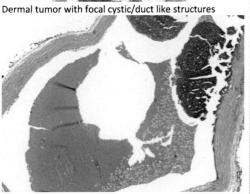
Dermal tumor with focal cystic/duct like structures

DIGITAL PAPILLARY ADENOCARCINOMA

CLINICAL FEATURES
- Solitary, painless cystic nodule on hand or feet
- Typically found between nail bed and distal interphalangeal joint
- Clinically can resemble PEA/TAA
- **Aggressive** with **risk of metastasis**

HISTOLOGIC FEATURES
- Large lobulated dermal tumor with **focal cystic/duct like structures**
- Cystic spaces filled with **eosinophilic material**, solid areas with variable **atypia**, **mitoses**, and **necrosis and back-to-back glands**
- "HPAP" gone wild

OTHER HIGH YIELD POINTS
- Even those lacking atypia are classified as aggressive and can metastasize
- Association with HPV42 has been documented

DIFFERENTIAL DIAGNOSIS

HIDRADENOMA PAPILLIFERUM
- Densely packed glands with papillary projections into cystic lumina (maze-like)

HIDRADENOMA
- Lack of papillary structures, diffuse positivity for p40 and P63, absence of S100 and SMA

Cystic spaces with eosinophilic material

Path Presenter

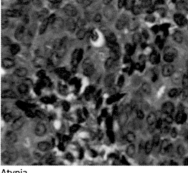
Atypia

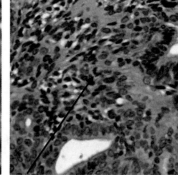
Mitoses

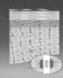

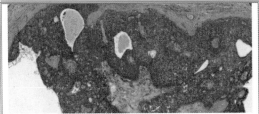

Hidradenoma

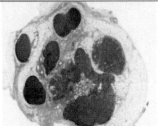

Spiradenoma

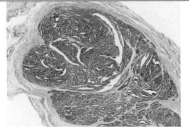

Hidradenoma papilliferum

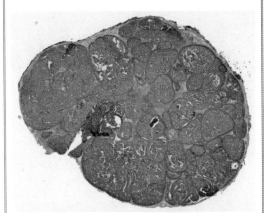

Well circumscribe with multiple nodules

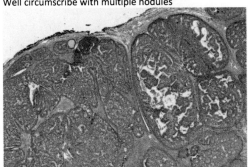

Nodules with solid, cystic, and papillary areas

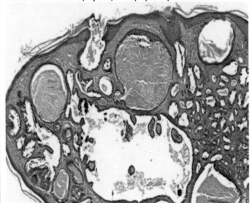

Tubular apocrine adenoma

ENDOCRINE MUCIN PRODUCING SWEAT GLAND CARCINOMA

CLINICAL FEATURES

- Commonly presents on **lower eyelid** or cheek of **elderly females**
- Can arise within **hidrocystoma** and progress to **mucinous carcinoma**

HISTOLOGIC FEATURES

- **Well circumscribed** and may have one or multiple **nodules of solid, cystic and papillary areas**
- Uniform medium **round cells** with **stippled chromatin** and **abundant cytoplasm**
- Moderate atypia and **mitoses**
- **Decapitation secretion** may be present
- Mucicarmine stains intracellular mucin
- Related to mucinous carcinoma where half of cases may have same features

OTHER HIGH YIELD POINTS

- Positive for neuroendocrine markers **synaptophysin** and **chromogranin**
- Positive **estrogen** and **progesterone** receptor

DIFFERENTIAL DIAGNOSIS

TUBULAR APOCRINE ADENOMA

- Variably sized well-formed tubules or glands with decapitation secretion

HIDROCYSTOMA

- Cystic cavity with simple lining one or two layers thick

MUCINOUS CARCINOMA

- Basaloid nests floating in a sea of snot

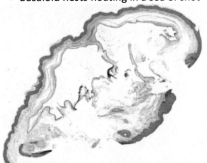

Hidrocystoma

Path Presenter

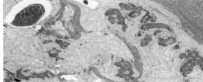

Mucinous carcinoma

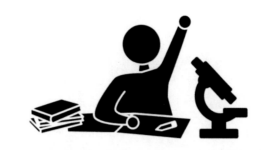

CHAPTER 6: MELANOCYTIC NEOPLASMS

CHRISTINE AHN, MD

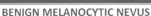
MELANOCYTIC NEOPLASMS

Oval nests limited to the DEJ (junctional nevus)

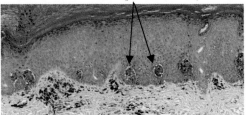

Maturation and dispersion of nests (compound nevus)

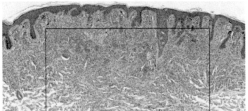

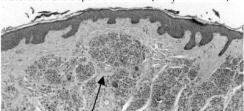

Uniform nests within the dermis beneath a Grenz zone (intradermal nevus)

Path Presenter

BENIGN MELANOCYTIC NEVUS

CLINICAL FEATURES

- **Junctional nevi** are smooth, symmetric, uniform, round to oval tan or brown macules ranging in 1 to 6 mm in size, usually appearing in teen years
- **Compound nevi** are uniform macules or papules that range in color from tan to reddish brown to dark brown
- **Intradermal nevi** are soft and fleshy papules that can be skin-colored or tan-brown

HISTOLOGIC FEATURES

- Round to oval melanocytic nests that are limited to the DEJ (**junctional**), in the epidermis and dermis with evidence of maturation (**compound**), or with nests within the dermis only (**intradermal**) without atypia in the epidermal or dermal components
- Architecture is symmetrical, composed of well circumscribed melanocytes
- Compound and intradermal nevi demonstrate maturation of nests with dispersion at the base as single cells
- No mitoses in the dermal component

OTHER HIGH YIELD POINTS

- Dermoscopy helpful adjunct tool – evaluate symmetry of pigment network, vascular patterns, colors

DIFFERENTIAL DIAGNOSIS

- Dysplastic nevus with mild/moderate atypia – nests bridging between adjacent rete ridges, shoulder phenomenon (junctional component extends three rete ridges beyond dermal component), papillary dermal fibrosis
- Spitz nevus – vertically oriented nests of epithelioid and spindled melanocytes
- Nevoid melanoma – resembles benign nevi on low power, high power reveals melanocytes with subtle pleomorphic features, lack maturation, fail to disperse, deep dermal mitoses present
- Mastocytosis – uniform dermal infiltrate of mast cells

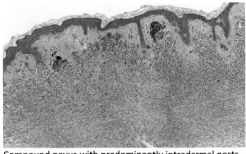

Compound nevus with predominantly intradermal nests

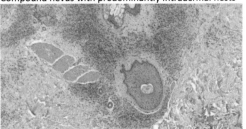

Intradermal nests tracking down adnexa

CONGENITAL NEVUS

CLINICAL FEATURES

- Macules, patches or plaques of varying shades of brown present at birth that grow proportionally with the child
- With time they often increase in thickness and may become papillomatous
- Occur anywhere on the body and are typically larger than acquired nevi
- Stratified into three groups according to size:
  - o Small: <15 cm in greatest diameter
  - o Medium: 15-19.9 cm in greatest diameter
  - o Large or giant: >20 cm in greatest diameter

HISTOLOGIC FEATURES

- Compound or predominantly intradermal nevus with dermal nests aggregating or tracking down adnexa

OTHER HIGH YIELD POINTS

- NRAS mutations present in majority of cases
- Large and giant congenital nevi have increased risk of malignant melanoma and can be associated with neurocutaneous melanosis – melanocytic proliferation within leptomeninges and brain parenchyma
- Can develop proliferative nodules which mimic melanoma histologically

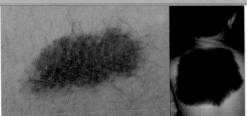

Congenital nevus (small and giant)

DIFFERENTIAL DIAGNOSIS
- Compound nevus – similar histologic features but clinical presentation and lack of tracking down adnexa can help differentiate the two
- Nevoid melanoma – subtly pleomorphic cells, dermal mitoses

Path Presenter

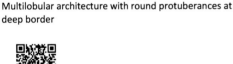

Spindled dendritic melanocytes in the dermis with collagenous stroma

Multilobular architecture with round protuberances at deep border

Path Presenter

BLUE NEVUS (COMMON, CELLULAR)
CLINICAL FEATURES
- Common blue nevi are usually solitary, gray-blue to black, smooth-surfaced macules, papules, or plaques
- Usually found on distal extremities, buttocks, scalp, and face
- Typically present in late childhood or later
- Cellular blue nevi are similar to common blue nevi but typically larger and present on the buttock, sacrococcygeal region and dorsal aspects of hand and feet in adulthood, more commonly in women

HISTOLOGIC FEATURES
- Common blue nevi composed of spindled dendritic melanocytes in the dermis with a surrounding collagenous stroma
- Cellular blue nevi consist of dense proliferation spindled to oval melanocytes in the dermis with admixed melanophages and variable pigment, no junctional component
- Multilobular architecture (dumbbell), rounded protuberances in lower border

OTHER HIGH YIELD POINTS
- Activating GNAQ and GNA11 mutations in >80%
- Multiple blue nevi associated with Carney complex

DIFFERENTIAL DIAGNOSIS
- Tattoo – melanophages containing pigment
- Malignant blue nevus – background of blue nevus but with cytologic atypia, pleomorphism, mitoses, and/or focal necrosis

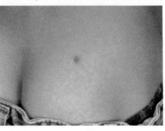
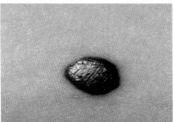

Solitary grey blue papule   Solitary black nodule

Wedge-shaped pattern, extending to subcutaneous fat

DEEP PENETRATING NEVUS (WNT-ACTIVATED MELANOCYTOMA)
CLINICAL FEATURES
- Well-circumscribed blue to black papule or nodule
- Most common in young adults on the face, neck, or shoulder

HISTOLOGIC FEATURES
- Symmetrical, compound melanocytic proliferation, extending to lower reticular dermis and/or subcutaneous fat usually in a wedge-shaped pattern
- Nuclei small with hyperchromasia, dispersed chromatin pattern and inconspicuous nucleoli, finely granular greyish-brown cytoplasmic pigment
- Surrounded by melanophages
- Tracks down adventitia of eccrine coils/follicles and neurovascular bundles

OTHER HIGH YIELD POINTS
- Distinct from blue nevus family due to lack of GNAQ/GNA11 mutation

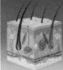
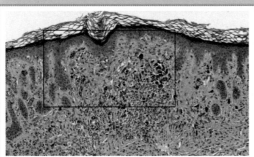

Junctional component present in DPN

- New terminology-WNT-activated melanocytoma
- Nuclear positivity for beta-catenin and p16 with lack of PRAME helpful

DIFFERENTIAL DIAGNOSIS
- Cellular blue nevus – lacks junctional component that is seen in DPN
- Malignant blue nevus - background of blue nevus but with cytologic atypia, pleomorphism, mitoses, and/or focal necrosis

Path Presenter

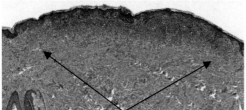

Compound nevus with overall symmetric architecture

Dense lymphocytic infiltrate admixed with intradermal melanocytes

Path Presenter

HALO NEVUS
CLINICAL FEATURES
- Central pigmented nevus with surrounding depigmentation
- Most common in young adults, most often on back
- Can present with multiple lesions
- With time the central nevus gradually loses its pigment and disappears

HISTOLOGIC FEATURES
- Symmetrical, usually compound melanocytic nevus with dense admixed lymphocytes in dermis
- No pagetoid spread, dermal mitosis or pleomorphism
- Some dysplastic features may be seen

OTHER HIGH YIELD POINTS
- May be associated with vitiligo, atypical nevi, or rarely melanoma

DIFFERENTIAL DIAGNOSIS
- Compound nevus – can have associated inflammation without clinical features of halo nevus
- Benign lichenoid keratosis – lichenoid infiltrate without melanocytes
- Melanoma – can have associated inflammation but lymphocytes form a lichenoid band around melanoma

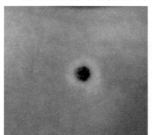
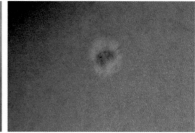

Central pigmented nevus with surrounding "halo" of depigmentation

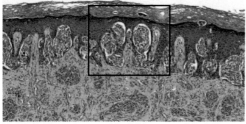

Verticall oriented nests with clefting around the DEJ

Path Presenter

SPITZ NEVUS
CLINICAL FEATURES
- Pink, smooth, dome-shaped papules most commonly on the face and extremities
- Usually seen in the first two decades of life

HISTOLOGIC FEATURES
- Symmetrical, well circumscribed melanocytic proliferation with overlying epidermal hyperplasia
- Vertically oriented nests of epithelioid and spindled cells (banana bunches)
- Artifactual clefting of nests around DEJ
- Pagetoid spread limited to center of lesion
- Melanocytes show abundant amphophilic cytoplasm, large regular oval vesicular nuclei and prominent central nucleoli (predominant in intradermal Spitz nevi)

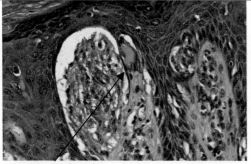

Kamino bodies (PAS+) near the DEJ

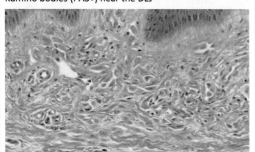

Melanocytes with abundant amphophilic cytoplasm in intradermal Spitz nevus

- Kamino bodies are pathognomonic - homogenous pale eosinophilic globules near DEJ
- Dermal component demonstrates maturation and dispersion, numerous deep or atypical mitoses should be absent (usually <2 mitosis/ mm^2)

OTHER HIGH YIELD POINTS
- Kamino bodies PAS+
- Associated with HRAS mutation/11p gains; gene fusion such as ALK, NTRK1
- HMB45 staining shows maturation; KI-67 is low (<5-10 %); no loss of p16

DIFFERENTIAL DIAGNOSIS
- Pigmented Spindle Cell Nevus of Reed – heavily pigmented variant of Spitz nevus
- Atypical Spitzoid neoplasms – expression of p16 often lost or diminished, FISH analysis helpful in risk stratification
- Spitzoid melanoma – pleomorphic features, deep or atypical mitoses present

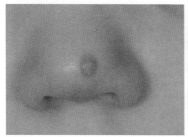

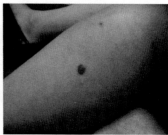

Tan to pink-red papules on the face and extremities

ATYPICAL SPITZ TUMOR (SPITZ MELANOCYTOMA)
CLINICAL FEATURES
- Describes spitzoid neoplasm with borderline histopathologic features and uncertain clinical outcome
- Dome-shaped papules that tend to be larger, asymmetric, and less well circumscribed as Spitz nevi
- Can occur anywhere on the body, seen in all ages but usually > 10 years old

HISTOLOGIC FEATURES
- May show epidermal effacement and ulceration
- Poorly circumscribed asymmetrical lesion of spindled and epithelioid cells with variable cytological atypia and lack of maturation
- Granular cytoplasm with prominent nucleoli
- 2-6 mitosis/mm^2 deep or marginal dermal mitoses may be present
- Increased cellularity with host response in the form of scattered lymphocytes

OTHER HIGH YIELD POINTS
- Often harbor kinase fusions (*ROS1, NTRK1, ALK, BRAF, RET*)

DIFFERENTIAL DIAGNOSIS
- Spitzoid melanoma – epidermal effacement, irregular extension with infiltrative growth pattern, higher proliferative index, increased cytologic atypia and pleomorphism
- Spitz nevus – symmetric growth with epidermal hyperplasia, maturation with dermal depth

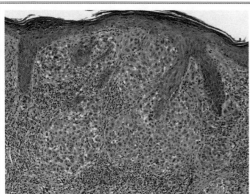

Asymmetric lesion with epithelioid cells with cytologic atypia

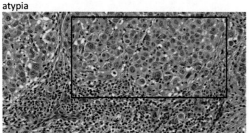

Abundant granular cytoplasm with prominent nucleoli and surrounding scattered lymphocytic infiltrate (*)

Path Presenter

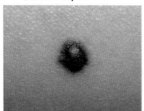

Red-brown papule with slightly asymmetric borders

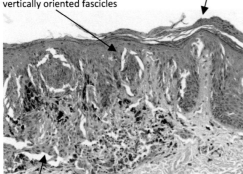

Conspicuous melanin with pigmented parakeratosis, vertically oriented fascicles

Compound nevus with dermal component limited to papillary dermis

PIGMENTED SPINDLE CELL NEVUS OF REED

CLINICAL FEATURES
- Considered a variant of Spitz nevi
- Heavily pigmented macules usually on the legs of young women

HISTOLOGIC FEATURES
- Junctional or compound (usually limited to papillary dermis) spindled melanocytes in vertically oriented fascicles
- Conspicuous melanin pigment, sometimes with pigmented parakeratosis
- Symmetrical configuration with sharp lateral borders
- No significant nuclear atypia

OTHER HIGH YIELD POINTS
- Classic dermoscopic feature is a starburst pattern

DIFFERENTIAL DIAGNOSIS
- Spitz nevus – similar to Spitz but confined to DEJ or papillary dermis

Path Presenter

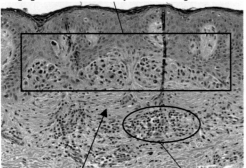

Bridging of nests between adjacent rete ridges

Concentric papillary fibrosis and scattered dermal inflammation

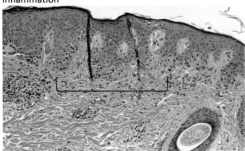

"Shoulder phenomenon" where junctional component extends beyond dermal component

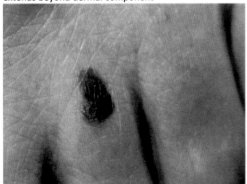

Asymmetric patch with central raised papule, variegated pigment

DYSPLASTIC NEVUS (MILD, MODERATE, SEVERE)

CLINICAL FEATURES
- Variegated tan, brown, and pink macules with or without a papular center
- Usually larger (>6 mm), more irregular, indistinct borders compared to nevi
- Most common site is on the back and scalp of adults

HISTOLOGIC FEATURES
- Graded as mild, moderate severe based on architectural and cytological atypia; some authors prefer a 2-tier grading system- low grade (mild and moderate) and high (severe) grade
- Composed predominantly of horizontally oriented nests, arranged near the DEJ near the tips and sides of elongated rete ridges
- Bridging of nests between adjacent rete and scattered single melanocytes
- Shoulder phenomenon seen in compound nevi, where junctional component extends to three rete ridges beyond dermal component
- Concentric papillary dermal or lamellar fibrosis
- Nuclear enlargement (twice the size of basal keratinocytes) with/without nucleoli throughout the lesion
- Predominantly nested at DEJ; proportion of confluent single melanocytes increase with severity
- Focal pagetoid spread in severe
- Sparse to dense dermal inflammation, usually evenly distributed

OTHER HIGH YIELD POINTS
- Patients with numerous dysplastic nevi should be evaluated for familial atypical multiple mole melanoma syndrome (FAMMM)- associated with CDKN2A mutations
- Patients with this syndrome are also at an increased risk for developing other malignancies, including pancreatic cancer

DIFFERENTIAL DIAGNOSIS
- Special site nevi – benign nevi that exhibit unusual histologic features due to anatomic site
- Melanoma – asymmetric, poorly circumscribed, dyscohesive nests with lentiginous growth along DEJ, epidermal consumption, cytologic atypia

Path Presenter

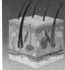

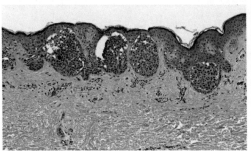

Large, irregular nests

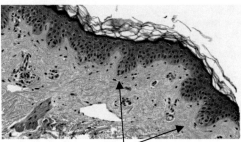

Poor lateral circumscription

NEVUS OF SPECIAL SITES

CLINICAL FEATURES

- These benign site-related nevi exhibit unusual clinical and histologic features
- Anatomic sites include: acral, genitalia, breast, ear, flexures, umbilicus, abdomen (along the milk lines), and scalp

HISTOLOGIC FEATURES

- Overlapping features of dysplastic nevus at DEJ and benign nevi in dermis
- Epidermal component shows large nests with poor cohesion, poor lateral circumscription, shoulder phenomenon, irregular nests, but should lack significant atypia or mitosis in dermal component
- Good maturation and dispersion

OTHER HIGH YIELD POINTS

- Developmental factors and/or hormonal changes thought to be contributing factors to development of special site nevi

DIFFERENTIAL DIAGNOSIS

- Dysplastic nevus – similar histologic features but clinical history and site can help differentiate
- Melanoma – lack maturation, more cytologic atypia

Path Presenter

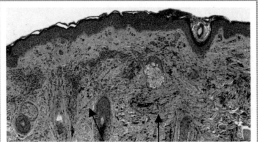

Nevus with congenital nevus and common blue nevus components

COMBINED NEVUS

CLINICAL FEATURES

- Usually in children or young adults involving the trunk, extremities, or face
- Most often darkly pigmented papule or nodule

HISTOLOGIC FEATURES

- Characterized by mixed cytologic patterns: two or more populations of nevi such as blue, common, Spitz, and/or congenital nevi

DIFFERENTIAL DIAGNOSIS

- Spitz nevus, blue nevus – often a component of the lesion, can be misdiagnosed if secondary component is missed

Path Presenter

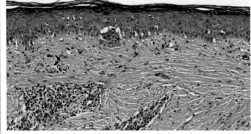

Dermal scar with irregular nests in the overlying epidermis with numerous single cells

Path Presenter

RECURRENT NEVUS

CLINICAL FEATURES

- Irregular, streaky pigmentation arising within a scar from prior partial removal of a nevus
- The back is the most common site

HISTOLOGIC FEATURES

- Melanocytic proliferation in association with dermal scar
- Can simulate melanoma because of areas of single cell predominance, and presence of mild to moderate cytological atypia particularly above the scar
- Periphery may demonstrate features of common nevus

OTHER HIGH YIELD POINTS

- Clinical history is paramount in evaluation of these lesions

DIFFERENTIAL DIAGNOSIS

- Dysplastic nevus with severe atypia – challenging to differentiate, presence of scar in recurrent nevus and relevant clinical history essential
- Melanoma – absence of dermal scar and clinical history of previously biopsied lesion important

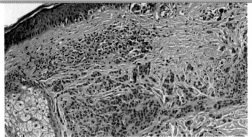

Periphery (beyond dermal scar) demonstrates features of a benign compound nevus

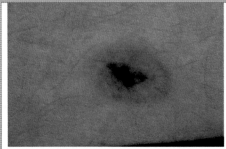

Scar with central dark, asymmetric pigmentation

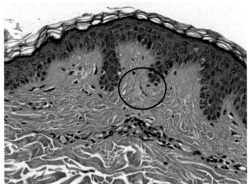

Scattered dendritic melanocytes with melanin granules in upper dermis

Gray-blue pigmentation with scleral involvement

NEVUS OF OTA/ITO

CLINICAL FEATURES

- Types of dermal melanocytosis that present has gray/blue macules and patches
- Nevus of Ota presents in infants or adolescents Gray blue macules and patches present at birth in the V1/V2 distribution, usually unilateral and with scleral involvement
- Nevus of Ito is a variant that is located on the shoulder, supraclavicular, and scapular region with no risk of progression to melanoma

HISTOLOGIC FEATURES

- Elongated dendritic melanocytes with melanin granules in the upper dermis

OTHER HIGH YIELD POINTS

- Nevus of Ota can have activating mutations in GNAQ and can be associated with uveal melanoma (rare)
- Mongolian Spots occur in buttock area of children and show similar histology

DIFFERENTIAL DIAGNOSIS

- Blue nevus – higher cellularity, more well-circumscribed

Path Presenter

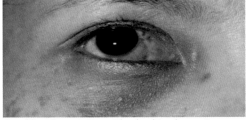

Melanocytic proliferation

Epidermal spongiosis, lymphocyte exostosis, and parakeratosis

MEYERSON'S NEVUS

CLINICAL FEATURES

- Tan to brown macule or papule with surrounding erythematous, scaly plaque (eczematous halo reaction)
- More common in males than females
- May co-exist with halo nevi; patients with or without history of eczema

HISTOLOGIC FEATURES

- Symmetric and uniform melanocytic proliferation with associated features of epidermal spongiosis, parakeratosis, lymphocyte exostosis, and scattered dermal lymphocytic inflammation

OTHER HIGH YIELD POINTS

- Etiology unknown but certain factors thought to be triggers like exposure to UV radiation, medications

DIFFERENTIAL DIAGNOSIS

- Halo nevus – similar features but more prominent epidermal spongiosis seen in Meyerson's nevus, central nevus remains unchanged in Meyerson's nevus

Path Presenter

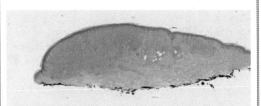

Dermal two cell population of small melanocytes and admixed epithelioid melanocytes

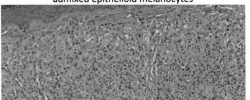

Variable cytologic atypia with large epithelioid melanocytes with glassy eosinophilic cytoplasm

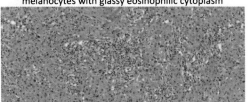

Admixed lymphocytc infiltrate

Path Presenter

BAP1-INACTIVATED MELANOCYTOMA/BAPOMA

CLINICAL FEATURES
- Well-circumscribed, dome-shaped, skin-colored to tan fleshy papules or nodules, mimic intradermal nevi
- Can appear at any age but most common in second and third decades of life
- Can be solitary or multiple

HISTOLOGIC FEATURES
- Composed of intradermal proliferation of epithelioid melanocytes with glassy eosinophilic cytoplasm, haphazard maturation, occasional lymphocytic infiltrate, arranged in a sheet-like growth pattern
- Two cell population-admixed benign nevic cells
- Occasional involvement of epidermis has been described
- Scattered epithelioid melanocytes with bi-nucleation
- Scattered lymphocytic infiltrate in dermis
- Low mitotic activity
- Absent BAP1 nuclear staining within large melanocytes

OTHER HIGH YIELD POINTS
- Most are sporadic but patients with AD-inherited *BAP1* germline mutation more likely to have multiple tumors
- *BAP1* germline mutation associated with multiple BIMT, increased risk of uveal melanoma and mesothelioma

DIFFERENTIAL DIAGNOSIS
- Spitz nevus – share similar features of large vesicular nuclei with prominent nucleoli but Kamino bodies, junctional supranest clefting, spindled melanocytes, and epidermal hyperplastic changes can help differentiate
- Nevoid melanoma – higher degree of cytologic atypia and presence of dermal mitotic figures

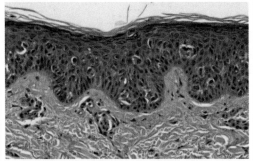

Atypical melanocytes with predominantly single melanocytes demonstrate pagetoid spread

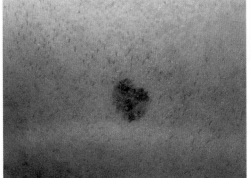

Uneven color and irregular, asymmetric borders

MELANOMA IN SITU

CLINICAL FEATURES
- Dark macules with uneven color and border
- Rarely amelanotic
- Seen in intermittently sun-exposed sites in adults
- When arising within a preexistent nevus, presents as a brown macule adjacent to a papule

HISTOLOGIC FEATURES
- Melanocytic proliferation confined to the epidermis with confluent population of single melanocytes, irregular distribution of junctional nests, and significant pagetoid spread of melanocytes
- Atypical melanocytes with abundant cytoplasm, may extend down follicles
- Skip zones may be present

OTHER HIGH YIELD POINTS
- Less than 0.1% of metastatic disease in some databases

DIFFERENTIAL DIAGNOSIS
- Junctional nevus – lacks nuclear atypia, pleomorphism, and pagetoid spread
- Dysplastic nevus – pagetoid spread should be largely absent
- Paget's disease – non-melanocytic, atypical cells are mostly suprabasal

Path Presenter

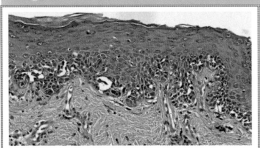

Proliferation of melanocytes in sun-damaged skin, mostly as single melanocytes and some as small nests

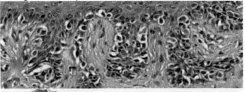

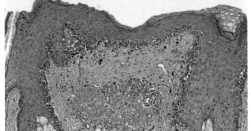

Extension down adnexa of confluent, atypical melanocytes

LENTIGO MALIGNA

CLINICAL FEATURES

- Subtype of melanoma in situ in heavily sun-damaged skin
- Most commonly presents as irregular brown macule or patch on chronic sun-exposed sites such as the face, forearms, and upper back in older individuals

HISTOLOGIC FEATURES

- Proliferation of atypical melanocytes at the basal layer with solar elastosis
- Melanocytes become confluent, composed of predominantly single cells and small nests with extension along adnexal structures common
- Pagetoid spread within epidermis can be seen
- Multinucleated melanocytes with peripheral rim of nuclei (starburst pattern) may be present
- Variable infiltrate of lymphocytes and melanophages

OTHER HIGH YIELD POINTS

- This form of melanoma in situ can remain in the in-situ phase for years

DIFFERENTIAL DIAGNOSIS

- Melanocytic hyperplasia – melanocytes regularly distributed along basal layer, equidistant without significant skip regions, does not extend to inferior segment of follicles and into sebaceous lobules
- Pigmented actinic keratosis – atypical keratinocytes not melanocytes

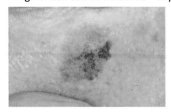

Tan to brown patch with irregular borders and variegated pigment

Path Presenter

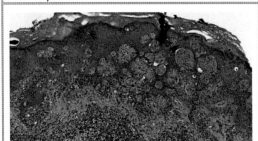

Pagetoid spread within the epidermis

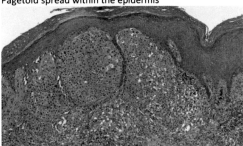

Proliferation of irregular nests at the DEJ with marked pleomorphism, necrotic melanocytes

Path Presenter

SUPERFICIAL SPREADING MELANOMA

CLINICAL FEATURES

- Describes lesions of melanoma during its radial growth phase
- Usually seen in adults, peak onset 40-60 years old
- Most common sites are the back in men and legs in women
- Characterized by variable color with black, blue, white or gray, and irregular borders that become more asymmetric as the lesion grows

HISTOLOGIC FEATURES

- Significant pagetoid spread within the epidermis with marked nuclear pleomorphism
- Necrotic melanocytes or mitotic figures in the epidermis, severe cytologic atypia of melanocytes
- Contiguous proliferation of single cells and irregular nests at DEJ

OTHER HIGH YIELD POINTS

- *BRAF (V600E)* most common mutation in superficial spreading melanoma

DIFFERENTIAL DIAGNOSIS

- Special site nevi – clinical history (age, site) important, lack cytologic atypia
- Paget's disease – IHC distinguishes from melanoma
- Recurrent nevus – presence of scar and atypia in junctional component primarily in the area above the scar, evidence of common nevus on periphery

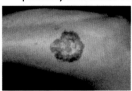

Large plaque with irregular, asymmetric borders, multiple colors (red, tan, brown, black)

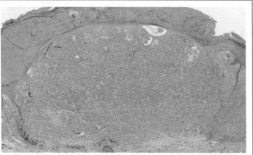

Exophytic nodule with ulcerated surface, vertical growth

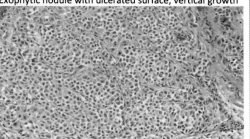

Large atypical, epithelioid melanocytes with abundant cytoplasm, pleomorphic nuclei, and mitotic figures

NODULAR MELANOMA

CLINICAL FEATURES

- Peak onset sixties, incidence higher in men
- Most commonly on head/neck and back
- Presents as exophytic blue-black papule, nodule, or polypod tumor, represents vertical growth phase

HISTOLOGIC FEATURES

- Bulky collection of atypical melanocytes in dermis, epithelioid with vesicular nuclei, abundant cytoplasm; no maturation
- Can have an epidermal component but limited to 3 rete ridges of dermal component
- Often ulcerated, numerous mitotic figures

OTHER HIGH YIELD POINTS

- Tend to present at more advanced stages
- Classical "ABCD" criteria often do not help identify this subtype of melanoma

DIFFERENTIAL DIAGNOSIS

- Spitz nevus – lack dermal mitoses, no sheets or nodules of tumor that compress adjacent cells
- Metastatic melanoma – more homogenous cytology, lymphatic invasion, often lack of pigment

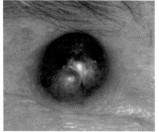

Black raised nodule with atypical border   Path Presenter

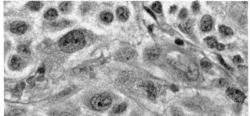

Lentiginous pattern of melanocytes on acral skin

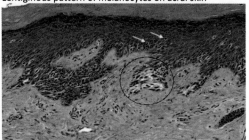

Plump melanocytes with halo (arrow) and formation of nests (circle)

ACRAL LENTIGINOUS MELANOMA

CLINICAL FEATURES

- 5-10% of cutaneous melanoma
- Palmar, plantar, subungual skin
- Most common subtype in darker skin types

HISTOLOGIC FEATURES

- Lentiginous pattern of atypical melanocytes, can have pagetoid spread
- Epidermal component can be subtle, melanocytes appear plump or heavily pigmented with dendritic processes
- Dermal component can show giant, nevoid, clear cells
- Presence of tumor-infiltrating lymphocytes favor melanoma over nevus

OTHER HIGH YIELD POINTS

- Often advanced at time of diagnosis
- Associated with parallel ridge pattern on dermoscopy

DIFFERENTIAL DIAGNOSIS

- Nevus of special site – site-related atypia important to distinguish

Path Presenter

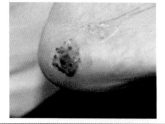

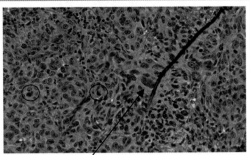

Large, atypical melanocytes with numerous mitotic figures (circles) and necrotic cells (*)

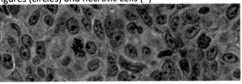

Path Presenter

METASTATIC MELANOMA
CLINICAL FEATURES
- Usually seen in patients with history of primary melanoma, but rarely can be first sign of disease or after entirely regressed melanoma
- Pigmented small macules or papules, black to gray/blue or amelanotic
HISTOLOGIC FEATURES
- Solid sheets or nodules of large, atypical melanocytes in the dermis or subcutis
- Usually inflammatory reaction sparse or absent
- Numerous mitotic figures and necrosis
OTHER HIGH YIELD POINTS
- In-transit metastases seen most frequently on extremities, scalp, and external ear - refers to metastases beyond 2 cm from primary lesion but within the skin area served by the same lymphatic drainage If within 2 cm-termed as satellite metastasis
- Epidermotropic metastatic melanoma can simulate primary melanoma with involvement of epidermis
DIFFERENTIAL DIAGNOSIS
- Melanotic schwannoma – nerve sheath tumor with melanin-producing Schwann cells, more spindled
- Metastatic carcinoma – sheets of neoplastic cells; immunostains helpful to distinguish origin of primary

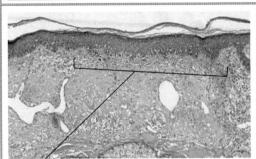

Lentiginous melanocytic proliferation in overlying epidermis

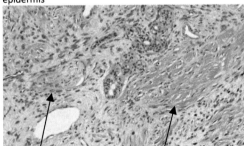

Perineural invasion, spindled proliferation in areas with fibrotic stroma

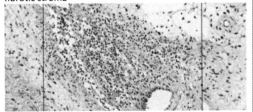

Focal host response of lymphocytes +/- plasma cell

DESMOPLASTIC MELANOMA
CLINICAL FEATURES
- Presents as a skin-colored, tan, or pink plaque or nodule on the head and neck of an older person
- Can be seen in association with lentigo maligna
HISTOLOGIC FEATURES
- Subtle proliferation of spindle cells in dermis with scattered atypical cells
- Spindle cells may form fascicles in a fibrotic stroma resembling a scar
- Focal host response of lymphocytes and/or plasma cells is frequently present
- Perineural invasion often seen
- Epidermis typically shows an atypical lentiginous melanocytic proliferation in greater than 50% of cases
- Classified sometimes into 2 categories-Pure desmoplastic melanoma-in which >90% of invasive tumor is desmoplastic and combined desmoplastic melanoma in which desmoplastic foci is <90% and has admixed non-desmoplastic foci
OTHER HIGH YIELD POINTS
- Spindled cells stain positive for SOX-10 and S100, negative for Melan A and HMB45
- Ki-67 shows greater than 5% proliferation index
- Around half have underlying mutations of NF1
DIFFERENTIAL DIAGNOSIS
- Desmoplastic Spitz nevus – more likely to have epidermal hyperplasia, lack the thin, wavy melanocytes of desmoplastic melanoma, p16(+)
- Scar – fibers more regularly parallel to epidermis, fibroblasts S100(-)
- Recurrent nevus – clinical history, lack of perineural invasion

Path Presenter

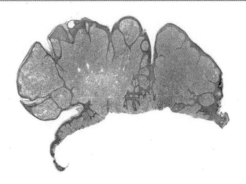
Low power polypod melanocytic proliferation resembling benign nevus

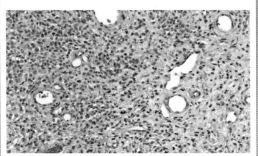
Pseudomaturation: large melanocytes with enlarged nuclei within the dermis

NEVOID MELANOMA

CLINICAL FEATURES
- Occur usually in older patients
- Papillomatous or dome-shaped papule or nodule on the trunk or extremities – often mistaken for benign nevus or seborrheic keratosis

HISTOLOGIC FEATURES
- Polypoid nested melanocytic proliferation filling the dermis with enlarged hyperchromatic nuclei
- Thinning or effacement of epidermis
- Deep mitotic features, lack of maturation and pseudo-maturation

IMMUNOHISTOCHEMISTRY
- Loss of p16 expression seen in 70% of nevoid melanoma (correlates to loss of CDKN2A gene)
- HMB45 usually strongly positive in dermal component
- Ki-67 strong nuclear staining

OTHER HIGH YIELD POINTS
- Dermoscopy can be misleading, frequently shows nevus-like pattern but presence enlargement or irregularly distributed dots and globules, irregular pigmentation, and atypical vascular pattern can be seen

DIFFERENTIAL DIAGNOSIS
- Benign nevi (mitotically active) – challenging to distinguish, p16 and molecular profiling used

Path Presenter

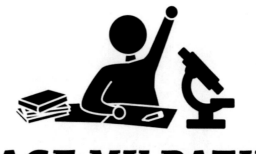

ACE MY PATH
Come Ace With Us!

CHAPTER 7: NEURAL TUMORS

NATHAN BOWERS, MD
JESUS ALBERTO CARDENAS DE LA GARZA, MD

CHAPTER 7: NEURAL TUMORS

NEURAL TUMORS

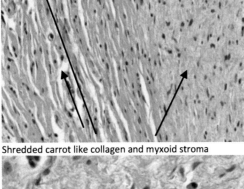
Dermal proliferation

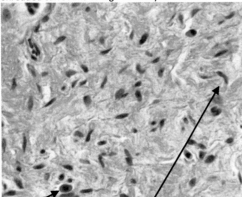
Shredded carrot like collagen and myxoid stroma

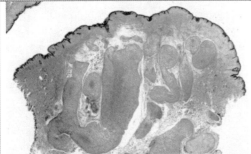
Mast cell   Spindled cells with wavy nuclei

NEUROFIBROMA
CLINICAL FEATURES
- Common superficial skin tumors that commonly present as solitary/localized skin-colored papule.
- Can be multiple
- Classic "buttonhole" sign (invagination with gently applied pressure)

HISTOLOGIC FEATURES
- Non encapsulated proliferation of **spindle shaped cells with wavy nuclei with scant cytoplasm**
- Loose haphazard arrangement of spindle cells with myxoid stroma
- Composition of Schwann cells, fibroblasts, and scattered **mast cells**
- Presence of mast cells can be a useful clue to differentiate from other dermal spindle-cell proliferation

IMMUNOFLUORESCENCE/IMMUNOHISTOCHEMISTRY
- S100 positive, SOX10 positive
- CD34 positivity is variable (fingerprint pattern)
- Negative for EMA (except in plexiform neurofibromas)

OTHER HIGH YIELD POINTS
- Multiple neurofibromas and/or plexiform and diffuse neurofibromas may be seen in association with **neurofibromatosis** (*NF1* mutations)

DIFFERENTIAL DIAGNOSIS
TRAUMATIC NEUROMA
- Proliferation of small bundles of well delineated nerve fibers scar-like stroma
- Haphazard arrangement of nerve fibers

DERMAL NEVUS
- Melanocytes arranged in nests within the dermis

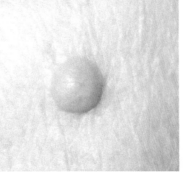
Neurofibroma - Soft, pink nodule

Path Presenter

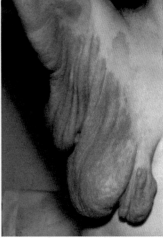
Plexiform Neurofibroma

PLEXIFORM NEUROFIBROMA
CLINICAL FEATURES
- Clinical plexiform neurofibromas start at a young age, usually before 5 years
- Large pendulous mass composed of thick tortuous nerves classically described as a "bag of worms"
- Commonly located on the head and neck

HISTOLOGIC FEATURES
- Dermal proliferation of **large nerve fascicles** with a snake-like pattern
- Often demonstrating a myxoid change within a background of diffuse neurofibroma

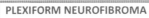

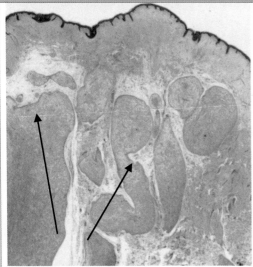

Large nerve fascicles

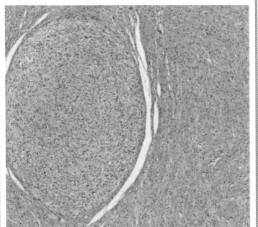

Large nerve fasicles with background of diffuse neurofibroma

- Cellular composition similar to neurofibroma with Schwann cells, mast cells, and fibroblasts

IMMUNOFLUORESCENCE/IMMUNOHISTOCHEMISTRY

- S100 positive **and** SOX10 positive
- Variable CD34 positivity
- EMA positive (negative in common neurofibromas)   Path Presenter

OTHER HIGH YIELD POINTS

- A **clinical plexiform neurofibroma is NOT equivalent to a histologic plexiform neurofibroma** (may see plexiform histology on non-plexiform neurofibroma)
- Strong association with clinical plexiform **neurofibromatosis type 1** (*NF1* mutation)
- Rapid growth of existing plexiform neurofibroma should raise concern for development of **malignant peripheral nerve sheath tumor**
- Imaging (MRI) if rapid growth of plexiform neurofibroma

DIFFERENTIAL DIAGNOSIS

NEUROTHEKEOMA

- Circumscribed nodular proliferation in dermis composed of nests and fascicles or epithelioid and spindle cells
- Nodules separated by a fibrous stroma

PLEXIFORM SCHWANNOMA

- Multinodular plexiform pattern of growth with individual fascicles composed of Schwann cells

NEUROTHEKEOMA	PLEXIFORM SCHWANNOMA

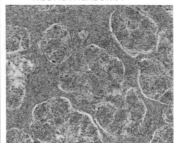 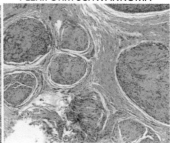

Nests of epithelioid and spindle cells separated by fibrous stroma | Multinodular plexiform pattern of fascicles composed of Schwann cells

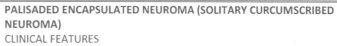

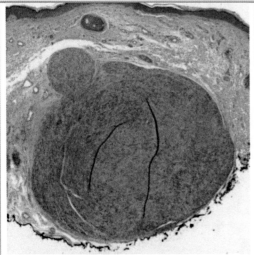

Lobular dermal proliferation

PALISADED ENCAPSULATED NEUROMA (SOLITARY CURCUMSCRIBED NEUROMA)

CLINICAL FEATURES

- Infrequent tumor that presents as a small and asymptomatic papule on the **head or neck**
- Often clinically thought to be a basal cell carcinoma or an intradermal nevus
- Also known as a **solitary circumscribed** neuroma

HISTOLOGIC FEATURES

- Presents as a lobular, plexiform, or fungating well-circumscribed dermal proliferation of **Schwann cells**, running in fascicles, often surrounded by **artifactual clefts**
- Surrounded by thin capsule which may have focal loss of continuity

IMMUNOFLUORESCENCE/IMMUNOHISTOCHEMISTRY

- **Diffuse S100** positivity
- GFAP negative

OTHER HIGH YIELD POINTS

- Few mast cells unlike neurofibroma
- **Palisading is uncommon or absent**

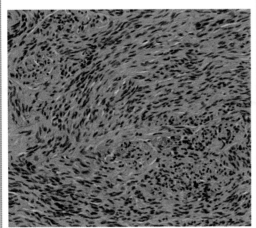

Surrounded by thin capsule

Proliferation of Schwannn cells

DIFFERENTIAL DIAGNOSIS
NEUROFIBROMA
- Not well circumscribed, no clefting
- Neurofibroma with haphazard arrangement of spindle cells with background of myxoid stroma

SCHWANNOMA
- Encapsulated and well-circumscribed collection of Schwann cells with Antoni A (parallel rows of nuclei separated by acellular areas) and Antoni B (loose edematous stroma)
- Typically very deep in dermis or subcutaneous tissue

NEUROFIBROMA

SCHWANNOMA

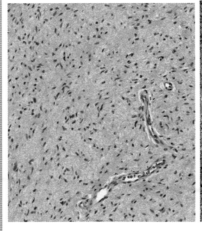

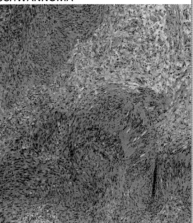

Path Presenter

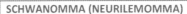

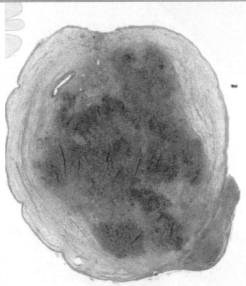

Encapsulated dermal proliferation of Schwann cells

SCHWANOMMA (NEURILEMOMMA)
CLINICAL FEATURES
- More common in middle-aged patients and presents as skin-colored nodule or tumor on the extremities
- Can have associated pain or paresthesia with larger tumors

HISTOLOGIC FEATURES
- **Encapsulated, deep** dermal or subcutaneous proliferation of **Schwann cells** with two distinct compositions (Antoni A and Antoni B areas)
- **Antoni A** areas are composed of **parallel rows of nuclei** separated by acellular areas (**Verocay bodies**)
- **Antoni B** areas are composed of loose **edematous stroma**
- Admixed **hyalinized vessels** are common

IMMUNOFLUORESCENCE/IMMUNOHISTOCHEMISTRY
- **S100** strong and diffusely positive
- **SOX-10** positive

OTHER HIGH YIELD POINTS
- Multiple tumors should raise suspicion of several different genodermatoses including **neurofibromatosis type 1 (NF1)** and **familiar schwannomatosis**
- Psammomatous melanocytic schwannomas contain melanin and Psammoma bodies and are associated with Carney complex (myxomas, lentigines, and endocrinopathy)

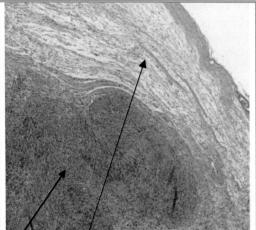

Antoni A and Antoni B areas

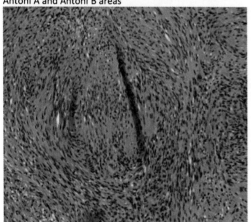

Verocay bodies

DIFFERENTIAL DIAGNOSIS

NEUROFIBROMA

- None encapsulated proliferation of spindle shaped cells with wavy nuclei with scant cytoplasm
- Loose haphazard arrangement of spindle cells with background of myxoid stroma

TRAUMATIC NEUROMA

- Proliferation of small bundles of well delineated nerve fibers in a fibrous stroma
- Haphazard arrangement of nerve fibers

NEUROFIBROMA   **TRAUMATIC NEUROMA**

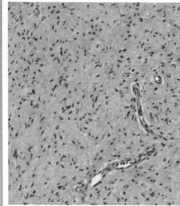   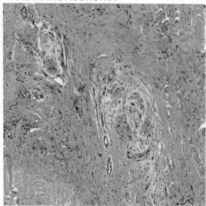

Path Presenter

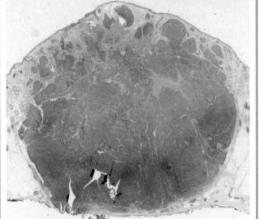

Dermal proliferation of monotanous appearing blue cells

Path Presenter

MERKEL CELL CARCINOMA (MCC)

CLINICAL FEATURES

- Presents as an asymptomatic fast-growing nodule on **sun exposed skin** with preference for the **head and neck**
- Most common in **elderly males** with skin phototypes 1 or 2
- Represents an aggressive neuroendocrine neoplasm of unknown cell origin
- Metastasis is common
- Two pathways of development proposed-de novo and Merkel cell polyomavirus associated

HISTOLOGIC FEATURES

- **Small, round blue cell** tumor with infiltrative pattern
- Dermal nodule, trabecular, and/or sheet-like proliferation of abundant monotonous looking blue cells
- Sometimes epidermal involvement and rarely only epidermal proliferation can be seen
- Cell with **high nuclear to cytoplasmic ratio**
- Typically show the **salt and pepper chromatin pattern**
- Nuclear **molding, mitosis,** and **necrosis** are frequent

IMMUNOFLUORESCENCE/IMMUNOHISTOCHEMISTRY

- **CK20** positive in a **paranuclear dot pattern**
- **Chromogranin** and **Synaptophysin** positive
- **INSMI** is the **most sensitive neuroendocrine marker**
- **CK7, TTF-1, S100, CD45 negative** in tumor cells

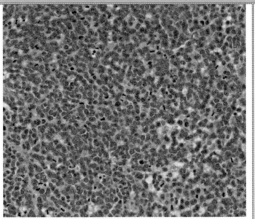

Tumor is composed of monotonous looking blue cells

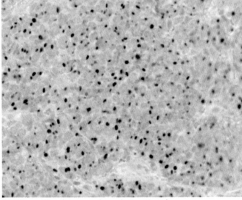

CK20 positive (paranuclear dot pattern)

OTHER HIGH YIELD POINTS
- Histology differential diagnosis includes small-cell carcinoma of the lung, melanoma, lymphoma, and less likely Ewing's sarcoma
- IHC with TTF-1 differentiates MCC (CK20+/TTF-1-) and small-cell carcinoma of the lung (TTF-1+/CK20-)
- Melanocytic and lymphocytic stains are negative
- More common in immunosuppressed patients
- Viral associated lesions can show presence of the MCPyV by immunohistochemistry targeting the MCPyV large T-antigen and/or by molecular studies
- MCPyV-positive tumors tend to lack mutations or show rare ones
- A high mutation burden frequently involving TP53 and RBI is typical of virus-negative tumors

DIFFERENTIAL DIAGNOSIS

Melanoma
- Atypical nests and sheets of melanocytes in the dermis
- May see areas of nesting as a clue to melanoma and not MCC
- Stains for melanocytic markers (MART-1, SOX-10, etc.)

Small Cell Carcinoma of the Lung
- Dermal proliferation of small blue cells
- Stain positive for TTF-1
- Stains negative for CK20

Ewing's Sarcoma
- Sarcoma composed of small round blue cells
- CD99 diffuse membranous expression
- Most common location is bone (diaphyseal/metaphyseal of long bones with only minority involving soft tissue

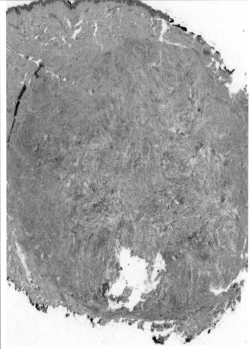

Well-circumscribed dermal nodule

NERVE SHEATH MYXOMA

CLINICAL FEATURES
- Presents as slow growing solitary superficial nodule or mass on the extremities with a **predilection for the fingers**
- More frequent in 3rd-4th decades

HISTOLOGIC FEATURES
- Well-circumscribed dermic **multilobulated** tumor composed of delineated nodules separated by collagenous septa
- Nodules are **myxomatous** and composed of **epithelioid and spindled Schwann cells**
- Frequent subcutaneous tissue involvement
- **Minimal or absent cellular pleomorphism or mitoses**

IMMUNOFLUORESCENCE/IMMUNOHISTOCHEMISTRY
- Diffuse **S100 positive**
- Glial Fibrillary Acidic Protein **(GFAP) positive**

OTHER HIGH YIELD POINTS
- **Formerly** known as **Myxoid Neurothekeoma**

DIFFERENTIAL DIAGNOSIS

CELLULAR NEUROTHEKEOMA
- Nests/fascicles of epithelioid and/or spindled cells with absent or sparse myxoid stroma
- Can have moderate cellular pleomorphism
- S100 negative
- CD63 (NKI/C3), S100A6 and PGP95 positive

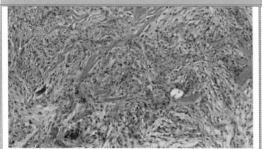
Schwann cells with background of myxoid stroma

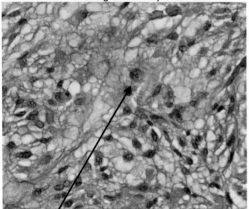
Epitheliod-appearing Schwann cells

Nodules separted by collagenous septa
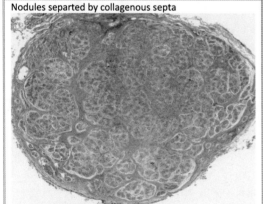
Well-circumsribed dermal nodule

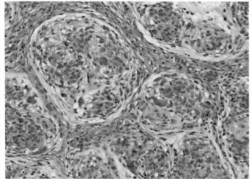
Nests of epetheliod/spindled cells with intervening fibrous stroma

SCHWANNOMA

- Encapsulated and well-circumscribed collection of Schwann cells with Antoni A (parallel rows of nuclei separated by acellular areas) and Antoni B (loose edematous stroma)

CELLULAR NEUROTHEKEOMA   SCWHANNOMA

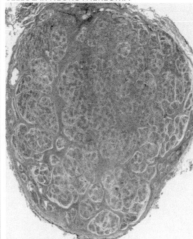
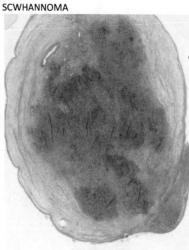

Path Presenter

CELLULAR NEUROTHEKEOMA

CLINICAL FEATURES

- Presents as slow growing, often asymptomatic, nodule or subcutaneous mass
- The most frequent location is the **head, neck, and upper extremities**
- Age of presentation is **2nd to 3rd decades**

HISTOLOGIC FEATURES

- Lobulated neoplasm composed of **nests of epithelioid and sometimes spindled cells, often separated by dense collagenous stroma**
- Absent or **sparse myxoid stroma**
- Can have **moderate cellular pleomorphism and scattered mitosis**

IMMUNOFLUORESCENCE/IMMUNOHISTOCHEMISTRY

- S100 negative
- **CD63 (NKI/C3), S100A6 and PGP95 positive**
- Can be MITF positive

OTHER HIGH YIELD POINTS

- Thought to **originate from fibrohistiocytic cells** as opposed to nerve sheath

DIFFERENTIAL DIAGNOSIS

NERVE SHEATH MYXOMA

- Well-circumscribed dermic multinodular collection of epithelioid appearing Schwann cells with background of abundant myxoid stroma
- S100 positive

MELANOMA

- Melanocytic markers are positive (MART-1, SOX-10, etc.)
- Typically without myxoid stroma

Path Presenter

CHAPTER 7: NEURAL TUMORS

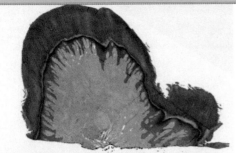

Acral papule with dermal collection of nerve bundles

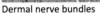

Dermal nerve bundles

SUPERNUMERARY DIGIT
CLINICAL FEATURES
- **Congenital** lesion that presents as a nodule or papule **classically** located on the **ulnar side** at the base of the **fifth digit**
- Synonym: Rudimentary Polydactyly
HISTOLOGIC FEATURES
- **Acral papule** with dermal collection of **nerve bundles** with **Meissner corpuscles**
IMMUNOFLUORESCENCE/IMMUNOHISTOCHEMISTRY
- S100 positive
- Factor XIIIa negative
DIFFERENTIAL DIAGNOSIS
AQUIRED DIGITAL FIBROKERATOMA
- Acral papule with longitudinal streaking collagen
- Lacks nerve bundles and contains large stellate factor XIIIa-positive dendrocytes

Path Presenter

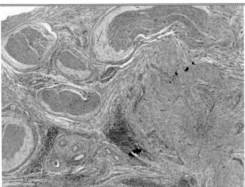

Haphazard proliferation of nerve fasicles with scar

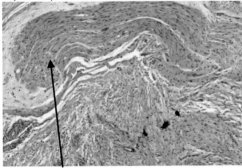

Distinct nerve fasicle

TRAUMATIC NEUROMA
CLINICAL FEATURES
- Etiology secondary to trauma, surgery, or amputation
- Present as painful or tender dermal or subcutaneous nodules
- Treatment of choice is surgical removal
HISTOLOGIC FEATURES
- Non-encapsulated, **haphazard proliferation** of distinct **nerve fascicles** surrounded by **scar tissue**
- Nerve **fascicles** are **enclosed by perineural cells**
IMMUNOFLUORESCENCE/IMMUNOHISTOCHEMISTRY
- S100 positive (Schwann cells)
- EMA and GLUT1 positive (surrounding perineurium)
OTHER HIGH YIELD POINTS
- Length-wise regenerative growth of nerve trunk results in complex folding that appears as multiple discrete fascicles in cross-section
DIFFERENTIAL DIAGNOSIS
NEUROFIBROMA
- Loose haphazard arrangement. No discrete nerve fascicles
SCHWANNOMA
- Encapsulated and well-circumscribed collection of Schwann cells
- No discrete nerve fascicles

Path Presenter

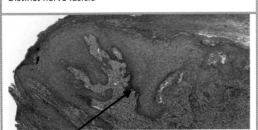

Pseudoepitheliomatous Hyperplasia

GRANULAR CELL TUMOR
CLINICAL FEATURES
- Arises most commonly in adults 30-60 years of age with a predilection for females. Appear on the tongue, trunk or limbs, particularly the arms
HISTOLOGIC FEATURES
- Ill-defined Sheets or trabeculae of large round-to-polygonal cells with **granular eosinophilic** cytoplasm and indistinct cellular borders
- Nuclei are small and centrally located; can be enlarged and hyperchromatic

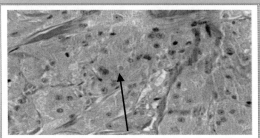

Granular cytoplasm with Pustulo-ovoid bodies of Milian

<u>Path Presenter</u>

- **Pseudoepitheliomatous hyperplasia (PEH)** may be present in the overlying epidermis. May have perineural invasion
- Presence of eosinophilic cytoplasmic granules (**Pustulo-ovoid bodies of Milian**), correspond to phagolysosomes and stain positive for PAS

IMMUNOFLUORESCENCE/IMMUNOHISTOCHEMISTRY
- Granular cells are S100 and CD68 positive

OTHER HIGH YIELD POINTS
- Overlying PEH can lead to misdiagnosis as squamous cell carcinoma
- Malignant variants have been described

DIFFERENTIAL DIAGNOSIS

ADULT RHABDOMYOMA
- Large polygonal cells with granular and eosinophilic cytoplasm
- Desmin and myoglobin positive

NON-NEURAL GRANULAR CELL TUMOR
- Lacks S100 expression and can exhibit greater nuclear atypia and mitotic activity

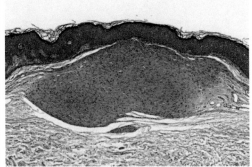

Well-demarcated, non-encapsulated tumor

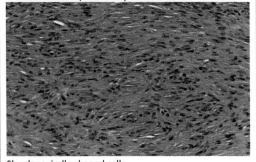

Slender spindle shaped cells

<u>Path Presenter</u>

PERINEURIOMA

CLINICAL FEATURES
- Tumor of peripheral nerve sheath origin on the **extremities or trunk**
- Typically affects adolescent or young adults
- **Sclerosing variant** usually presents on the **hands**

HISTOLOGIC FEATURES
- Arise in dermis, subcutis, or soft tissue
- Well-demarcated, **non-encapsulated** tumor composed of elongated slender **spindle-shaped** cells, sometimes with a myxoid background
- Nuclei are pale and wavy with inconspicuous eosinophilic cytoplasm
- **Sclerosing variant** presents with **plump epithelioid or fusiform cells** in a **whorled pattern** with dense **hyalinized stroma** and thin walled vessels

IMMUNOFLUORESCENCE/IMMUNOHISTOCHEMISTRY
- **EMA, Claudin-1, GLUT-1 positive**
- S100 and cytokeratin negative
- CD34 positivity is variable

OTHER HIGH YIELD POINTS
- Cutaneous perineuriomas are usually smaller than their soft tissue counter parts

DIFFERENTIAL DIAGNOSIS

NEUROFIBROMA
- Neurofibromas with scattered mast cells and classic 'bubble-gum' pink stroma
- S100 positive

FIBROMA OF TENDON SHEATH
- Well circumscribed tumor of bland spindle cells in a collagenous background
- Admixed thin walled slit-like vessels
- No mitosis or necrosis
- May see scattered giant cells

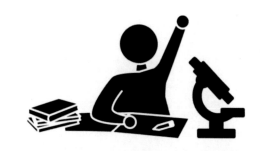

ACE MY PATH

Come Ace With Us!

CHAPTER 8: VASCULAR NEOPLASMS

SNEHAL SONAWANE, MD

VASCULAR TUMORS - BENIGN

Single, large dilated vascular space in upper dermis

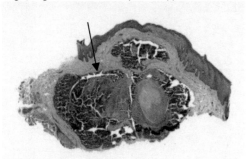

Dilated vascular space in upper dermis lined by flattened endothelial cells and thin fibrosis

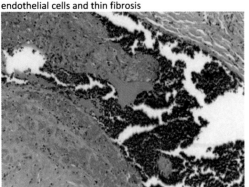

VENOUS LAKE
CLINICAL FEATURES
- Common vascular ectasia
- Small, dark blue compressible blebs
- Located on the face, ears, lips, and dorsal hands-on sun damaged skin

HISTOLOGIC FEATURES
- Single dilated vascular space in upper dermis lined by flattened endothelial cells and thin fibrosis
- May show thrombosis

OTHER HIGH YIELD POINTS
- Benign but minor trauma can produce bleeding
- Treatment options include electrosurgery, laser therapy, infrared coagulation, cryotherapy, and intralesional polidocanol injection

DIFFERENTIAL DIAGNOSIS
- Lymphangioma – dilated lymphatic spaces in loose stroma, lacks erythrocytes within space
- Angiokeratoma – multiple superficial dermal vessels in close contact with epidermis

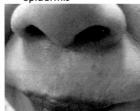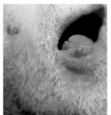

Small, dark blue blebs are located on the face, ears, lips   Path Presenter

---

Tightly grouped, well circumscribed proliferation of capillaries and venules in papillary dermis

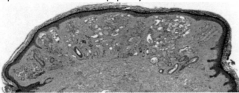

Proliferation of capillaries   Elevated ruby-red papules

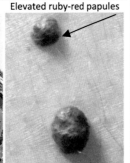

CHERRY ANGIOMA
CLINICAL FEATURES
- Common, benign vascular tumor
- Most frequently on the trunk
- Small, elevated bright red to purple papules
- Increase in incidence with age

Path Presenter

HISTOLOGIC FEATURES
- Tightly grouped, well-circumscribed proliferation of capillaries and venules in the papillary dermis, often surrounded by an epidermal collarette
- Some of the endothelial cell nuclei may be protuberant
- Thickened basement membrane is seen around some of the vessels

OTHER HIGH YIELD POINTS
- Removal for cosmetic purposes can be achieved by various modalities (e.g., shave excision, electrosurgery, laser ablation)

DIFFERENTIAL DIAGNOSIS
- Angiokeratoma – thin ectatic vessels in close contact with epidermis
- Pyogenic granuloma – epidermal collarette with lobular arrangement of capillary-sized vessels

---

Dilated vessels surrounded by the epidermis giving appearance of intraepidermal vessels

ANGIOKERATOMA
CLINICAL FEATURES
- Verrucous, dull, red to purple papules
- Numerous variants: Mibelli (dorsal fingers and toes, elbows, and knees), Fordyce (genitalia), caviar spots (tongue) and angiokeratoma circumscriptum (lower extremity or trunk)
- Angiokeratoma corporis diffusum seen in Fabry disease, presents as angiokeratomas concentrated between the umbilicus and the knees

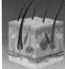
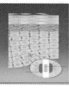

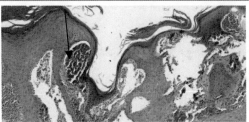

Verrucous dull red or purple papule

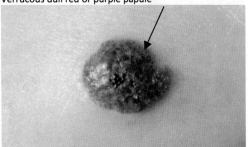

HISTOLOGIC FEATURES

- Acanthotic epidermis with hyperkeratosis
- Intermixed dilated vessels in the papillary dermis, surrounded by epidermis giving the appearance of intraepidermal vessels

OTHER HIGH YIELD POINTS

- Angiokeratoma corporis diffusum typically associated with Fabry's disease (X-linked disorder) and other inherited metabolic disorders
- If treatment is desired, options include shave excision, electrocautery, laser ablation, fulguration

DIFFERENTIAL DIAGNOSIS

- Seborrheic keratosis – hyperkeratotic, acanthotic, lacks vessels
- Capillary hemangioma – small, capillary-sized vessels within the dermis
- Lymphangioma – channels of lymphatic spaces in close contact with epidermis but spaces filled with lymph, blood, or thrombus

Path Presenter

Dilated lymphatics at all levels of the dermis

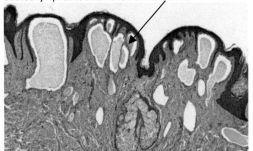

Dilated lymphatics in deep dermis

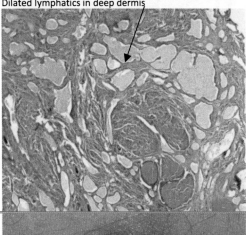

LYMPHANGIOMA

CLINICAL FEATURES

- Superficial lymphangioma (lymphangioma circumscriptum): scattered or grouped translucent papules and vesicles, predilection for the abdomen, axillae, genitalia, and tongue
- Deep lymphangioma: include cavernous lymphangioma and cystic hygroma, characterized by soft swellings in skin and subcutaneous tissue with normal overlying epidermis

HISTOLOGIC FEATURES

- Superficial irregular ectatic lymphatics in the papillary dermis, in close contact with overlying epidermis, contain lymph, blood, and/or thrombus
- Deep lymphangioma have dilated lymphatics at all levels of the dermis with possible extension into subcutaneous tissue and muscle (unfavorable sign)

OTHER HIGH YIELD POINTS

- Cystic hygroma associated with Turner syndrome (45, XO karyotype), hydrops fetalis, and fetal death, can coexist with nevus flammeus
- Imaging for deep lymphangioma necessary to determine extent of involvement of deeper structures

DIFFERENTIAL DIAGNOSIS

- Angiokeratoma - thin ectatic vessels in close contact with the epidermis filled with erythrocytes

Path Presenter

TARGETOID HEMOSIDEROTIC HEMANGIOMA (HOBNAIL HEMANGIOMA)

CLINICAL FEATURES

- Occurs in young to middle-aged patients
- Predominantly seen on the trunk or extremities as a brown or violaceous papule with a halo

HISTOLOGIC FEATURES

- Ectatic vessels with hob nailing of endothelial cells in superficial dermis
- Vascular channels dissecting collagen bundles in deep dermis and occasional intraluminal papillary projections

Brown or violaceous papule with an ecchymotic halo

Ectatic vessels and vascular channels dissecting collagen bundles in deep dermis

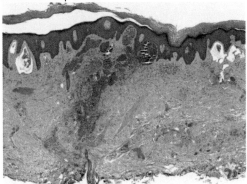

Path Presenter

- Perivascular lymphocytic inflammation with red cell extravasation and interspersed hemosiderin deposits

DIFFERENTIAL DIAGNOSIS

- Kaposi sarcoma – spindled endothelial cells, irregular, jagged vascular spaces
- Papillary intralymphatic angioendothelioma – intraluminal proliferation with papillary processes associated with thrombus
- Retiform hemangioendothelioma – hobnail endothelial cells line the vessels but arborizing pattern is distinctive of this entity

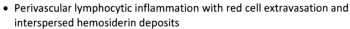
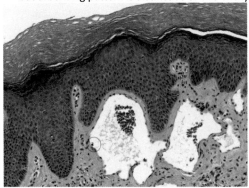

Ectatic vessels with hobnailing of endothelial cells

PYOGENIC GRANULOMA/LOBULAR CAPILLARY HEMANGIOMA

CLINICAL FEATURES

- Acquired, friable, pedunculated papule or nodule
- Most common in children, but can occur at any age
- Predilection for hands, forearm, and face (gingival seen in pregnancy)

HISTOLOGIC FEATURES

- Polypoid lesion showing lobulated proliferation of capillaries with epidermal collarette
- Often ulcerated with associated admixed acute and chronic inflammation and edematous stroma
- Less frequently, proliferations can be intravenous and subcutaneous

OTHER HIGH YIELD POINTS

- Linked to trauma, medication (isotretinoin, capecitabine, indinavir), pregnancy
- Treatment options include curettage or shave excision with destruction of base with silver nitrate or fulguration, topical imiquimod, sclerotherapy with monoethanolamine oleate, laser therapy, and intralesional steroids

DIFFERENTIAL DIAGNOSIS

- Kaposi sarcoma – characteristic interlacing spindle cells and split-like vessels
- Bacillary Angiomatosis -admixed aggregates of neutrophils and Warthin starry positive clumps of bacteria

Lobulated proliferation of capillaries

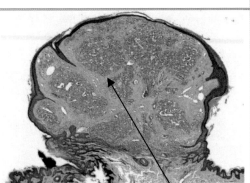
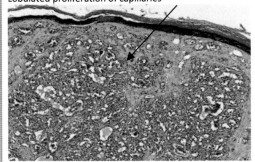
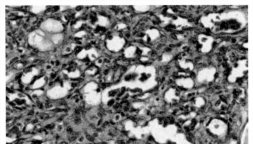

Path Presenter

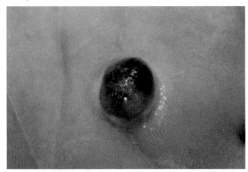

Pedunculated nodule with epidermal collarette

Solid, well circumscribed nodular proliferation

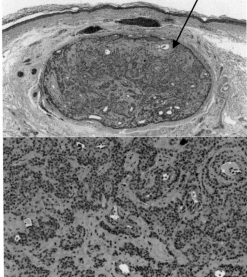

Small monotonous cells around dilated blood vessels

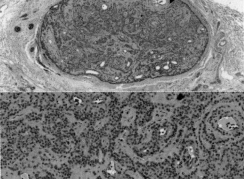

GLOMUS TUMOR

CLINICAL FEATURES
- Solitary blue-purple dermal nodule, predilection for fingers and toes
- Subungual tumors can present as longitudinal erythronychia, located on nail matrix
- Almost always painful

HISTOLOGIC FEATURES
- Solid, well circumscribed nodular proliferation of small monotonous cells with round central nucleus and eosinophilic cytoplasm around dilated blood vessels; no atypia

IMMUNOHISTOCHEMISTRY
- Positive for α-smooth muscle actin (SMA)

OTHER HIGH YIELD POINTS
- Glomus cells derived from Sucquet-Hoyer canal, function in thermoregulation
- Plain radiography can demonstrate bony erosions, especially in the case of subungual lesions

DIFFERENTIAL DIAGNOSIS
- Hidradenoma – sweat gland differentiation, ductal structures present
- Intradermal nevus – nested appearance with round monomorphic cells
- Solitary mastocytosis – composed of mast cells, IHC can differentiate

Path Presenter

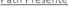

Subungual tumor with erythronychia

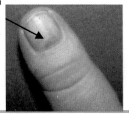

GLOMUVENOUS MALFORMATION (GVM) / GLOMANGIOMA

CLINICAL FEATURES
- Blue-violaceous partially compressible papules or nodules, painful to touch
- Typically multiple or segmental distribution (mosaicism)

HISTOLOGIC FEATURES
- Large vascular channels surrounded by few layers of glomus cells, poorly circumscribed and unencapsulated

IMMUNOHISTOCHEMISTRY
- Positive for α-smooth muscle actin (SMA)

OTHER HIGH YIELD POINTS
- Previously known as glomangioma, considered variant of glomus tumor
- Glomangiomatosis refers to diffuse angiomatosis with associated glomus cells

DIFFERENTIAL DIAGNOSIS
- Hemangioma – dilated vascular spaces, lack glomus cells
- Deep lymphangioma – dilated lymphatic spaces, lack glomus cells

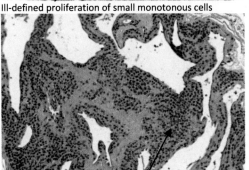

Ill-defined proliferation of small monotonous cells

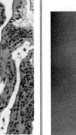

Proliferation of small monotonous cells with round central nucleus and eosinophilic cytoplasm around dilated blood vessels

Path Presenter

Blue-purple partially compressible papules

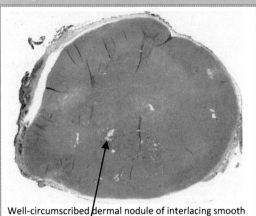

Well-circumscribed dermal nodule of interlacing smooth muscle cells around interspersed vessels

ANGIOLEIOMYOMA 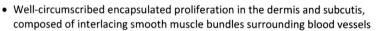 Path Presenter

CLINICAL FEATURES
- Solitary nodule
- Favors extremities, particularly lower legs

HISTOLOGIC FEATURES
- Well-circumscribed encapsulated proliferation in the dermis and subcutis, composed of interlacing smooth muscle bundles surrounding blood vessels
- Rounded or slit-like vessels with muscular walls are identified within the lesion

IMMUNOHISTOCHEMISTRY
- Positive for α-smooth muscle actin (SMA), calponin, h-caldesmon
- Vessels highlighted by vascular markers (CD31, CD34)

DIFFERENTIAL DIAGNOSIS
- Leiomyoma – lack vascular component, less circumscribed
- Angiomyolipoma – admixed foci of mature adipocytes between muscle bundles and blood vessels

---

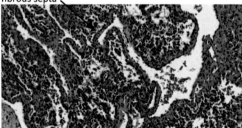

Capillaries arranged in defined lobules separated by thin fibrous septa

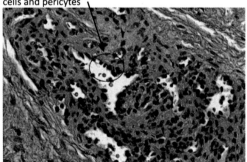

Capillaries with tiny luminal and plump endothelial cells and pericytes

INFANTILE HEMANGIOMA (HEMANGIOMA OF INFANCY)

CLINICAL FEATURES
- Most common tumors of infancy, female predominance, favor head and neck
- Present within first few weeks of life, evolve and enlarge over months to bright red, raised nodule or plaque
- Total or partial regression occurs in most lesions

HISTOLOGIC FEATURES
- Three stages-Proliferation, Partial involution, Complete involution
- Early lesions are highly cellular with proliferation of small, slit-like capillaries with plump endothelial cells and pericytes with abundant cytoplasm and enlarged nuclei
- Established lesions have larger and more obvious vascular lumina, flatter endothelial cells lining the vessels. Diminishing vessels with interstitial fibrosis, replacement if vascular tissue with lobules of fat in regressing lesions
- Normal mitotic figures present, often accompanied by mast cells and dermal dendrocytes within the stroma

IMMUNOHISTOCHEMISTRY
- Positive for GLUT-1, CD31, SMA (pericytes), shares markers specific for placental vessels

OTHER HIGH YIELD POINTS
- Multiple disseminated cutaneous hemangiomas can be associated with visceral hemangiomas
- PHACES syndrome: Posterior fossa malformations, hemangiomas (large facial), arterial anomalies, cardiac anomalies, eye abnormalities, sternal cleft and/or supraumbilical raphe

DIFFERENTIAL DIAGNOSIS
- Vascular malformation – large, dilated vessels lined by flat endothelium
- Congenital non-progressive hemangioma (RICH, NICH)- present at birth, negative for GLUT1   Path Presenter

ANGIOLYMPHOID HYPERPLASIA WITH EOSINOPHILIA (EPITHELIOID HEMANGIOMA)

CLINICAL FEATURES
- Affects young to middle-aged adults
- Grouped pink to red–brown, dome-shaped, papules or nodules on the head and neck, especially around the ears or on the scalp

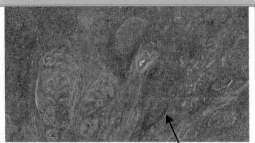
Moderate to dense lymphocytic infiltrate

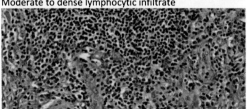
Lymphocytic infiltrate & numerous eosinophils

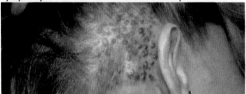
Pink to red–brown, dome-shaped, papules or nodules

HISTOLOGIC FEATURES
- Dermal or subcutaneous circumscribed collection of capillary vessels lined by prominent epithelioid endothelial cells, focal vacuolization
- Sometimes centered around large central vessels
- Moderate to dense lymphocytic infiltrate with numerous eosinophils, fibrous or myxoid stroma
- Reactive germinal centers may sometimes be seen

OTHER HIGH YIELD POINTS
- Reported in association with pregnancy, HIV infection, lichen amyloidosis, nephrotic syndrome
- Can be treated with excision, laser, cryosurgery, intralesional corticosteroids

DIFFERENTIAL DIAGNOSIS
- Arthropod bite – dense inflammatory infiltrate with eosinophils, without vascular proliferation and vacuolization
- Epithelioid angiosarcoma – more prominent atypia
- Epithelioid hemangioendothelioma – epithelioid endothelial cells with cytoplasmic vacuoles, nests, and cords growth pattern
- Eosinophilic lymphogranuloma (Kimura's disease) – reactive lymphoid follicles with eosinophils, associated with regional lymphadenopathy, peripheral eosinophilia, IgE hyperglobulinemia, lack epithelioid endothelial cells
- IgG4-related disease – nodular infiltrates of venules with lymphocytes, eosinophils, plasma cells

---

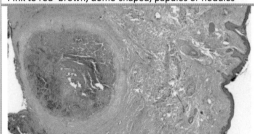
Papillary projections of loose connective tissue lined by endothelial cells within a vascular structure

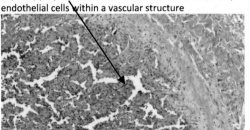

INTRAVASCULAR PAPILLARY ENDOTHELIAL HYPERPLASIA (MASSON'S TUMOR)
CLINICAL FEATURES
- Single or multiple firm, blue or purple dermal nodule, can be painful
- Most common on fingers, head, neck, and trunk. More often in women

HISTOLOGIC FEATURES
- Proliferation within the lumen of a vessel with an organizing thrombus and papillary projections of loose connective tissue lined by endothelial cells
- Occasionally fibrous capsule only remains, vessel wall absent or ruptured

DIFFERENTIAL DIAGNOSIS
- Papillary intralymphatic angioendothelioma – irregular vascular channels, lumen contain papillary structures with fibrous cores
- Glomeruloid hemangioma – dilated dermal vascular spaces containing small capillary vessels with eosinophilic globules

Path Presenter

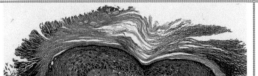
Solid sheets of epithelioid cells

CUTANEOUS EPITHELIOID ANGIOMATOUS NODULE
CLINICAL FEATURES
- Clinical-solitary papule/nodule in young to middle-aged adults

HISTOLOGIC FEATURES
- Well circumscribed nodule in superficial to mid dermis with epidermal collarette
- Composed of solid sheets of epithelioid cells, often showing intracytoplasmic vacuoles
- Scattered mitosis may be seen but lacks nuclear pleomorphism or atypical mitosis

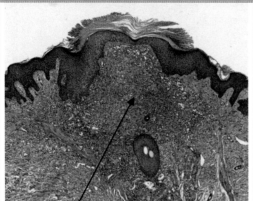

Well circumscribed nodule in superficial to mid dermis

- Admixed inflammation may be noted

IMMUNOHISTOCHEMISTRY
- Positive for vascular markers, CD31 positive, HHV 8 negative

DIFFERENTIAL DIAGNOSIS
- Pyogenic granuloma
- Bacillary angiomatosis- characterized by neutrophilic infiltrate, and aggregates of eosinophilic material (clusters of Bartonella henselae organisms)
- Epithelioid hemangioendothelioma

Path Presenter

Poorly circumscribed proliferation of irregularly branching thin walled blood vessels

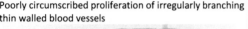

Path Presenter

MICROVENULAR HEMANGIOMA
CLINICAL FEATURES
- Red to purple small, slow-growing papules or nodules seen on the trunk and extremities
- Predominantly affects young and middle-aged adults

HISTOLOGIC FEATURES
- Poorly circumscribed proliferation of thin, uniform, flattened vessels throughout the dermis
- Extension into pilar erector muscle is common
- Surrounded by a single layer of pericytes, highlighted by SMA
- No multilayering of endothelial cells
- Collagenous stroma

IMMUNOHISTOCHEMISTRY
- Positive for CD31, ERG negative for GLUT-1, D2-40

DIFFERENTIAL DIAGNOSIS
- Kaposi Sarcoma – eosinophilic globules present, HHV-8 positive
- Diffuse dermal angiomatosis – hyperplastic endothelial cells, often spindled, small vascular lumen

Band like proliferation of capillaries in mid dermis running parallel to epidermis

ACQUIRED ELASTOTIC HEMANGIOMA
CLINICAL FEATURES
- Papule/plaque in sun-exposed areas

HISTOLOGIC FEATURES
- Band-like proliferation of capillaries in mid dermis running parallel to epidermis in a background of solar elastosis

IMMUNOHISTOCHEMISTRY
- Usually not required
- Positive for vascular markers such as CD31 and CD34

DIFFERENTIAL DIAGNOSIS
- Low grade angiosarcoma
- Capillary hemangioma

Path Presenter

Path Presenter

ACROANGIODERMATITIS
CLINICAL FEATURES
- Reactive vasoproliferative disorder occurring in chronic venous insufficiency
- Violaceous to brown papules and plaques, most frequently affects lower

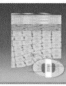

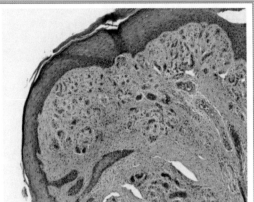

Increased thick-walled blood vessels

extremities, can be bilateral

HISTOLOGIC FEATURES

- Proliferation of small thick-walled blood vessels with extravasation of erythrocytes, scattered hemosiderin in edematous dermis

DIFFERENTIAL DIAGNOSIS

- Kaposi sarcoma – spindled endothelial cells, HHV-8 positive

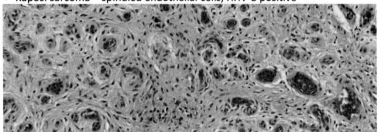

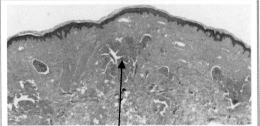

Proliferation of vessels in upper and mid dermis

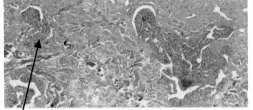

Tufts of proliferating coiled capillaries projecting within walls of ectatic vessels mimicking renal glomeruli

Path Presenter

GLOMERULOID HEMANGIOMA

CLINICAL FEATURES

- Benign vascular tumor, present as multiple eruptive, red, or purple papules on the trunk and limbs in the setting of POEMS syndrome

HISTOLOGIC FEATURES

- Tufts of proliferating coiled capillaries projecting within the walls of ectatic sinusoidal dermal vessels mimicking renal glomeruli
- Endothelial cells lining vessels contain PAS-positive eosinophilic globules

IMMUNOHISTOCHEMISTRY

- Capillary-type endothelial cells positive for CD31, CD34
- Sinusoidal endothelial cells positive for CD31, CD68, negative for CD34

OTHER HIGH YIELD POINTS

- Associated with **POEMS syndrome** (*p*olyneuropathy, *o*rganomegaly, *e*ndocrinopathy, *M*-protein, and *s*kin changes) and **TAFRO syndrome**, variant of idiopathic multicentric Castleman's disease (*t*hrombocytopenia, *a*nasarca, *f*ever, *r*eticulin fibrosis or *r*enal dysfunction, *o*rganomegaly)
- When multifocal termed as papillary hemangioma

DIFFERENTIAL DIAGNOSIS

- Tufted angioma – multiple cellular lobules in the dermis and subcutis, no PAS-positive globules
- Intravascular papillary endothelial hyperplasia – proliferation within a vessel with thrombus

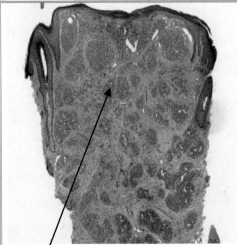

Cannon ball like aggregates of endothelial cells

TUFTED HEMANGIOMA

CLINICAL FEATURES

- Usually solitary, slowly spreading erythematous macule, plaque, or nodule
- Predominantly seen in children and young adults, rarely congenital

HISTOLOGIC FEATURES

- Cannon ball-like aggregates of tightly packed capillaries with endothelial cells showing spindled and oval nuclei, dilated crescentic thin-walled vessels within lobules or at the periphery
- Endothelial cells may occasionally show intracytoplasmic hyaline structures
- Stroma can be desmoplastic and may show lymphatic channels
- IHC show positivity for CD31, CD34, negative for GLUT-1
- Dilated vessels show focal staining with D2-40, proliferative capillaries are negative

OTHER HIGH YIELD POINTS

- Associated with Kasabach-Merritt phenomenon (platelet trapping and consumptive coagulopathy)

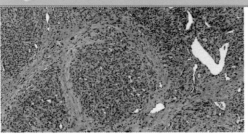

Small capillary lumina are identified within the aggregates of endothelial cells

DIFFERENTIAL DIAGNOSIS

- Glomeruloid hemangioma – proliferating coiled capillaries within vessels
- Kaposiform hemangioendothelioma – similar features but extension into the deep dermis and subcutis

Path Presenter

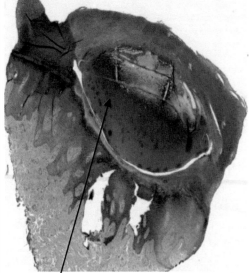

Hyperkeratosis, epidermal acanthosis, and inspissated hemorrhage within the stratum corneum

TALON NOIR

CLINICAL FEATURES

- Blue/black macule on acral site, usually on the posterior or posterolateral heel, or can be seen on metatarsals
- Horizontally arranged petechiae formation

HISTOLOGIC FEATURES

- Located on acral skin
- Characterized by hyperkeratosis, epidermal acanthosis, and inspissated hemorrhage within the stratum corneum
- Telangiectatic vessels and extravasation of erythrocytes may be noted in the papillary dermis

DIFFERENTIAL DIAGNOSIS

- Verruca vulgaris – epidermal hyperkeratosis and acanthosis with hypergranulosis
- Melanoma – atypical melanocytes present

Path Presenter

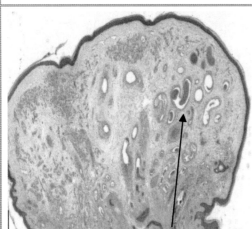

Well circumscribed proliferation of thick and thin vessels

Path Presenter

ARTERIOVENOUS HEMANGIOMA

CLINICAL FEATURES

- Asymptomatic, solitary red or purple papule, most commonly on the lips, perioral skin, nose, eyelids

HISTOLOGIC FEATURES

- Well-circumscribed proliferation of thin-walled angiomatous capillaries and thick-walled vessels in the upper and mid-dermis
- Vessels lined by endothelium and muscular wall with elastic fibers

DIFFERENTIAL DIAGNOSIS

- Arteriovenous malformation – admixed veins, capillaries, and arteries that is not a discrete neoplasm but rather a congenital malformation
- Pyogenic granuloma – lobular proliferation of small capillary-sized vessels which are much smaller in size than AV hemangioma

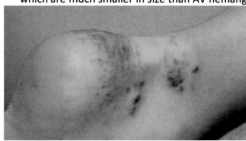

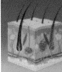
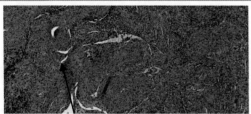
Proliferation of cavernous blood vessels admixed with cellular spindle cell proliferation

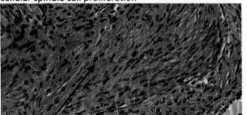
Spindle cells with elongated nuclei and eosinophilic cytoplasm

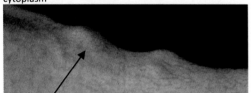
Subcutaneous bluish nodules

SPINDLE CELL HEMANGIOMA

CLINICAL FEATURES

- Single or multiple firm, blue, or hemorrhagic nodules most commonly on the hands, feet, or trunk
- Can occur at any age, up to 50% seen in children and young adults

HISTOLOGIC FEATURES

- Well-circumscribed vascular tumor in the dermis and subcutis
- Composed of proliferation of thin-walled cavernous blood vessels lined by a single layer of flattened endothelial cells
- Admixed with cellular spindle cell proliferation and solid areas of plump endothelial cells that have intracytoplasmic vacuoles
- Minimal nuclear atypia and mitotic figures

OTHER HIGH YIELD POINTS

- Associated with Maffucci syndrome and Klippel-Trenaunay syndrome

DIFFERENTIAL DIAGNOSIS

- Kaposi Sarcoma – eosinophilic globules, more atypical vascular spaces
- Angiosarcoma – nuclear atypia, mitotic figures, bizarre and irregular vascular spaces

Path Presenter

VASCULAR TUMORS- ATYPICAL

ATYPICAL VASCULAR LESION

CLINICAL FEATURES

- Erythematous to violaceous macules or papules, usually smaller than angiosarcoma
- Most commonly involves breast after radiation

HISTOLOGIC FEATURES

- Dilated vascular spaces in an anastomosing pattern situated in the upper dermis
- Lined by hyperchromatic endothelial cells with plump or flattened nuclei
- Absence of severe cytologic atypia, mitotic activity, multilayering of endothelial cells and infiltration into subcutaneous fat

IMMUNOHISTOCHEMISTRY

- Endothelial cells positive for CD31, CD34, D2-40

DIFFERENTIAL DIAGNOSIS

- Angiosarcoma – FISH analysis for *MYC* amplification and IHC for MYC can help distinguish
- Kaposi sarcoma – atypical, spindled cells, HHV-8 positive

Path Presenter

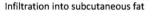

KAPOSI SARCOMA

CLINICAL FEATURES

- Four clinicopathologic types:
  (1) **Classic type** affects middle-aged Mediterranean men, presents as violaceous papules or nodules usually on the lower extremities;
  (2) **African (endemic) type** is endemic to areas of topical Africa, can be more

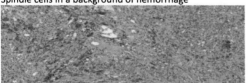

Anastomosing pattern of vessels with hyperchromatic endothelial cells

Infiltration into subcutaneous fat

Spindle cells in a background of hemorrhage

Proliferation of interlacing bundles of spindle cells

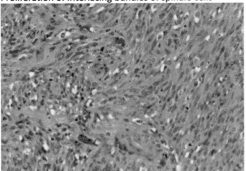

Red-brown patch of patch-stage

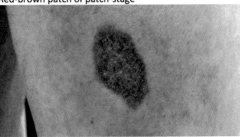

Path Presenter

aggressive with extensive fungating tumors;

(3) **HIV-associated (epidemic) type** presents as an AIDS-defining illness, brown to red macules or patches in early stages, can become violaceous nodules;

(4) **KS associated with immunosuppressive therapy** is a complication of iatrogenic immunosuppression, may be more aggressive than classic KS

HISTOLOGIC FEATURES

- **PATCH STAGE**: subtle proliferation of small, irregularly shaped vessels partly surrounding ectatic vessels known as "promontory sign", dissects between collagen bundles, extravasated erythrocytes and hemosiderin deposition
- **PLAQUE STAGE**: more prominent proliferation of interlacing bundles of spindle cells n a hemorrhagic background, slit-like vascular spaces, scattered plasma cells and hyaline eosinophilic globules
- **NODULAR STAGE**: Proliferation of spindle cells in a hemorrhagic background, apoptosis of endothelial cells seen

IMMUNOHISTOCHEMISTRY

- Positive for HHV-8 (causative agent in all types)

OTHER HIGH YIELD POINTS

- HIV testing indicated if status is unknown
- Imaging evaluation and other studies to determine extent of disease

DIFFERENTIAL DIAGNOSIS

- Low-grade angiosarcoma – negative for HHV-8
- Aneurysmal dermatofibroma – spindle cell proliferation with background of hemorrhage but with features of dermatofibroma (collagen trapping on periphery)
- Spindle cell hemangioendothelioma – more cavernous vessels, epithelioid and vacuolated endothelial cells, no eosinophilic globules
- Kaposiform hemangioendothelioma – may have more epithelioid endothelial cells, similar hyaline eosinophilic globules are present, HHV-8 negative

EPITHELIOID HEMANGIOENDOTHELIOMA

CLINICAL FEATURES

- Painful lesion
- If the lesion is arising from vein, it can lead to symptoms of vascular occlusion
- Potential for local recurrence
- Rarely metastasize

HISTOLOGIC FEATURES

- Two different subtypes of epithelioid hemangioendothelioma (EHE), namely the WWTR1-CAMTA1 subtype (classic EHE) and the YAP-TFE3 subtype

WWTR1-CAMTA1 Subtype (Classic EHE):

- Histological Features: Cords, strands, or small nests of large endothelial cells with abundant eosinophilic cytoplasm embedded in a myxohyaline stroma
- Vesicular, round to oval, sometimes indented nuclei
- Some tumor cells have intracytoplasmic, round, clear vacuoles representing small vascular lumina, which may contain erythrocytes
- Behavior: Typically exhibits minimal mitotic activity, atypia, or necrosis. Not as aggressive as the YAP-TFE3 subtype

YAP-TFE3 Subtype:

- Histological Features: Solid nests or pseudo-alveolar arrangement of epithelioid cells enmeshed in a fibrous stroma. Tumor cells can form vascular spaces
- Tumor cells have abundant, densely eosinophilic cytoplasm
- Intracytoplasmic vacuoles are rare compared to the WWTR1-CAMTA1 subtype
- Behavior: Usually minimal mitotic activity, atypia, or necrosis. However, up to 10% of cases may exhibit frank malignant features, such as prominent nuclear pleomorphism, increased mitotic activity, solid growth, or necrosis. These

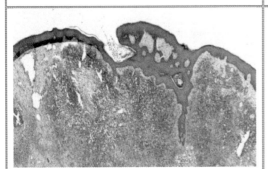

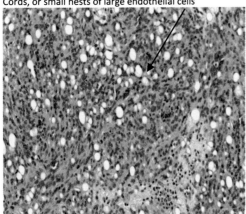

Cords, or small nests of large endothelial cells

Intracytoplasmic, round, clear vacuoles representing small vascular lumina

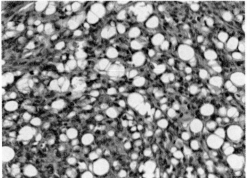

Path Presenter

aggressive cases resemble epithelioid angiosarcoma and have more aggressive behavior

IMMUNOHISTOCHEMISTRY
- Positive Stains: ERG, CD31, podoplanin (D2-40), FLI1, von Willebrand factor
- Negative Stains: CD34 (can be negative), S100, SOX10, desmin, EMA (usually negative)
- Variable Stains: Keratin (positive up to 40%), SMA (positive up to 45%)

MOLECULAR:
- Characterized by recurrent WWTR1-CAMTA1 or YAP1-TFE3 gene fusion

DIFFERENTIAL DIAGNOSIS
- Epithelioid sarcoma-positive for epithelial markers
- Epithelioid angiosarcoma-atypical endothelial cells lining vessels, infiltrative
- Melanoma-positive for melanocytic markers
- Metastatic carcinoma-immunostains depend on origin of primary

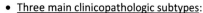

VASCULAR TUMORS- MALIGNANT

ANGIOSARCOMA

CLINICAL FEATURES
- Three main clinicopathologic subtypes:

  (1) **Idiopathic cutaneous angiosarcoma**: common locations include head and neck of elderly adults, presents as single or multifocal blue to violaceous patches, plaques, or nodules, rarely can present as recurrent angioedema of face, alopecia, or rosacea-like eruption

  (2) **Lymphedema-associated angiosarcoma**: most frequently seen as Stewart-Treves syndrome, red to violaceous raised nodules arise after radical mastectomy within chronic lymphedema of the arm; can rarely occur in setting of other chronic lymphedematous states (Milroy's disease, filarial lymphedema)

  (3) **Post irradiation angiosarcoma**: after radiotherapy of malignancy tumors such as breast carcinoma, median latent period ~20 years

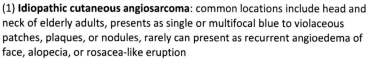

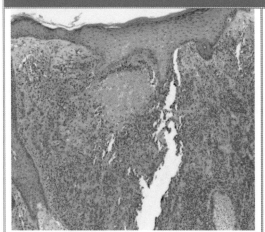

infiltrating anaplastic cells derived from blood vessels and lining irregular blood-filled spaces

HISTOLOGIC FEATURES
- Poorly demarcated proliferation of anastomosing blood vessels (cracked collagen pattern) and solid areas
- Infiltrating anaplastic cells derived from blood vessels and lining irregular blood-filled spaces with variable spindled or epithelioid appearance, papillary processes extending into the lumina
- Luminal formation may be absent

IMMUNOHISTOCHEMISTRY
- Positive for endothelial markers: CD34, CD31 and lymphatic markers: D2-40
- Radiation associated AS- Positive for MYC
- Poorly differentiated tumors may show variable staining

OTHER HIGH YIELD POINTS
- FISH demonstrates *MYC* amplification

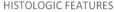

DIFFERENTIAL DIAGNOSIS
- Atypical vascular lesion – occurs in setting of irradiated skin, *MYC* amplification absent, no multilayering of endothelial cells
- Poorly differentiated carcinoma or melanoma – share features with poorly differentiated angiosarcoma, immunohistochemical profile helps to differentiate
- Kaposi Sarcoma – atypical slit-like vascular spaces with spindle cells, negative for *MYC*, positive for HHV-8

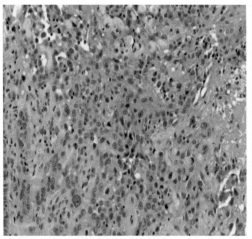

Epithelioid endothelial cells with significant atypia

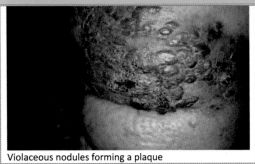

Violaceous nodules forming a plaque

Path Presenter

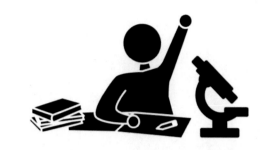

ACE MY PATH
Come Ace With Us!

CHAPTER 9: FIBROUS NEOPLASMS

TERRANCE LYNN, MD

FIBROUS NEOPLASMS

Dense collagenous stroma   Mature adipose

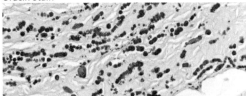

Abnormal elastic fibers

Von Gieson stain   Abnormal elastic fibers
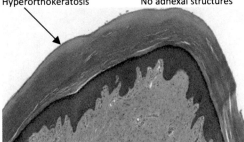

Oracin Stain

Image Credit: Raul Perret, MD, MSc @kells108

ELASTOFIBROMA DORSI
CLINICAL FEATURES
- Ill-defined, slow-growing, painless, firm deep soft tissue tumor
- Female predominance, **older age** (>50 years)
- Usually occurs at **posterior margin of scapula** but has been seen in stomach, omentum, rectum, and oral cavities
- Most often is solitary but can be bilateral

HISTOLOGIC FEATURES
- **Dense collagenous stroma** and mature adipose with interspersed **beaded elastic fibers** of various sizes
- Stroma can be edematous or have myxoid change
- Can infiltrate into skeletal muscle and entrap the muscle fibers

OTHER HIGH YIELD POINTS
- **Von Gieson** or Orcin stains highlight abnormal elastic fibers
- **Gross examination**: Tan-**white to yellow firm mass** with poorly defined margins
- Pathogenesis is hypothesized to be from repetitive trauma
- Molecular alterations include:
  - Nonrandom X-inactivation or gains of Xq
  - Recurrent rearrangements in 1p and 7q

DIFFERENTIAL DIAGNOSIS
- **Desmoid fibromatosis**: increased cellularity, sweeping fascicles of myofibroblasts with parallel alignment, positive nuclear β-catenin
- **Nuchal-type fibroma**: predominantly composed of dense collagen, lacks abnormal elastic fibers, located in different anatomic locations
- **Fibrolipoma**: elastic fibers are normal

Path Presenter

Hyperorthokeratosis   No adnexal structures

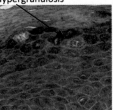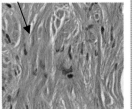

Hypergranulosis   Vertically oriented

More than two cells thick   Thickened collagen bundles

ACQUIRED DIGITAL FIBROKERATOMA
CLINICAL FEATURES
- **Solitary, skin-colored, dome-shaped papules** located on acral surfaces
- Most lesions are small and do not exceed 15 cm in height or diameter
- May have a **collarette** surrounding the papule
- Usually presents in **adults** and more commonly in **males**

HISTOLOGIC FEATURES
- Epidermis is **acanthotic** and has overlying **hyperorthokeratosis**
- Granular cell layer shows **hypergranulosis**
- Thickened collagen bundles that are vertically oriented to epidermis
- No adnexal structures in core
- Often have dilated capillaries in papillary dermis
- Dermal fibroblast proliferation is present but hypocellular

OTHER HIGH YIELD POINTS
- Small proportion of cases are associated with **Tuberous Sclerosis**
  - Mutations of **TSC1** or **TSC2**
  - Will be ungual located, have multiple papules, frequently in clusters
  - Begin developing in adolescence
- Positive for FXIIIA; Negative for CD34 (Spindle cell variant is CD34 positive)

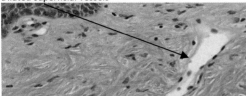

Dilated superficial vessels

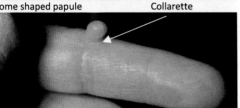

Dome shaped papule   Collarette

DIFFERENTIAL DIAGNOSIS

- **Supernumerary digit (accessory digit):** usually present at base of 5-th digit, has Meissner corpuscles and disorganized nerves
- **Cellular digital fibroma:** lacks vertically-oriented collagen fibers, more cellular and has spindle cells in bland fascicles
- **Superficial acral fibromyxoma:** loose storiform or fascicular pattern, lacks vertically oriented collagen fibers, matrix can be myxoid to collagenous, spindle cells positive for CD34
- **Infantile digital fibromatosis (Inclusion Body Fibromatosis):** fibroblasts arranged in fascicles, eosinophilic perinuclear inclusions that are positive on trichrome or PTAH

Path Presenter

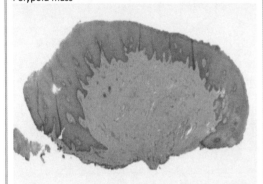

Polypoid mass

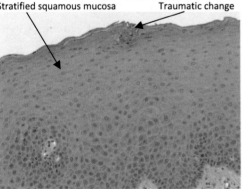

Stratified squamous mucosa   Traumatic change

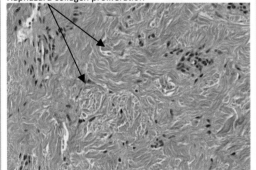

Haphazard collagen proliferation

ORAL FIBROMA

CLINICAL FEATURES

- **Solitary, mucosal-colored, polypoid mass** on the buccal occlusal line, lip, tongue, or gingiva
- Most lesions are small and do not exceed 20 cm
- **May or may not be painful** and have associated ulceration
- Most common lesion of the oral cavity and occurs in **middle-aged**
- **Females** are twice as affected as males

HISTOLOGIC FEATURES

- **Stratified squamous mucosa** which may exhibit atrophy, hyperkeratosis, or have mucosal ulceration
- **Haphazard arrangement** of a **dense collagenous proliferation**
- Fibroblasts can have nucleomegaly → "giant cell fibroma"
- Unencapsulated

OTHER HIGH YIELD POINTS

- **Benign, reactive process** caused by trauma or repetitive localized irritation. These can include biting of lips or cheek, accumulation of dental plaque, orthodontic appliances, or dentures

DIFFERENTIAL DIAGNOSIS

- **Peripheral ossifying fibroma:** stroma is cellular and has calcified spicules or bone
- **Granular cell tumor:** granular eosinophilic cells that are positive for CD68 and S100 protein
- **Pyogenic granuloma:** lobular vascular proliferation with inflammatory infiltrate and overlying ulceration/erosion
- **Peripheral giant cell granuloma:** multinucleated giant cells
- **Gingival parulis:** acute inflammatory infiltrate and granulation tissue
- **Mucocele:** Extravasated extracellular mucin into stroma

Path Presenter

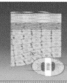
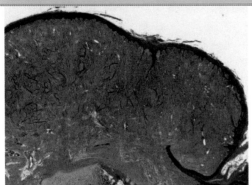

Spindle cells   Whorl   Fascicle

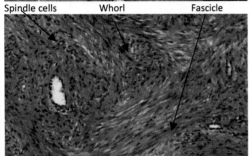

Eosinophilic inclusion

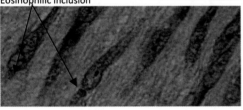

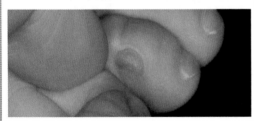

INFANTILE DIGITAL FIBROMA
CLINICAL FEATURES
- A **solitary dome-shaped swelling** over the **dorsal or lateral aspects** of **digits**
- Patients present in the **first year of life** with a rapidly growing, nontender swelling on dorsal or lateral aspects of digits
- Few cases have spontaneous regression
- No sex predilection
- Usually never seen on the thumb or big toe

HISTOLOGIC FEATURES
- Epidermis with **flattened** or **absence** of **rete ridges**
- **Entrapped adnexal structures** are frequently seen
- **Cytologically bland spindle cells** arranged in a "criss-cross", fascicular, whorled, or sheets
- **Spherical paranuclear eosinophilic inclusions** (inclusion body)
- No necrosis or mitosis is present
- As lesion ages, inclusions are less conspicuous

IMMUNOHISTOCHEMISTRY
- **Phosphotungstic acid hematoxylin (PTAH)** or **Masson Trichrome** stains the paranuclear inclusions
- **Positive**: SMA and calponin
- **Negative**: CD34, desmin, β-catenin, S100 protein

OTHER HIGH YIELD POINTS
Path Presenter
- Electron microscopy demonstrates
  - Cytoplasmic inclusions composed of **filament aggregates** with cytoplasmic filaments extending onto the inclusion
  - Rough endoplasmic reticulum
  - Scattered **dense bodies**

DIFFERENTIAL DIAGNOSIS
- **Superficial/desmoid fibromatosis:** Lacks paranuclear cytoplasmic inclusions
- **Dermatofibroma:** lacks paranuclear cytoplasmic inclusions, has peripheral collagen trapping, variable inflammatory infiltrate
- **Pilar leiomyoma:** Lacks paranuclear cytoplasmic inclusions, positive for SMA
- **Neurofibroma:** Lacks paranuclear cytoplasmic inclusions, no fascicular growth, positive for S100 protein and negative for SMA
- **Perineurioma:** Lacks paranuclear cytoplasmic inclusions, positive for EMA, Claudin-1, negative for SMA
- **Dermatomyofibroma:** Lacks paranuclear cytoplasmic inclusions
- **Calcifying aponeurotic fibroma:** Lacks paranuclear cytoplasmic inclusions
- **Acral fibromyxoma:** Lacks paranuclear cytoplasmic vacuoles

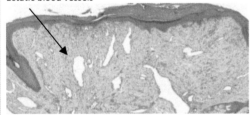

Ectatic blood vessels

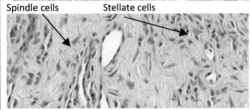

Spindle cells   Stellate cells

ANGIOFIBROMA
CLINICAL FEATURES
- Clinical presentation varies based on the location
- **Fibrous Papule**
  - Solitary, **flesh-colored dome shaped papule** that occurs on nose or face
  - Most often seen in middle-aged individuals
  - Can clinically mimic basal cell carcinoma
  - **Variants:** Clear cell, granular cell, epithelioid, inflammatory
- **Pearly Penile Papules**
  - Clustered or linear, **while papules** that are on the sulcus or coronal margin of the **penis**
- **Adenoma Sebaceum**
  - Clustered/grouped papules or nodules on the **central face** in a **butterfly distribution**
  - Term is a misnomer, no association with sebaceous glands
  - Associated with **Tuberous Sclerosis**

Small, skin colored papule

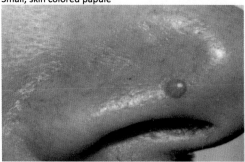

Path Presenter

- **Mutations** in **TSC1** or **TSC2**

HISTOLOGIC FEATURES

- Superficial hypocellular dermal proliferation of **cytologically bland spindle and stellate cells**
- Densely **eosinophilic collagen** without elastic fibers
- **Ectatic blood vessels** with or without **concentric perivascular fibrosis, also sometimes seen around adnexa**
- Perivascular lymphocytes may be seen around vessels
- Absence of solar elastosis

IMMUNOHISTOCHEMISTRY

- Not generally needed; variable CD34, Factor XIIIA, and CD68 staining

DIFFERENTIAL DIAGNOSIS

- **Dermatofibroma:** spindle cells in storiform arrangement, basal hyperpigmentation, epidermal hyperplasia, peripheral collagen trapping
- **Pleomorphic fibroma:** Scattered sparse fibroblasts with cytological atypia
- **Xanthogranuloma:** Touton giant cells, foamy histocytes
- **Intradermal nevus:** Melanocytes in cohesive nests with congenital features
- **Cellular neurothekeoma:** cellular nested epithelioid-spindled cells and fibrous septae

---

Unencapsulated   Flattened rete

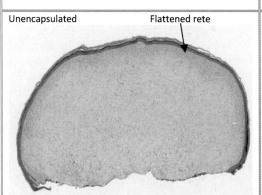

Storiform   bland spindle cells

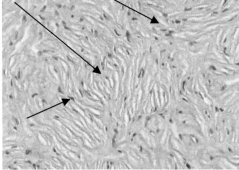

Clefting   Solitary nodule

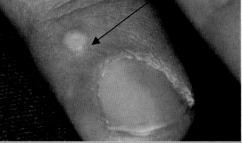

SCLEROTIC FIBROMA (STORIFORM COLLAGENOMA)

CLINICAL FEATURES

- Solitary, **flesh-colored nodule** or papule presents at any age and any sex
- Usually seen on the **trunk**, **face**, or **extremities**
- Multiple lesions should raise suspicion for **Cowden's disease**

HISTOLOGIC FEATURES

- Dermally located unencapsulated lesion composed of **cytologically bland spindle or stellate fibroblasts**
- Characteristic **hyalinized collagen bundles** with **conspicuous clefting and arranged in a storiform** or **plywood/Starry night** appearance
- Spindle cells whorl around vessels
- **Flattened rete ridges**

OTHER HIGH YIELD POINTS

- May be from regressed dermatofibromas, trauma, or associated with Cowden Syndrome
- Cowden Syndrome
  - **Germline mutation** of **PTEN** tumor suppressor gene on chromosome 10q23
  - **Presents as** sclerotic fibromas, many trichilemmomas, AV malformations, skeletal defects, endocrine dysfunctions, cardiorespiratory lesions, breast and thyroid cancers

DIFFERENTIAL DIAGNOSIS

- **Pleomorphic fibroma:** lacks storiform pattern
- **Dermatofibroma:** peripheral collagen trapping, lacks storiform pattern
- **Collagenous fibroma:** fibromyxoid stroma or dense collagenous, lacks storiform pattern
- **Subungual or periungual fibroma:** acanthosis and hyperkeratosis, thick collagen bundles with variable vertical orientation

Path Presenter

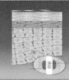
Dome shaped   Epidermal flattening

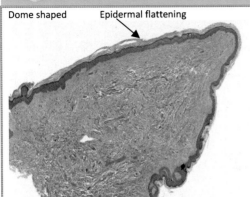

Pleomorphic cells

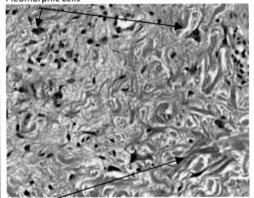

Hyalinized collagen

Path Presenter

PLEOMORPHIC FIBROMA (PSEUDOSARCOMATOUS POLYP)

CLINICAL FEATURES

- **Slow-growing** dome-shaped or nodular lesion that may **resemble a skin tag**
- Occurs in **adults** most often on the **extremities**, **trunk**, or **head** and **neck**

HISTOLOGIC FEATURES

- **Well circumscribed**, dome-shaped, or nodular lesion
- **Epidermal flattening** and absence of rete
- **Hypocellular** dermal proliferation of multi-nucleated, **pleomorphic fibroblasts** with nuclear hyperchromasia, small nucleoli, and minimal cytoplasm
- **Stromal collagen is** often **hyalinized**
- Mitotic activity should be rare to none
- May have myxoid areas (myxoid pleomorphic fibroma)

IMMUNOHISTOCHEMISTRY

- Positive: CD34 (strong), and SMA (focal or weak); variable Factor XIIIA
- Negative: **Loss of RB1** (similar to pleomorphic lipomas)

DIFFERENTIAL DIAGNOSIS

- **Fibrous papule:** increased telangiectatic blood vessels
- **Dermatofibroma:** lacks same degree of pleomorphism, peripheral collagen trapping
- **Sclerotic fibroma:** storiform pattern of thick, hyalinized collagen bundles
- **Atypical fibroxanthoma:** cellular and composed of atypical cells, solar elastosis, atypical mitotic figures

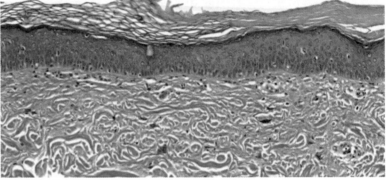

Flattened epidermis with scattered pleomorphic fibroblasts

Rete flattening

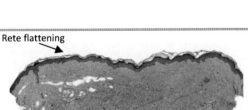

Spindle cells   Collagen trapping

DERMATOFIBROMA

CLINICAL FEATURES

- **Single, round papule**, usually **reddish brown, or flesh-colored** with a darker rim at periphery
- Usually firm and characteristically show dimpling when pinched by fingers
- There are several clinical variants

HISTOLOGIC FEATURES

- Proliferation of cytologically bland **spindle cells** set within a slightly **collagenous stroma**
- Spindle cells surround groups of **keloidal collagen** at the periphery ("**collagen trapping**
- Acanthotic epidermis and fibrosis separated by a Grenz zone
- Overlying epidermal changes include **flattening of rete (table topping)** with **increased pigmentation** of **basal layer**
- Varying number of foamy histiocytes, may have admixed lymphocytes
- May have **epidermal induction** and **adjacent adnexal hyperplasia**
- As the lesion ages, it becomes more fibrotic

IMMUNOHISTOCHEMISTRY

- Positive: FXIIIA, Stromelysin, CD163, CD68

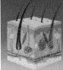

Reddish-brown papule

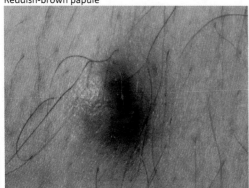

- Negative: CD34

DIFFERENTIAL DIAGNOSIS

- **Dermatofibrosarcoma protuberans:** prominent storiform pattern, extends along septae and demonstrates fat entrapment, **CD34(+), FXIIIA (-)**, CD10(-), CD163(-)
- **Atypical Fibroxanthoma:** highly atypical and spindled-epithelioid cells
- **Kaposi Sarcoma:** spindle cell lesion proliferating through collagen fibers, slit-like vascular spaces
- **Superficial-multicentric basal cell carcinoma:** CK20 negative as BCC usually lacks Merkel cells, which distinguish from follicular induction in DF

Path Presenter

Acanthosis   Grenz Zone

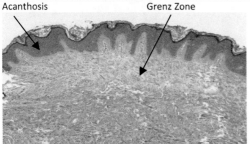

Increased cellularity   Multinucleated cells

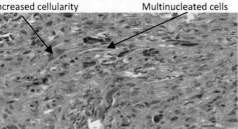

Skin-colored nodule

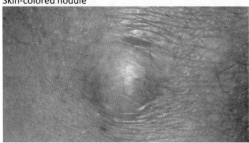

CELLULAR DERMATOFIBROMA

CLINICAL FEATURES

- Variant is typically slightly larger than common dermatofibroma
- Most often seen on the extremities or head and neck of young men
- Increased propensity for recurrence

HISTOLOGIC FEATURES

- **Hypercellular proliferation** of cytologically bland **spindle cells** set within a slightly **collagenous stroma**
- Spindle cells surround groups of **keloidal collagen** at the periphery ("**collagen trapping**") but not involving adipose
- Acanthotic epidermis and fibrosis separated by a Grenz zone
- Overlying epidermal changes include **flattening of rete (table topping)** with **increased pigmentation** of basal layer
- Occasional mitotic figures and multinucleated cells, or central necrosis

IMMUNOHISTOCHEMISTRY

- **Positive: FXIIIA, CD163, CD68; negative** for **CD34**

DIFFERENTIAL DIAGNOSIS

- **Dermatofibrosarcoma protuberans:** prominent storiform pattern, extends along septae, demonstrates fat entrapment, **CD34(+), FXIIIA (-)**, CD10(-), CD163(-)
- **Atypical Fibroxanthoma:** highly atypical and spindled-epithelioid cells
- **Kaposi Sarcoma:** spindle cell lesion proliferating through collagen fibers, slit-like vascular spaces
- **Superficial-multicentric basal cell carcinoma:** CK20 negative as BCC usually lacks Merkel cells, which distinguish from follicular induction in DF

Path Presenter

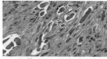

Collagen trapping

Spindle cells   Giant cells

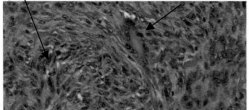

ANEURYSMAL DERMATOFIBROMA (HEMOSIDEROTIC TYPE)

CLINICAL FEATURES

- Presents as a **blue-brown nodule** on the limbs
- Predominantly seen in **middle-aged females**
- Mimics angiosarcoma or Kaposi sarcoma

HISTOLOGIC FEATURES

- Dermatofibroma with **hemorrhage** and **hemosiderin** deposition
- Multinucleated **siderophages** mimicking Touton type giant cells
- **Pseudovascular spaces** that lack **endothelial cells**
- Can show cytologic atypia but does not have high-grade atypia

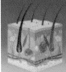

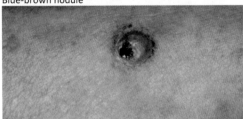

Pseudovascular spaces   No endothelial cells

Blue-brown nodule

- Mitotic activity is rare

IMMUNOHISTOCHEMISTRY

- Positive: FXIIIA, CD163, CD68; negative for CD34

DIFFERENTIAL DIAGNOSIS

- **Kaposi Sarcoma:** spindle cell lesion proliferating through collagen fibers, slit-like vascular spaces, HHV8 (+)
- **Angiosarcoma:** Poorly demarcated proliferation of anastomosing blood vessels (cracked collagen pattern) and solid areas

Path Presenter

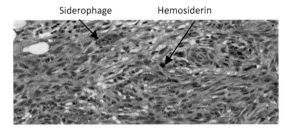

Siderophage   Hemosiderin

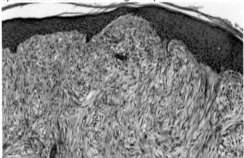

Spindled dermal cells abutting the epidermis

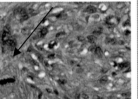

Multinucleated cells   Mitosis

Eroded and crusted lesion

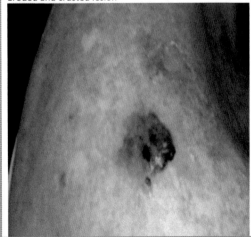

ATYPICAL FIBROXANTHOMA

CLINICAL FEATURES

- **Rapid growing tumor** of the **head and neck** that **ulcerates** or **bleeds**
- Seen in **sun-damaged areas** in **elderly patients**
- Recurrence is low

HISTOLOGIC FEATURES

- Dermal proliferation of **highly atypical** and **pleomorphic spindled to epithelioid cells**
- Scattered bizarre and large multinucleated cells
- Usually, **unencapsulated** but may have an **epidermal collarette**
- **Mitoses frequently seen** and are **highly atypical**
- Prominent **solar elastosis**
- No necrosis, lymphovascular invasion, or involvement of subcutaneous adipose tissue
- If involving deep reticular dermis or subcutis-better classified as Undifferentiated Pleomorphic Sarcoma (UPS)

IMMUNOHISTOCHEMISTRY

- Utility is to exclude all other differential diagnoses
- **Positive: CD10**, CD68 (weak), CD99
- Negative: CD34, melanocytic markers, cytokeratins

DIFFERENTIAL DIAGNOSIS

- **Spindle cell melanoma:** usually has junctional component, S100(+), SOX10(+)
- **Leiomyosarcoma:** cigar-shaped nuclei, abundant eosinophilic cytoplasm, SMA(+), MSA(+), desmin (+)
- **Squamous cell carcinoma (spindle variant):** positive for cytokeratins, p63, p40
- **Fibrosarcoma:** prominent herringbone pattern
- **Malignant peripheral nerve sheath tumor:** S100(+), rarely involves dermis

Path Presenter

Grenz zone

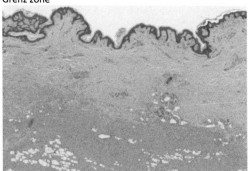

Honeycomb   Monomorphous   Storiform Pattern

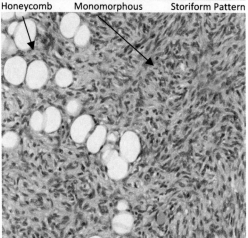

Multinodular indurated mass

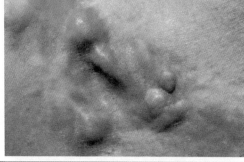

Melanin pigment   Spindle cells

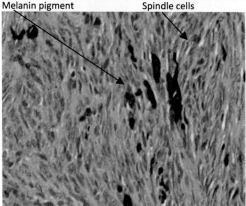

DERMATOFIBROSARCOMA PROTUBERANS

CLINICAL FEATURES

- Slow growing, **indurated plaque-like or multinodular mass** with associated areas of flattening and atrophy
- Trunk or extremities
- Usually seen in **young adults with a male predominance**
- As size increases, tend to become more painful
- Very low rate of metastasis

HISTOLOGIC FEATURES

- **Poorly circumscribed** and composed of a **hypercellular monomorphous proliferation** of **spindle cells** which lack cytologic atypia
- Spindle cells have **cartwheel or storiform patterns**
- **Honeycomb infiltrative pattern** with cells encircling around individual adipocytes or adnexal structures but are not obliterated
- Perineural invasion may be seen
- Mitotic figures are relatively infrequent
- May have myxoid change that can be very prominent
- Can have focal areas of significant atypia-termed as fibrosarcomatous transformation-tend to behave more aggressively
- Giant cell fibroblastoma-considered as a variant of DFPS presenting in childhood. Usually, hypocellular spindle cell proliferation with scattered wreath-like arrangement of nuclei around pseudovascular spaces

IMMUNOHISTOCHEMISTRY

- Positive: CD34 (most reliable)
- Negative: FVIIIa, CD68, CD10, S100, and chymotrypsin

OTHER HIGH YIELD POINTS

- **Rearrangements of *COL1A1-PDGFRB* resulting in a t (17;22) translocation**
- Can detect via next generation sequencing (NGS), FISH, or PCR

DIFFERENTIAL DIAGNOSIS

- **Cellular dermatofibroma:** increased pleomorphic cells, FXIIIA (+), CD68(+), CD163(+), lacks honeycombing fat entrapment
- **Leiomyosarcoma:** fascicles of spindle cells, SMA/MSA (+)
- **Fibromatosis:** nuclear β-catenin (+), SMA (+)
- **Solitary fibrous tumor:** STAT6(+), staghorn vessels, patternless pattern
- **Atypical fibroxanthoma:** Spindled/epithelioid cells, tumor giant cells

Path Presenter

PIGMENTED DERMATOFIBROSARCOMA PROTUBERANS (BEDNAR TUMOR)

CLINICAL FEATURES

- Presents as a slow growing **multi-nodular plaque** most often on the trunk
- **Pigmentation** may or **may not be seen clinically**

HISTOLOGIC FEATURES

- **Poorly circumscribed** and composed of a **hypercellular monomorphous proliferation** of **spindle cells** which lack cytologic atypia
- Spindle cells have **cartwheel or storiform patterns**
- **Honeycomb infiltrative pattern** with cells encircling around individual adipocytes or adnexal structures but are not obliterated
- Perineural invasion may be seen
- Scattered **benign melanocytes** containing **melanin pigment**

IMMUNOHISTOCHEMISTRY

- Positive: CD34 (most reliable) S100 (dendritic cells)

Pigmented Nodule

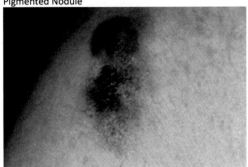

- Negative FVIIIa, CD10, CD68, lysozyme

OTHER HIGH YIELD POINTS
- **Rearrangements of COL1A1-PDGFRB** resulting in a **t (17;22) translocation**
- Can detect via next generation sequencing (NGS), FISH, or PCR

DIFFERENTIAL DIAGNOSIS
- **Cellular dermatofibroma:** increased pleomorphic cells, FXIIIA (+), CD68(+), CD163(+), lacks honeycombing fat entrapment

Path Presenter

[QR code]

Myoid areas   Hemangiopericytoma-like

Epithelioid   Myxoid   Spindle cells

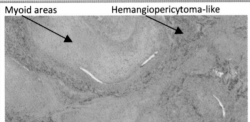

MYOFIBROMA
CLINICAL FEATURES
- **Multicentric form:** usually involves bone, soft tissue, or visceral organs
- **Solitary form:** usually involves **head and neck** subcutaneous tissues
- Most common to be **seen in first two years** and has a **male predominance**

HISTOLOGIC FEATURES
- Well marginated, multinodular proliferation of spindle cells that may resemble a "naked granuloma"
- Has a "biphasic" appearance with **myoid nodules** that have **spindle to epithelioid cells** with **round to tapered nuclei** and **eosinophilic cytoplasm**
- **Hemangiopericytoma-like** areas are cellular with **round blue cells** that **mimic glomus cells** and have **staghorn-like vessels**
- Minimal mitotic activity and atypia is seen

IMMUNOHISTOCHEMISTRY
- Positive: SMA, Calponin
- Negative: Desmin, caldesmon, CD34, and S100

OTHER HIGH YIELD POINTS
- Myofibromatosis: *PDGFRB, NOTCH3,* or *NDRG4* mutations

DIFFERENTIAL DIAGNOSIS
- **Hemangiopericytoma:** lacks myoid areas, more cellular
- **Myoepithelioma:** small round-oval cells, positive for SMA, S100, SOX10, epithelial markers
- **Myofibroblastoma:** lacks biphasic pattern, CD34(+), Desmin (+)

Path Presenter

[QR code]

Solitary mass

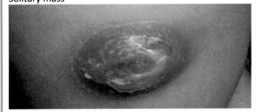

Bands of myofibroblasts   Immature cells   Adipose

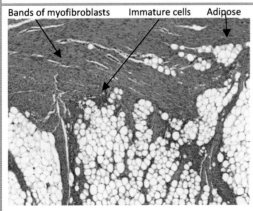

FIBROUS HAMARTOMA OF INFANCY
CLINICAL FEATURES
- **Slow or fast growing, non-tender** deep nodule is **present at or shortly after birth**
- Usually on the upper trunk, axilla, shoulder, or groin
- **Male predominance**
- Usually has **overlying skin changes:** Hypertrichosis, pigmentation

HISTOLOGIC FEATURES
- **Organoid growth pattern** of three distinct components:
  - Sheets and bands of **myofibroblasts:** spindle cells with eosinophilic cytoplasm
  - **Nests of Immature mesenchymal cells:** cells with plump round to ovoid nuclei and pale staining cytoplasm in a myxoid matrix
  - Numerous **mature adipocytes** in "islands"

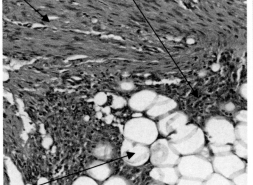

Myofibroblasts   Immature mesenchymal cells

Adipose
Pigmentation   Hypertrichosis

- May have hypocellular areas with conspicuous stromal collagen
- Mitotic activity is rare to absent

IMMUNOHISTOCHEMISTRY
- Positive: SMA (fibroblastic component) and CD34 (myxoid, collagenous areas)
- Negative: No nuclear β-catenin

OTHER HIGH YIELD POINTS
- *EGFR* exon 20: insertions or duplications
- Lack of *PLAG1*, *PDGFB*, or *NTRK1* mutations

DIFFERENTIAL DIAGNOSIS
- **Lipofibromatosis-like neural tumor:** *NTRK1* gene rearrangements
- **Lipoblastoma:** Lacks organoid growth pattern, has lipoblasts
- **Fibrolipoma:** absence of fascicles, organoid growth, or immature mesenchyma
- **Infantile fibrosarcoma:** *ETV6-NTRK3* fusion, lacks organoid growth pattern
- **Rhabdomyosarcoma:** Myogenin (+), Desmin (+)
- **Calcifying aponeurotic fibroma:** cartilage or calcification formation

Path Presenter

Immature mesenchymal cells

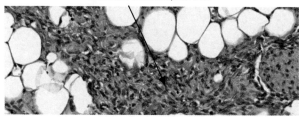

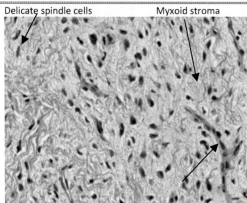

Delicate spindle cells   Myxoid stroma

Minimal atypia   Thin vessels
Exophytic nodule near nail bed

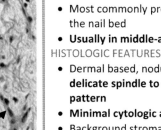

SUPERFICIAL ACRAL FIBROMYXOMA

CLINICAL FEATURES
- Most commonly presents as a slow growing, solitary, **exophytic nodule** near the nail bed
- **Usually in middle-aged adult males**

HISTOLOGIC FEATURES
- Dermal based, nodular lesion composed of hypocellular population of **delicate spindle to stellate fibroblasts** arranged in a **fascicular or storiform pattern**
- **Minimal cytologic atypia** is present
- Background stroma is usually **myxoid to collagenous**
- Scattered **mast cells**; thin-walled vessels are seen in the background
- No necrosis and minimal mitotic activity, rarely infiltrates bone

IMMUNOHISTOCHEMISTRY
- Positive: CD34, CD99, Nestin
- Negative: SMA, desmin, STAT6, MUC4, **loss of RB1**

OTHER HIGH YIELD POINTS
- **RB1 deletion** seen on fluorescence in situ hybridization (FISH)

DIFFERENTIAL DIAGNOSIS
- **Dermatofibrosarcoma Protuberans:** t (17;22) fusion, CD34(+)
- **Dermatofibroma:** CD34(-), FXIIIA (+)
- **Perineurioma:** whorled growth pattern, EMA (+), Claudin-1 (+)
- **Superficial angiomyxoma:** blood vessels with fibrotic walls

Path Presenter

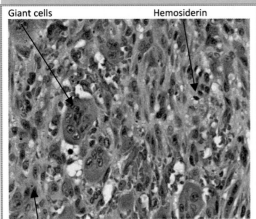

Giant cells   Hemosiderin
Epithelioid cells
Nodule on flexural surface

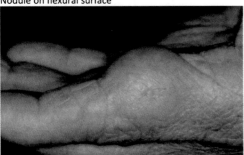

GIANT CELL TUMOR OF TENDON SHEATH (TENOSYNOVIAL GIANT CELL TUMOR- LOCALIZED TYPE)

CLINICAL FEATURES
- Deep **firm, fixed nodule on tendon sheath or fascia of flexural fingers, hands, or wrist**
- Peak incidence is in **young to middle-aged adults** with **slight female predominance**

HISTOLOGIC FEATURES
- **Well demarcated**, multinodular neoplasm composed of a polymorphous cellular population of **osteoclast-like giant cells**, monomorphic **epithelioid cells**, and **histiocytes**
- Background **hyalinized fibrous stroma**
- Small deposits of **hemosiderin**

IMMUNOHISTOCHEMISTRY
- Not generally needed

OTHER HIGH YIELD POINTS
- **Balanced translocation of 1p13** (*CSF1* gene) and often with ***COL6A3* fusion**

DIFFERENTIAL DIAGNOSIS
- **Fibroma of tendon sheath:** no hemosiderin or giant cells, show *USP6* rearrangement
- **Plexiform fibrohistiocytic tumor:** plexiform architecture, osteoclast-like GC
- **Dermatofibroma:** peripheral collagen entrapment, lacks osteoclast-like GC

Path Presenter

Dermal based lesion

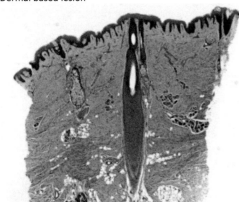

East-west configuration   Streaming

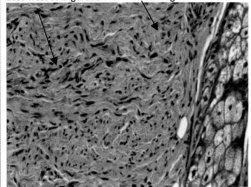
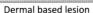

DERMATOMYOFIBROMA (PLAQUE-LIKE DERMAL FIBROMATOSIS)

CLINICAL FEATURES
- Slow growing, red-brown plaques, or nodules
- Usually occurs on the **shoulders of young females** or on **posterior neck** of **young males**

HISTOLOGIC FEATURES
- Dermal based proliferation of **delicate spindle cells** with **"wavy nuclei,"** uniform chromatin, inconspicuous nucleoli, and poorly defined cytoplasmic borders
- Cells are arranged in an **'east-west'** parallel configuration with well-circumscribed superficial and deep margins
- **Adnexal structures are uninvolved,** but spindle cells go around them
- Frequently has overlying epidermal hyperplasia
- Can resemble a cicatrix but elastic fibers are chunky on a Von Gieson

IMMUNOHISTOCHEMISTRY
- Variable positivity for SMA
- Negative: MSA, S100, desmin, CD34, and Factor XIIIA

DIFFERENTIAL DIAGNOSIS
- **Dermatofibroma:** peripheral collagen trapping
- **Hypertrophic scar:** dense collagen, vertically oriented vessels
- **Leiomyoma:** fascicles of spindle cells, SMA(+), MSA(+), Desmin (+)

Path Presenter

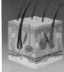

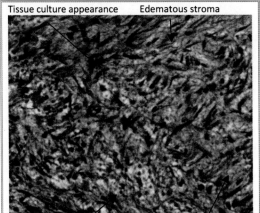

Tissue culture appearance   Edematous stroma

Extravasated erythrocytes   Myxoid change
Subcutaneous nodule

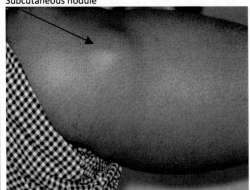

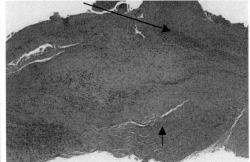

NODULAR FASCIITIS
CLINICAL FEATURES
- Presents as a sudden, rapidly growing, **tender firm, deep nodule** on the arms
- Most common in **young adults** with no specific sex predilection
- **Regresses** over a period of months
HISTOLOGIC FEATURES
- Proliferation of **plump myofibroblasts** and **pyramidal fibroblasts** (stellate fibroblasts) impart a **"tissue culture"** appearance
- May have scattered keloid-like collagen
- Frequently has **increased mitotic activity**
- May be locally infiltrative, have alternating hyper and hypocellular areas
- **Extravasated erythrocytes** are seen throughout
- **Hemosiderin** is seen throughout
- Variants:
  - **Skull of infants:** cranial fasciitis
  - **Extending into vascular lumen:** Intravascular fasciitis
IMMUNOHISTOCHEMISTRY
- Variable positivity for SMA; negative for MSA, S100, desmin, CD34
OTHER HIGH YIELD POINTS
- *MYH9-USP6* fusion detected by molecular methods
DIFFERENTIAL DIAGNOSIS
- Neurofibroma: S100 protein (+), SMA (-)
- **Inflammatory myofibroblastic tumor:** ALK (+), lacks *USP6* rearrangements
- **Cellular dermatofibroma:** SMA (-)
- **Fibromatosis:** nuclear β-catenin (+), evenly distributed stromal collagen

Path Presenter

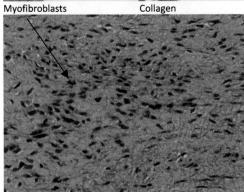

Sweeping fascicles at low power

Myofibroblasts   Collagen

FIBROMATOSIS
CLINICAL FEATURES
- **Variable presentation**, recurrence common
  - **Palmar (Dupuytren Contracture):** volar surface nodular myofibroblastic proliferation, predominantly male adults >50 years old, no metastasis, rare in non-white individuals
  - **Plantar:** plantar surface of foot nodular myofibroblastic proliferation, middle-aged individuals, slight male predominance, no metastasis
  - **Penile (Peyronie Disease):** Fibrous proliferation/lesion which causes penile deformities and painful erections and often reports of erectile dysfunction; occurs in white adult males >50
  - **Deep (Desmoid tumor):** myofibroblastic proliferation in deep soft tissue, can cause skeletal muscle atrophy
- Associated with **Familial Adenomatous Polyposis Syndrome** → dramatically increased risk (~1000x general population) → associated with cicatricial variant of fibromatosis
HISTOLOGIC FEATURES
- Infiltrative **proliferation of myofibroblasts in sweeping fascicles**
- Myofibroblasts have **regularly spaced nuclei** with **smooth** nuclear **contours**, small **conspicuous nucleolus**, and lack atypia; **cytoplasm** can be **stellate**
- **Collagen in the background** (can be keloidal-like) with **small vessels** and occasional lymphocytic infiltrate and scattered giant cells
- Can have **osseous metaplasia**
IMMUNOHISTOCHEMISTRY
- **Nuclear Beta Catenin+,** SMA+; variable CD117, calretinin expression; Negative

Plantar Fibromatosis
Myofibroblasts   Collagen

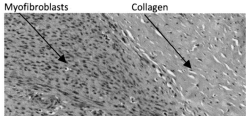

Depuytren contracture

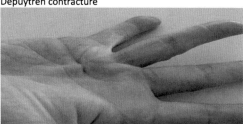

for keratin, desmin

OTHER HIGH YIELD POINTS
- Testing for APC or CTNNB1 mutations
  - **Familial/FAP → APC**
  - **Sporadic → CTNNB1**

DIFFERENTIAL DIAGNOSIS
- **Monophasic synovial sarcoma:** cellular and monomorphic, *SS18*(SYT) fusions, nuclear TLE1(+)
- **Leiomyoma:** SMA (+), Desmin (+)
- **Malignant Peripheral Nerve Sheath Tumor:** loss of H3K27me3 expression, SMA (-), Desmin (-)

Path Presenter

Dermal based proliferation

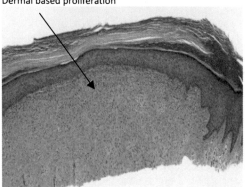

Epithelioid cells

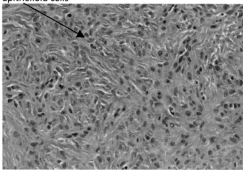

EPITHELIOID CELL HISTIOCYTOMA (EPITHELIOID FIBROUS HISTIOCYTOMA)

CLINICAL FEATURES
- Usually seen in **young adults** and presents as an **erythematous nodule** on the **upper extremities**, can occur on head, neck, or trunk
- No malignant potential

HISTOLOGIC FEATURES
- **Dermal proliferation** of **monomorphic epithelioid to polygonal cells, usually with epidermal collarette**
- Epithelioid to polygonal cells have **round to ovoid nuclei, vesicular chromatin, small nucleoli**, and **abundant eosinophilic cytoplasm**
- Dermal **fibrosis** and scattered conspicuous vascularity
- May have a background **inflammatory infiltrate**

IMMUNOHISTOCHEMISTRY
- Positive for CD10, CD68, Factor XIIIA, and ALK

DIFFERENTIAL DIAGNOSIS
- **Dermatofibroma:** ALK (-), collagen trapping
- **Spitz nevus:** Melanocytic markers (+), spindled-epithelioid cells
- **Cutaneous Epithelioid Angiomatous Nodule:** epithelioid endothelial cells, CD31/CD34(+), ERG (+)

Path Presenter

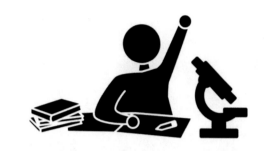

ACE MY PATH

Come Ace With Us!

CHAPTER 10: FAT, MUSCLE, AND
BONE NEOPLASMS

TERRANCE LYNN, MD

FAT, MUSCLE, BONE LESIONS

LIPOMA
MORPHOLOGY
- Mature adipocytes with single large fat droplet and eccentric nuclei

OTHER HIGH YIELD POINTS
- Common benign tumor composed of mature adipocytes
- Clinically presents as **painless** mass and are superficial/subcutaneous
- Most common mesenchymal tumor in adults, M=F
- Gross exam: well circumscribed, homogenous cut surface, <5 cm
- If retroperitoneal/large, **must** exclude well-differentiated liposarcoma
- Recurrence uncommon, slightly higher risk if incompletely resected
- Difficult to identify margins intraoperatively
- **IHC:** Usually not indicated
- **FISH:** Absence of MDM2 amplification
- **Molecular:** Rearrangements of *HMGA1, HMGA2*

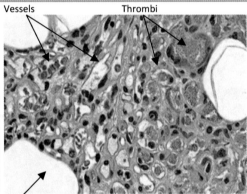

Vessels   Thrombi

Adipocyte
Subcutaneous nodule

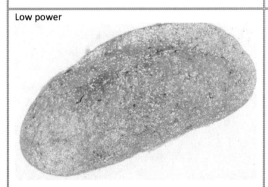

ANGIOLIPOMA
CLINICAL FEATURES
- **Painful, lobulated subcutaneous** soft tissue mass that is most commonly present on the forearm, trunk, or upper arm
- Most common in **young adult males**

HISTOLOGIC FEATURES
- **Mature adipocytes**
- Branching **vascular network** with peripheral prominence
- **Fibrin thrombi** frequently seen within the lumen of vessels
- **No cytological atypia** in the adipocytes or endothelial cells

IMMUNOHISTOCHEMISTRY
- **Positive:** S100 (adipocytes), ERG, CD31, CD34 (endothelial cells), SMA (pericytes)

OTHER HIGH YIELD POINTS
- *PRKD2* mutations (>80%), activating *PIK3CA* seen also

DIFFERENTIAL DIAGNOSIS
- **Lipoma:** lacks microthrombi
- **Intramuscular hemangioma:** large vessels with thick walls, organizing thrombi
- **Kaposi sarcoma:** HHV8(+), slit-like spaces, extravasated red blood cells
- **Angiomyolipoma:** MART1(+)/HMB-45(+), large vessels with thick walls
- **Spindle cell hemangioma:** large, cavernous vascular spaces, spindled and epithelioid cells, phleboliths, no small vessels in clusters

Path Presenter

Low power

PLEOMORPHIC/SPINDLE CELL LIPOMA
CLINICAL FEATURES
- **Uncommon** tumor with **cape-like distribution**: Neck, shoulder, back
- Mainly **middle-age** to **elder men**

HISTOLOGIC FEATURES
- **Mature adipocytes** with bland **spindle cells** and **ropey collagen**
- Variable myxoid background and mast cells
- **Can have a spectrum of histology**: can be largely fatty with minimal spindle cells, or can have minimal fat and composed of largely spindle cell component which mimics DFSP
- **Pleomorphic lipoma**: ropey collagen, pleomorphic spindle & **floret** cells, myxoid background

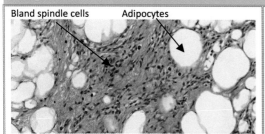
Bland spindle cells   Adipocytes

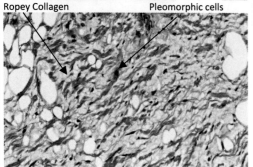
Ropey Collagen   Pleomorphic cells

Floret Cell

Path Presenter

- **Floret cells**: giant cells with multiple nuclei arranged along peripheral edge and central eosinophilic cytoplasm

IMMUNOHISTOCHEMISTRY
- Spindle & floret cells → CD34+, loss of nuclear RB1

OTHER HIGH YIELD POINTS
- Molecular alterations identified
  ➢ Monoallelic or Biallelic deletion of *RB1*

DIFFERENTIAL DIAGNOSIS
- **Atypical lipomatous tumor/Well differentiated liposarcoma:** ropey collagen, *MDM2* amplification, CDK4(+)
- **Neurofibroma:** CD34(+) fibroblastic cells, S100(+) spindle cells, may have plexiform pattern which may suggest plexiform neurofibroma
- **Cellular angiofibroma:** CD34(+), hyalinized vessels, loss of *Rb1* expression, morphologically similar
- **Mammary-type myofibroblastoma:** CD34(+), hyalinized vessels, loss of *Rb1* expression, monomorphic spindle cells in short fascicles, collagenous stroma
- **Solitary fibrous tumor:** STAT6(+), staghorn vessels, no ropey collagen
- **Myxoid Liposarcoma:** *DDIT3::FUS* fusion, CD34(-), uni- or multivacuolated lipoblasts, plexiform capillary network
- **Dermatofibrosarcoma Protuberans:** *COL1A1::PDGFB* fusion, CD34(+), storiform pattern
- **Giant Cell Fibroblastoma:** CD34(+), also has *COL1A1::PDGFB* fusion, multinucleated stromal giant cells lining vascular spaces
- **Schwannoma:** Antoni A and B foci, nuclear palisading, lacks intertumoral adipose

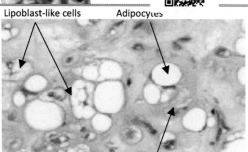
Lipoblast-like cells   Adipocytes

Myxochondroid background

Path Presenter

CHONDROID LIPOMA
MORPHOLOGY
- Nests/cords of "lipoblast-like" or chondrocyte-like vacuolated cells
- Chondromyxoid background
- Prominent vascular network +/- hemorrhage
- Absence of pleomorphism, atypia, mitoses, necrosis

OTHER HIGH YIELD POINTS
- Predominantly in females, 2nd decade and older
- Mostly seen in limb girdles/proximal extremities
- No metastasis, no recurrence
- **Molecular:** t(11;16) (q13;p12-13) translocation → fusion of C11*orf*95 and *MKL2* genes

DIFFERENTIAL DIAGNOSIS
- Soft tissue chondroma: True hyaline cartilage is present
- Chondrolipoma: Lipoma with admixed hyaline cartilage

Polygonal cells   Univacuolated adipocytes

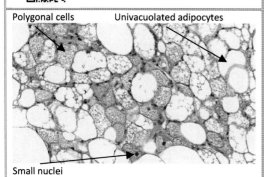

Small nuclei

HIBERNOMA
CLINICAL FEATURES
- Slow growing, painless mass, most common on the neck, trunk, and thigh
- Usually seen in adults in the 2nd-4th decade of life

HISTOLOGIC FEATURES
- **Polygonal eosinophilic cells** with **granular** and **vacuolated cytoplasm** and small bland centrally located nuclei with or without nucleoli
- **Univacuolated adipocytes** and **multivacuolated adipocytes**
- Scattered stromal vessels
- Morphologic variants include: myxoid, spindle cell, and lipoma-like

IMMUNOHISTOCHEMISTRY
- **S100 positive**

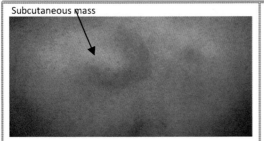

Subcutaneous mass

OTHER HIGH YIELD POINTS
- 11q13-21 rearrangements

DIFFERENTIAL DIAGNOSIS
- **Normal brown fat:** no discrete mass
- **Lipoma:** no granular or multivacuolated cells
- **Lipoblastoma:** myxoid stroma, lipoblasts, *PLAG1* gene rearrangements
- **Granular cell tumor:** lacks multivacuolated cells, S100(+)

Path Presenter

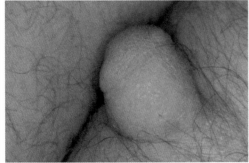

Polypoid lesion   No adnexal structures

Immature lipocytes   Mature adipose

Polypoid lesion

NEVUS LIPOMATOSUS SUPERFICIALIS
CLINICAL FEATURES
- **Solitary or cluster of papules** or polypoid lesions usually seen on **posterior surfaces** (back, upper thighs, and buttocks)
- The classical form occurs in **children** and **young adults** while the solitary form is seen in adults
- Can **mimic a skin tag** (acrochordon)

HISTOLOGIC FEATURES
- **Polypoid fragment** of tissue
- **Mature adipose** with occasional small immature-appearing lipocytes
- Increase in **delicate blood vessels**
- **No adnexal structures** are present
- No atypia
- May have **hyperkeratosis or erosion** due to trauma

DIFFERENTIAL DIAGNOSIS
- **Acrochordon:** lacks mature adipose tissue, typically has a thin stalk
- **Lipoma:** circumscribed nodule of adipose, no dermal collagen
- **Fibrolipoma:** fibrous tissue, collagen bundles and mature adipose tissue
- **Spindle cell lipoma:** CD34(+) short fascicles of spindle cells, "ropey" collagen, myxoid stroma, mast cells
- **Focal dermal hypoplasia (Goltz syndrome):** diminished reticular dermis

Path Presenter

Immature cells surrounding vessels

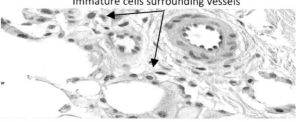

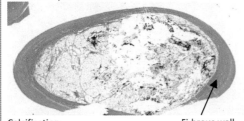

Round encapsulated lesion

Calcification   Fi-brous wall

ENCAPSULATED FAT NECROSIS (TRAUMATIC PANNICULITIS)
CLINICAL FEATURES
- Occurs at **sites of trauma** and may be seen in the **breast or extremities**
- Usually, **patients do not recall trauma** to the area
- Can occur at any age

HISTOLOGIC FEATURES
- **Rupture of adipocytes** and **necrotic** adipocytes, **foamy histiocytes, lymphocytes,** and **eosinophils**
- Foreign body **giant cells**
- **Fibrous capsule** surrounds the fat necrosis
- Late changes include **lipomembranous change**
  - Fern-like **"frost on a window"** appearance at the periphery of cystic spaces
- **Calcification**
- **Metaplastic ossification** may be seen

DIFFERENTIAL DIAGNOSIS

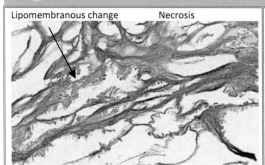
Lipomembranous change   Necrosis

- **Cold panniculitis:** no needle-like crystals, has lymphocytic panniculitis
- **Sclerema neonatorum:** has needle-like crystals, lacks necrosis, calcification, and inflammation
- **Post-steroid panniculitis**: needle-like crystals in adipose

Foamy histiocytes

Path Presenter

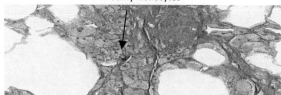

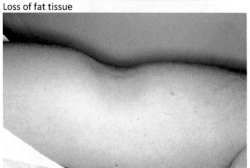
Loss of adipocyte volume   Fibrosis

Loss of fat tissue

LIPOATROPHY/LIPODYSTROPHY
CLINICAL FEATURES
- Localized **loss of adipose tissue**, which is usually in the **face, hands,** and **trunk**
- Most commonly is seen as a **side effect using certain medications** which may be **injected** or taken **orally, or can be congenitally acquired**
- Fat loss is **largely irreversible**

HISTOLOGIC FEATURES
- **Decrease in size** of the **adipocytes, decrease** in the **intracytoplasmic vacuoles**
- **Fat necrosis** and **loss of adipocytes** with or without inflammatory response
- May have focal calcification
- **Fibrosis with** dense collage

OTHER HIGH YIELD POINTS
- Conditions and/or medications
  - **Multiple sclerosis: Copaxone** injections
  - **HIV**-Associated: **Due to** antiretroviral medications (Protease inhibitors), and older medications, Zidovudine (AZT), Stavudine (d4T), and Didanosine (ddI)
  - **Diabetes:** Insulin injections

DIFFERENTIAL DIAGNOSIS
- **Lipoatrophic diabetes:** syndrome characterized by insulin resistant diabetes, acanthosis nigricans, generalized lipoatrophy, and other metabolic disturbances
- **Barraquer-Simons Disease**: Also called acquired partial lipodystrophy, characterized by loss of fat from the face, neck, shoulders, arms, forearms, chest, and abdomen. Onset usually begins in childhood following a viral illness
- **Congenital Lipodystrophy**: characterized by near total loss of adipose tissue and extreme muscularity; often present at birth or immediately after thereafter

Path Presenter

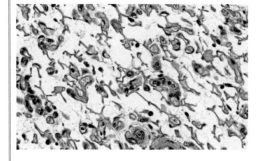
Necrosis, Atrophy

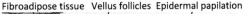
Fibroadipose tissue Vellus follicles Epidermal papilation

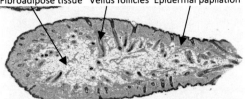
Vellus hairs

ACCESSORY TRAGUS
CLINICAL FEATURES
- **Single or multiple** polypoid papules or nodules in the preauricular space
- May be **soft** or **firm** and are **skin colored** and may be **surfaced with tiny hair**
- Can be **present at birth** and develop over life
- May **appear anywhere along** the **1st branchial arch migratory pathway**
- It is **painless**, **no pruritis**, and lacks any distinct or unusual pigmentation

HISTOLOGIC FEATURES
- **Polypoid** fragment of tissue with overlying **papilations of the epidermis**
- **Vellus follicles** and **small sebaceous glands** are present
- Subcutis is composed of **mature adipose** and **fibrovascular tissue**
- May have some **cartilage** which is present in the central aspect

OTHER HIGH YIELD POINTS
- Associated with multiple various **genetic syndromes** Oculoauriculovertebral syndrome (Goldenhar syndrome), Treacher Collins syndrome (Mandibulofacial dysostosis), VACTERL syndrome

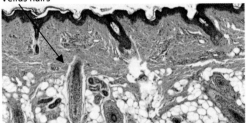
Preauricular   Along arch migration   Multiple

DIFFERENTIAL DIAGNOSIS
- **Acrochordon:** lacks vellus hair proliferation, fat, and/or cartilage
- **Hair follicle nevus:** epidermal hyperplasia with papillations, hair follicles, no fat or cartilage
- **Chondrocutaneous vestige:** cartilaginous core, subcutaneous tissue envelope

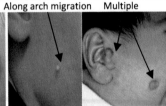

Path Presenter

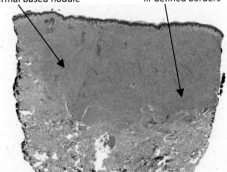
Dermal based nodule   Ill-defined borders

PILAR LEIOMYOMA
CLINICAL FEATURES
- Multiple **painful, red-brown papules** or **nodules** that may **coalesce into** large **plaques**
- Spread in a **dermatomal distribution**
- **Pain can be induced** or worsen upon exposure to stimuli such as **pressure, cold temperatures,** or **certain emotional states**
- Usually is seen in **children**

HISTOLOGIC FEATURES
- **Dermal based nodule** composed of haphazardly arranged smooth muscle bundles that dissect collagen fibers
- Smooth muscle fibers have **spindled bland nuclei** with **blunt ends** and abundant **eosinophilic cytoplasm**
- **Rare atypia** or **mitotic figures**

IMMUNOHISTOCHEMISTRY
- **Positive:** S100, SMA, MSA

OTHER HIGH YIELD POINTS
- Hereditary leiomyomatosis and renal cell cancer syndrome
  - ➤ Autosomal dominant inheritance of fumarate hydratase (FH) mutation
  - ➤ Multiple leiomyomata, some develop renal cell cancers

DIFFERENTIAL DIAGNOSIS
- **Smooth muscle hamartoma:** haphazard smooth muscle bundles in a band-like configuration
- **Angioleiomyoma:** smooth muscle with admixed vessels with thick walls, sharply circumscribed
- **Myofibroma:** cellular spindled foci, ectatic vessels, myoid and pseudochondroid areas
- **Leiomyosarcoma:** prominent cytologic atypia, increased mitotic activity

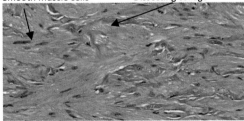
Smooth muscle cells   Dissecting collage

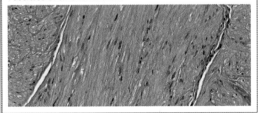
Fascicles of smooth muscle

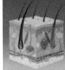

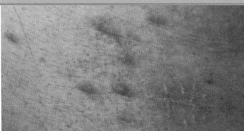

Path Presenter

ANGIOLEIOMYOMA

CLINICAL FEATURES

- **Solitary, slow growing** subcutaneous **nodule/mass** that may be painful
- Typically seen in **extremities of males** (upper) and **females (lower)**
- Wide age distribution
- Can be **exacerbated** by **menstrual cycle, pregnancy,** and **temperature**

HISTOLOGIC FEATURES

- **Sharply circumscribed** nodule of smooth muscle and vessels

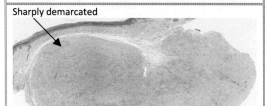
Sharply demarcated

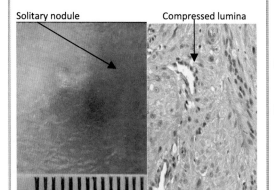
Solitary nodule   Compressed lumina

- Vessels are **medium to large** and have **compressed lumina** that have **concentric perivascular muscle cells**
- **Lacks atypia** and mitotic activity
- **Different patterns**: solid (most common), cavernous, and venous

IMMUNOHISTOCHEMISTRY

- **Positive**: SMA, h-caldesmon, desmin
- **Negative**: HMB45

DIFFERENTIAL DIAGNOSIS

- **Myopericytoma**: perivascular growth, no smooth muscle-like cells, SMA(+) and desmin (-)
- **Hemangioma**: increased vascularity of capillaries or cavernous vessels, no increase in smooth muscle cell proliferation
- **PEComa**: stroma is sclerotic, variable tumor cytoplasm features, variable adipose, SMA(+), MART1(+)

Path Presenter

GENITAL LEIOMYOMA

CLINICAL FEATURES

- **Solitary, slow growing** subcutaneous **papule/nodule** that is **asymptomatic**
- May be located in nipple, vulvar, penis, or scrotal regions
- Usually seen in middle-aged adults

HISTOLOGIC FEATURES

- **Well-circumscribed** nodule of smooth muscle that is usually hypercellular
- May have **myxoid change,** epithelioid morphology, or hyalinization
- Smooth muscle fibers have **spindled bland nuclei** with **blunt ends** and abundant **eosinophilic cytoplasm**
- **Lacks atypia** and mitotic activity

IMMUNOHISTOCHEMISTRY

- **Positive**: S100, SMA, MSA

DIFFERENTIAL DIAGNOSIS

- **Smooth muscle hamartoma**: haphazard smooth muscle bundles in a band-like configuration

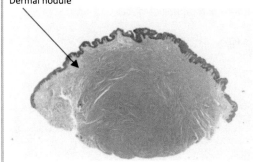
Dermal nodule

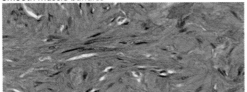
Smooth muscle bundles

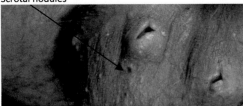
Scrotal nodules

- **Angioleiomyoma**: smooth muscle with admixed vessels with thick walls, sharply circumscribed
- **Leiomyosarcoma**: cytologic atypia that is prominent, increased mitotic activity
- **Myofibroma:** cellular spindled foci, ectatic vessels, myoid and pseudochondroid areas

Path Presenter

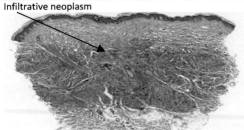
Infiltrative neoplasm

CUTANEOUS LEIOMYOSARCOMA
CLINICAL FEATURES
- Usually presents as a **single nodule** or **plaque** on the **extremities** or **trunk** of middle-aged males (**male predominance**)
- May **ulcerate** and have serum crusting

HISTOLOGIC FEATURES
- **Infiltrative neoplasm** of spindle cells
- **Spindle cells** have abundant eosinophilic cytoplasm, **elongated** and **blunt-ended nuclei**, often conspicuous nucleoli, and **moderate pleomorphism**

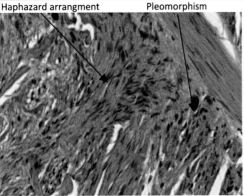
Haphazard arrangment   Pleomorphism

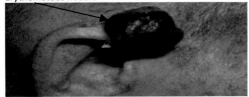
Erythematous nodule

- Bundles of **fascicles are arranged in perpendicular orientation**
- Often has **coagulative necrosis** and **variable mitotic activity**
- **Morphologic variants**: myxoid, epithelioid, and inflammatory patterns

IMMUNOHISTOCHEMISTRY
- **Positive**: S100, SMA, MSA, caldesmon; variable cytokeratin expression

DIFFERENTIAL DIAGNOSIS
- **Leiomyoma:** lacks mitotic activity, no cytologic atypia
- **Sarcomatoid squamous cell carcinoma:** HMWCK (+), desmin (-), caldesmon(-)
- **Cellular dermatofibroma:** no smooth muscle, CD10(+), FXIIIA (+), desmin (-), caldesmon(-)
- **Nodular fasciitis:** storiform pattern, no cytologic atypia or pleomorphism, has *USP6* gene rearrangements
- **Atypical fibroxanthoma:** atypical and cytologically bizarre morphology, desmin (-), caldesmon (-)
- **Spindle cell/desmoplastic melanoma:** SOX10(+), S100(+), often has associated in situ component

Path Presenter

Well circumscribed

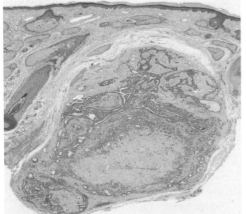

Epithelial cells   Chondromyxoid stroma

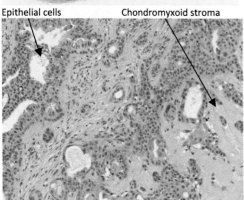

CHONDROID SYRINGOMA (CUTANEOUS MIXED TUMOR)

CLINICAL FEATURES

- **Asymptomatic**, skin-colored nodule is seen in **middle-aged to elderly males**
- Most common to be identified in the **head and neck**, or extremities and trunk

HISTOLOGIC FEATURES

- **Well circumscribed, biphasic** tumor with an **epithelial** component and **stroma**
- Epithelial component has **epithelial cells in small clusters**, **tubules** or **ducts**, or **cords** and are often surrounded by **myoepithelial cells**
- Epithelial cells may exhibit **metaplastic changes** which include squamous metaplasia, mucinous, columnar, oxyphilic, hobnail metaplasia, or clear cell changes
- **Stromal** component may be **myxoid**, **hyalinized**, **chondroid**, or **mixed**

IMMUNOHISTOCHEMISTRY

- **Positive**:
  - ➤ **Cuboidal cells:** Cytokeratin, EMA, CEA
  - ➤ **Myoepithelial cells:** p63/p40, Cytokeratin, SOX10, NSE

DIFFERENTIAL DIAGNOSIS

- **Malignant mixed tumor (malignant chondroid syringoma):** cytologic atypia of epithelial cells, necrosis, atypical mitotic figures
- **Myoepithelioma:** cytologically bland plasmacytoid cells, no ductal differentiation
- **Chondroid lipoma:** multivacuolated lipoblast-like cells, mature adipocytes, chondromyxoid stroma, no epithelial cells, no staining with epithelial markers
- **Extraskeletal chondroma:** cystic degeneration, largely hypocellular but mature hyaline cartilage, no epithelial or glandular differentiated components
- **Pleomorphic adenoma of salivary gland:** morphologically the same, location is key

Path Presenter

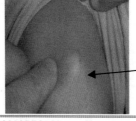

Circumscribed skin-colored nodule

Muscle fibers   Horizontal band-like arrangement

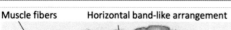

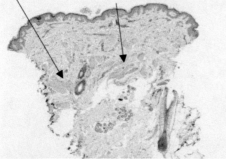

Bundles of smooth muscle

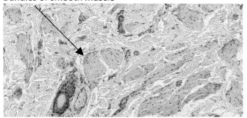

SMOOTH MUSCLE HAMARTOMA

CLINICAL FEATURES

- Usually seen in **infants** in the **lumbosacral region** or **proximal extremities**
- May be **hyperpigmented** and has associated **coarse hair**
- **Pseudo-Darier sign:** temporary induration or piloerection with rubbing
- **Michelin-Tire Baby Syndrome:** Diffuse cutaneous smooth muscle hamartoma, intellectual disabilities, and developmental abnormalities

HISTOLOGIC FEATURES

- **Haphazardly** arranged **bundles** of **smooth muscle** fibers in a **horizontal band-like configuration**
- Resembles arrector pili muscle bands
- May have **cleft artifact**
- **Epidermal hyperplasia** with **basal hyperpigmentation**
  - ➤ If lentiginous melanocytes in the junction are present: **Becker Nevus**

DIFFERENTIAL DIAGNOSIS

- **Cutaneous leiomyoma:** muscle bundles with irregular borders and forming a solid nodule
- **Cutaneous leiomyosarcoma:** smooth muscle cells with cytologic atypia, intersecting fascicles, increased mitotic activity
- **Acquired smooth muscle hamartoma of scrotum:** reactive hyperplasia of smooth muscle, possibly dilated lymphatic channels

Hyperpigmentation

- **Combined blue nevus with smooth muscle hamartoma:** smooth muscle bundles haphazardly arranged in dermis, pigmented spindled melanocytes and melanophages, variable epithelioid melanocytes
- **Normal special skin site:** smooth muscle bundles are increased in scrotum, vulva, and nipple

Path Presenter

Papillomatosis

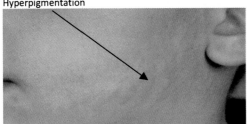

Increased pilosebaceous units

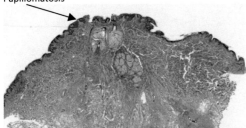

Acanthosis

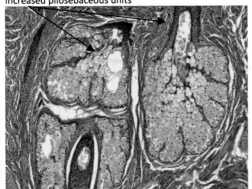

SUPERNUMERARY NIPPLE (ACCESSORY NIPPLE)

CLINICAL FEATURES

- Well demarcated **papule** or **macule** that is either skin colored or hyperpigmented
- Can be **unilateral** or **bilateral** and occurs anywhere along the mammary chain
  - ➤ Occurs due to failure of embryologic structures to regress
  - ➤ Occurs from axilla to groin
- **Most common** location is **immediately inferior to normal** breast
- Can **include areola** or **nipple only (Polythelia)**
  - ➤ Nipple only is the most common variant

HISTOLOGIC FEATURES

- Epidermis has **acanthosis, papillomatosis** and minimal hyperkeratosis
- Basal layer cells have **hyperpigmentation**
- **Increased** number of **pilosebaceous units (sebaceous glands, hair follicles),** and **smooth muscle bundles**

DIFFERENTIAL DIAGNOSIS

- **Leiomyoma:** proliferation of fascicles of smooth muscle
- **Becker nevus:** acanthosis of epidermis, melanocyte hyperplasia, increased basal-layer pigmentation, smooth muscle hamartoma (hair follicles, sebaceous glands, smooth muscle bundles), hypertrichosis
- **Lentigo:** lacks acanthosis, papillomatosis, and smooth muscle proliferation

Hyperpigmented basal cell layer   Minimal hyperkeratosis

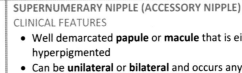

Path Presenter

Increased smooth muscle bundles

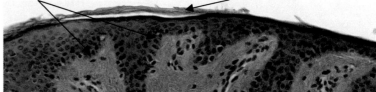

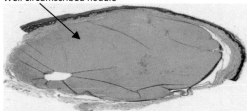
Well circumscribed nodule

Chondrocytes   Myxoid

Nodule on digit

CHONDROMA
CLINICAL FEATURES
- **Non-tender solitary nodule** that is rubbery, firm, and bosselated
- Usually located on the **acral surfaces** of **hands** and **feet**
- Most common in **middle-aged individuals**; can be seen at all ages
HISTOLOGIC FEATURES
- **Well-circumscribed** tumor composed of **mature chondrocytes** in a benign **cartilaginous matrix**
- Chondrocytes located in lacunae and may have **mild to moderate pleomorphism**, but have a **low mitotic rate**
- Majority of tumor is **mature hyaline cartilage**
- Variable amount of **calcification** is seen
- May have **myxoid degeneration**
IMMUNOHISTOCHEMISTRY
- **Positive:** S100, ERG
DIFFERENTIAL DIAGNOSIS
- **Tophaceous pseudogout:** has rhomboid shaped calcium pyrophosphate crystals, positive birefringence
- **Tumoral calcinosis:** psammomatous calcium hydroxyapatite crystals
- **Phosphoturic mesenchymal tumor:** evidence of osteomalacia
- **Synovial chondromatosis:** intra-articular loose bodies, *ACVR2A* gene rearrangements

Path Presenter

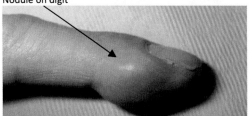
Lamellar bone   Marrow fat

Osteoblasts   Cement lines of new bone formation

Round papules

Path Presenter

OSTEOMA CUTIS
CLINICAL FEATURES
- **Well circumscribed**, solitary, or multiple, firm **dermal papules, plaques**, or **subcutaneous nodules**
- May be seen in **Albright Hereditary Osteodystrophy**
- May present as **progressive osseous heteroplasia**, **miliary osteomas of the face**, or as cutaneous osteomas
- **Primary** osteoma cutis is due to **primary ossification**
- **Secondary** osteoma cutis is due to **trauma, inflammatory**, or **neoplastic processes**
HISTOLOGIC FEATURES
- **Mature lamellar bone** which is located in the dermis or subcutaneous fat
- May have normal osteoblasts or normal marrow spaces
OTHER HIGH YIELD POINTS
- **Albright Hereditary Osteodystrophy**
  - **Autosomal dominant** inheritance
  - **Clinical:** Multiple osteomas, obesity, pseudohypoparathyroidism, brachydactyly, intellectual disabilities, short statures, and round facies
DIFFERENTIAL DIAGNOSIS
- **Osteochondroma:** mature cartilage with lamellar bone
- **Extraskeletal osteosarcoma:** multinucleated giant cells, pleomorphic cells, osteoblasts
- **Secondary ossification:** folliculitis, or neoplastic
- **Calcinosis cutis:** no mature bone formation, calcium deposition

Arising from follicle

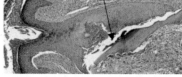

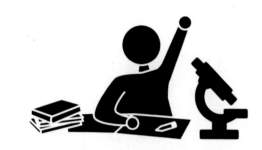

ACE MY PATH
Come Ace With Us!

CHAPTER 11: METASTASES

TERRANCE LYNN, MD

METASTASES

Cannonball metastasis

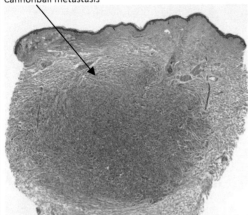

Nests of tumor cells   Small lumen

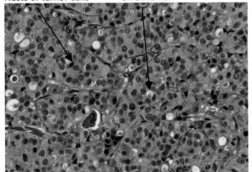

Lobular carcinoma   Single file

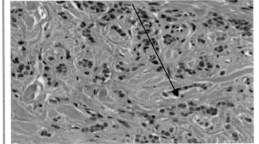

Cutaneous findings

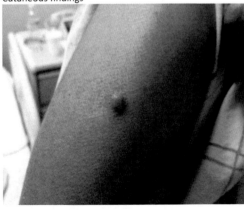

METASTATIC BREAST CARCINOMA

CLINICAL FEATURES

- Clinical presentation is variable and may include:
  - ➢ Sclerotic plaque (carcinoma en cuirasse)
  - ➢ Carcinoma telangiectaticum
  - ➢ Localized hair loss of the scalp (alopecia neoplastica)
  - ➢ Cellulitis-like erythema (carcinoma erysipeloides)

HISTOLOGIC FEATURES

- Metastatic breast cancer presents as a **dermal neoplasm** with **ductal (glandular) differentiation** and appears like a "**cannonball**" metastasis
- May be found within the lymphatic spaces of the skin
- The nuclei have **mild to moderate pleomorphism**, **conspicuous nucleoli**, and **variable eosinophilic cytoplasm**
- Cells can have any of the following features (depending on original tumor) and display **comedo-type necrosis**, **cribriform architecture**, cell clusters lying in pools of **mucin**, or micropapillary features
- **Lobular carcinoma** will infiltrate in **single file** formation

SPECIAL STAINS

- **Mucicarmine positive** intracytoplasmic lumens in **lobular carcinoma**

IMMUNOHISTOCHEMISTRY

- **Positive**: TRPS1 (sensitive and specific), **CK7**, **GATA3**, GCDFP15
- **Negative**: for **CK20**, **CDX2**, SATB2, TTF1, E-cadherin (Lobular carcinoma)
- If triple negative, GATA3 staining can be variable, do TRPS1

OTHER HIGH YIELD POINTS

- **Most common carcinoma** that **metastasizes to the skin** in women
- Variable clinical and histological appearances
- Accounts for **69% of cutaneous metastases** in female
- Prognostic markers **must be performed** on all metastases
  - ➢ Includes: ER, PR, and HER2

DIFFERENTIAL DIAGNOSIS

- **Acute myelomonocytic leukemia**: myeloid markers (+)
- **Syringoid eccrine carcinoma, metastatic salivary duct carcinoma**: clinical correlation

TRPS1 Immunohistochemistry   GATA3 in Triple Negative BC

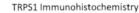
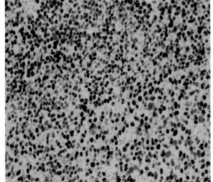

Path Presenter

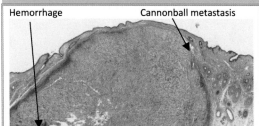
Hemorrhage   Cannonball metastasis

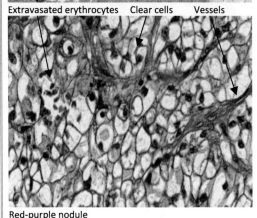
Extravasated erythrocytes   Clear cells   Vessels

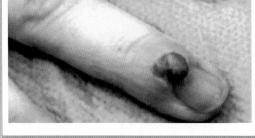
Red-purple nodule

METASTATIC RENAL CELL CARCINOMA

CLINICAL FEATURES
- **Deep red-purple friable nodules that may resemble pyogenic granuloma**
- Rare but if seen, usually is within 2-3 years of primary diagnosis

HISTOLOGIC FEATURES
- Cohesive **groups** and **lobules** of **cytologically bland** clear cells
- **Clear cells** have round to ovoid nuclei with focally irregular nuclear contours, **variable nucleoli, clear cytoplasm,** and **distinct** eosinophilic **cell borders**
- **Stroma is highly vascular** and contains thin-walled vessels that separate the cohesive nests of tumor cells
- **Extravasated erythrocytes** are common
- May have scattered **hemosiderin** due to hemorrhage

IMMUNOHISTOCHEMISTRY
- **Positive**: PAX8, CAIX, RCC, CD10, and EMA
- **Negative:** CK7, CK20, CDX2, SATB2, TTF1, GATA3

OTHER HIGH YIELD POINTS
- **Not a common** metastasis, about 6% of all cutaneous metastasis
- Survival is very poor, and death is frequent within 6 months
- Metastasis is usually through hematogenous spread

DIFFERENTIAL DIAGNOSIS
- **Adnexal tumors of skin:** p63(+), podoplanin (+), CK5/6(+)
- **Lobular carcinoma of breast:** E-cadherin (-), TRPS1(+), GATA3(+)
- **Hidradenocarcinoma:** HER2(-), p63/p40(+), CK5/6(+), variable poroid, squamoid, or clear cells
- **Hemangioma:** cavernous or capillary vascular spaces
- **Pyogenic granuloma:** circumscribed lobules of capillaries, granulation tissue, epidermal erosion, or ulceration, collarette

Path Presenter

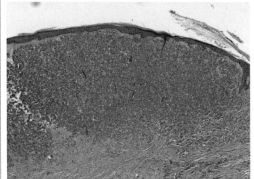
Blue nodule of metastatic tumor

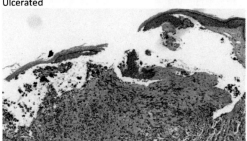
Ulcerated

METASTATIC LUNG ADENOCARCINOMA

CLINICAL FEATURES
- **Deep red firm nodule** with ulceration, usually on the head, neck, or chest
  - ➤ **Females:** Anterior chest wall and abdomen
  - ➤ **Males:** head, neck, and chest wall
- Rare but if seen, usually is within 2-3 years of primary diagnosis

HISTOLOGIC FEATURES
- Cohesive **groups** of **pleomorphic** or **poorly differentiated** epithelial cells
- May form **glandular structures, solid sheets, trabeculae, cords,** or **nests** if there is a more differentiated component
- Can have mucinous features or micropapillary configuration
- Malignant cells have **enlarged nuclei, irregular nuclear contours, conspicuous nucleoli, coarse chromatin,** and variable amounts of cytoplasm
- Mitotic activity is usually high, and necrosis is variable
- All histologic subtypes can metastasize to the skin

IMMUNOHISTOCHEMISTRY
- **Positive**: TTF1, CK7, MOC31, CEA (very non-specific)
- **Negative: CK20**, CDX2, SATB2, GATA3, TRPS1, PAX8, NKX 3.1, Uroplakin II
- If patient has history of adenosquamous carcinoma of lung, will have expression of both adenocarcinoma and squamous cell markers

OTHER HIGH YIELD POINTS
- Next generation sequencing should be done for primary or post therapy recurrent cases for treatment options and/or clinical trials

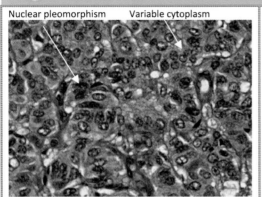

Nuclear pleomorphism   Variable cytoplasm

Stromal desmoplasia   Cords of tumor cells

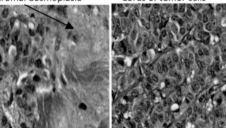

- Largest risk factors for lung cancer: **Smoking**
- Chest wall metastasis can occur through direct extension and/or invasion through chest wall in pleural based lung cancer
- **Survival is approximately 3-5 months** when there is cutaneous metastasis

DIFFERENTIAL DIAGNOSIS

- **Adnexal tumors of skin:** p63(+), podoplanin (+), CK5/6(+)
- **Lobular carcinoma of breast:** E-cadherin (-), TRPS1(+), GATA3(+)
- **Hidradenocarcinoma:** HER2(-), p63/p40(+), CK5/6(+), variable poroid, squamoid, or clear cells
- **Pyogenic granuloma:** circumscribed lobules of capillaries, granulation tissue, epidermal erosion or ulceration, collarette

Nodule with ulceration

Path Presenter

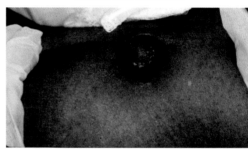

Blue sheets and nests of tumor

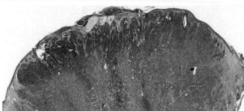

Many mitotic figures   Organoid

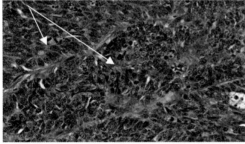

Apoptotic debris   Salt and pepper chromatin

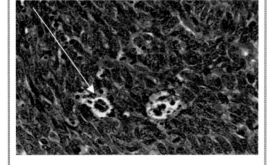

METASTATIC SMALL CELL CARCINOMA
CLINICAL FEATURES

- **Deep red firm nodule** with ulceration, usually on the head, neck, or chest
  - ➢ **Females:** Anterior chest wall and abdomen
  - ➢ **Males:** head, neck, and chest wall
- Rare but if seen, usually is within 2-3 years of primary diagnosis

HISTOLOGIC FEATURES

- Diffuse sheet-like or **organoid proliferation** of epithelial cells
- Epithelial cells have enlarged round to oval nuclei, **dense granular ("salt and pepper") chromatin pattern**, inconspicuous nucleoli, and **scant cytoplasm**
- Epithelial cells exhibit nuclear molding and have irregular nuclear contours
- High level of **mitotic activity**
- **Necrosis** is seen around vessels; there is increased basophilic debris which is composed of DNA material (**Azzopardi Effect/Phenomenon**)

IMMUNOHISTOCHEMISTRY

- **Positive:** CKAE1/AE3, **CD56, INSM1**, synaptophysin, TTF1, CK7
- KI-67 proliferation index is high (>70%)
- **Note:** TTF1 does **NOT** guarantee that this is of lung origin; small cell carcinoma of the pancreas and stomach (and other sites) are TTF1 positive

OTHER HIGH YIELD POINTS

- Next generation sequencing should be done for primary or post therapy recurrent cases for treatment options and/or clinical trials
- Largest risk factors for lung cancer: **smoking**

Synaptophysin

Path Presenter

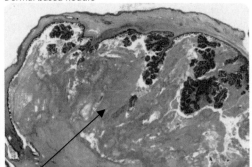
Dermal based nodule

Dirty necrosis

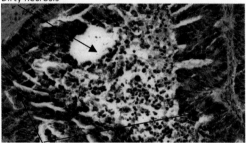
Nuclear pleomorphism
Scalp with erythema, ulceration and bleeding

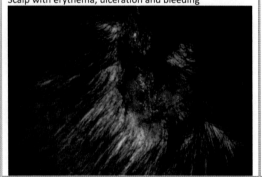

METASTATIC COLORECTAL ADENOCARCINOMA
CLINICAL FEATURES

- **Pink-red firm nodule** with or without ulceration and bleeding and is most commonly seen at the umbilicus ("**Sister Mary Joseph nodule**")
- Other sites include the perineum, head/neck, or extremities
- Uncommon but if seen, usually is within 2-3 years of primary diagnosis

HISTOLOGIC FEATURES

- Usually composed of **well-differentiated** to **moderately differentiated glands** with **central luminal necrosis** ("dirty necrosis")
- Malignant epithelial cells are columnar with nuclear elongation, nuclear stratification, coarse chromatin, and moderate amount of cytoplasm
  - ➢ Some cells may have more vacuolated and mucinous cytoplasm
- **Dirty necrosis** is composed of **neutrophils** and **necrotic cellular debris**
- Can also be in a papillary, micropapillary, solid, signet-ring, cribriform, or tubular pattern

IMMUNOHISTOCHEMISTRY

- **Positive: CK20, CDX2, SATB2**
- **Negative:** CK7, TTF1, NKX 3.1, GATA3, and PAX8

OTHER HIGH YIELD POINTS

- Testing for microsatellite instability is important
- Next generation sequencing should be done for primary or post therapy recurrent cases for treatment options and/or clinical trials

DIFFERENTIAL DIAGNOSIS

- **Proliferative pilar tumor:** cystic spaces with abundant eosinophilic keratin debris, lack of a granular cell layer, can have mitotic figures but not atypical mitoses or high-grade atypia, squamous cells with hyperchromatic and mildly enlarged nuclei

Path Presenter

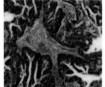
Papillary

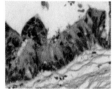
Mucinous cytoplasm, nuclear stratification

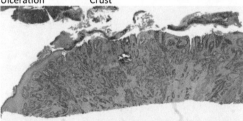
Ulceration   Crust

Necrosis   Nuclear pleormorphism   Mitosis

Squamous differentiation   Transition point

METASTATIC UROTHELIAL CARCINOMA
CLINICAL FEATURES

- **Urticarial** or **macular-like rash** on the **abdomen or trunk** or involving a **prior surgical site**
- May be due to **direct invasion** of tumor or **lymphovascular spread**
- Poor survival

HISTOLOGIC FEATURES

- **High grade epithelial malignancy** composed of epithelial cells
- Epithelial cells are atypical or bizarre and have **enlarged hyperchromatic nuclei**, conspicuous **nucleoli**, coarse irregular chromatin, and variable **amphophilic cytoplasm**
- **Binucleation** or **eccentric cytoplasm** is frequently seen
- May have squamous differentiation which will have intercellular bridges and focal keratinization or be **sarcomatoid** with **spindle-like cells**
- May be seen as small **nests, sheets, single cells, cords,** or **papillary architecture**
- **Necrosis is common** and **may mimic colorectal adenocarcinoma**

IMMUNOHISTOCHEMISTRY

- **Positive: GATA3, CK7,** CK20 (focal), p40, p63, **Uroplakin II,** CK903
- **Negative: PAX8,** TTF1, **TRPS1, RCC**

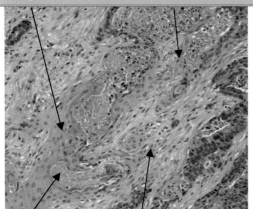

Keratinization   Sarcomatoid-like

OTHER HIGH YIELD POINTS
- *FGFR3* mutations and chromosome 9 deletions
- Male patients with high-grade urothelial carcinoma may have **microsatellite instability (MLH1** and **MSH2 loss)**

DIFFERENTIAL DIAGNOSIS
- **Other Metastatic carcinoma:** IHC markers

Path Presenter

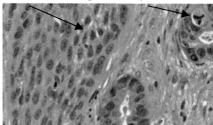

Intercellular bridges   Tripolar mitosis

Irregularly shaped glands   Stromal desmoplasia

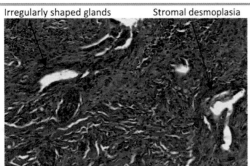

Nuclear pleomorphism

METASTATIC PANCREATIC ADENOCARCINOMA
CLINICAL FEATURES
- **Pink-red firm nodule** with or without ulceration and bleeding and is most commonly seen at the umbilicus ("**Sister Mary Joseph nodule**")
- Other sites include the perineum, head/neck, or extremities
- Uncommon but if seen, usually is within 2-3 years of primary diagnosis

HISTOLOGIC FEATURES
- Composed of **moderately** to **well differentiated glands** with angulated or irregular borders
- Malignant epithelial cells have **nuclear pleomorphism, irregular nuclear contours, conspicuous nucleoli,** loss of nuclear polarity, and variable amounts of cytoplasm
- **Desmoplastic stromal response** to infiltrative glands
- **Mitotic activity** is seen throughout
- Necrosis is variable

IMMUNOHISTOCHEMISTRY
- **Positive: KOC, Maspin, S100p,** CK7, CK19, CEA (non-specific)
- **Negative: VHL,** CK7, TTF1, NKX 3,1, GATA3, and PAX8

OTHER HIGH YIELD POINTS
- *SMAD4* deletion/loss of heterozygosity
- Next generation sequencing for targeted therapy or clinical trials

DIFFERENTIAL DIAGNOSIS
- **Metastatic carcinoma of another primary**: IHC markers

Path Presenter

Cannonball metastatic deposit

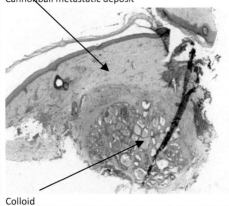

Colloid

METASTATIC FOLLICULAR THYROID CARCINOMA
CLINICAL FEATURES
- **Pink-red firm nodule** with or without ulceration and eschar
- Can be seen in the scar line from prior thyroidectomy, or other locations

HISTOLOGIC FEATURES
- Composed of **moderate** to **well differentiated glands** with colloid
- Malignant epithelial cells may have **variable nuclear pleomorphism, irregular nuclear contours, inconspicuous nucleoli,** and variable clear to eosinophilic cytoplasm
- Minimal desmoplastic stromal response

IMMUNOHISTOCHEMISTRY
- **Positive: PAX8, TTF1**
- **Negative:** NKX 3.1, GATA3, CDX2, SATB2

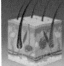
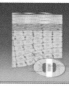
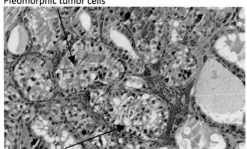

Pleomorphic tumor cells

Glandular architecture

- Risk factors include **radiation exposure** (increases relative risk by 52x) or Iodine deficiency
- *PTEN* Hamartoma tumor syndrome, Werner Syndrome, Carney Complex, *DICER1* syndrome, McCune-Albright syndrome, Li-Fraumeni syndrome
- Other molecular findings include RAS mutations, PPARG fusions, TERT promoter mutations

Path Presenter

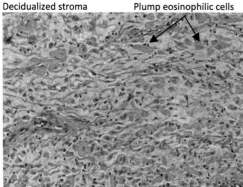

Endometrial glands   Endometrial stroma

Decidualized stroma   Plump eosinophilic cells

CUTANEOUS ENDOMETRIOSIS

CLINICAL FEATURES

- **Solitary firm rubbery nodule** that can be **red-blue** or **black-brown** and is usually **at the umbilicus** or nearby
- Majority of cases occur over a cicatrix
- Lesion may **bleed**, be **tender**, or have **changes in size** and will be synchronized to the menstrual cycle

HISTOLOGIC FEATURES

- Composed of **endometrial glands** that range in size from small to large
- **Morphology** of glands will depend on the stage of the menstrual cycle
  - ➢ **Proliferative: Round** or **tubular glands** with **pseudostratified** columnar cells and **numerous mitotic figures**
  - ➢ **Secretory:** Convoluted, irregularly shaped glands with increased eosinophilic cytoplasm and luminal secretions
  - ➢ **Menstrual:** hemorrhagic and central necrosis
- Associated **endometrial stroma** that is composed of **spindle cells** that have **basophilic cytoplasm**
  - ➢ **Decidualized stroma**: cells become plump and eosinophilic and suspended in a myxoid stroma
- Associated **vascular network** and may have **extravasated erythrocytes** or **hemosiderin** deposition

IMMUNOHISTOCHEMISTRY

- **Positive: CD10 (stroma), ER, PR, CK7 (glands)**

DIFFERENTIAL DIAGNOSIS

- **Metastatic endometrioid adenocarcinoma:** lacks stroma

Path Presenter

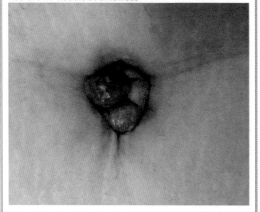

Red-brown nodule at umbilicus

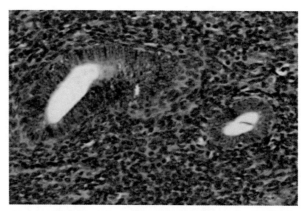

Endometrial glands in proliferative phase (pseudostratified)

Immunohistochemical Assays for Working up a Metastasis of Unknown Origin

Primary Origin/Lesion	Useful IHC Staining Panel
Adrenocortical carcinoma	SF1, calretinin, inhibin, Melan-A
Bladder (Urothelial)	CK5/6, p40, CK7, CK20 (+/-), GATA3 (+/-), p63
Breast	CK7, GATA3, TRPS1, ER, PR, mammaglobin, BRST2/GCDFP15, HER2
Colorectal	CK20, CDX2, SATB2
Endometrial	CK7, CK8/18, CK19, vimentin, ER, PR, PTEN, p16 (patchy)
Endocervical	P16 (diffuse), CK7; negative for ER, PR, CD10
Hepatocellular carcinoma	Arginase1, HepPar1
Lung - Adenocarcinoma	TTF1, CK7, napsin-A
Lung - Squamous Cell carcinoma	p40, p63, CK5/6
Lung – Small Cell Carcinoma	INSM1, synaptophysin, chromogranin, TTF1, CK7, AE1/AE3, ki-67 (very high)
Melanoma	SOX10, S100, Melan A, HMB45
Merkel cell carcinoma	CK20, INSM1, synaptophysin, MCPyV
Mesothelioma	Calretinin, CK5/6, WT1, D2-40, BAP1 (+/-)
Neuroendocrine neoplasms	INSM1, Synaptophysin, Chromogranin
Ovary & Fallopian Tube	PAX8, WT1, CK7, p53, ER (+/-), PR (-/+)
Pancreaticobiliary	CK7, CK19, Maspin, KOC, S100P, SMAD4/DPC4 (loss), VHL (loss), ARID1A, BAP1
Prostate	NKX 3.1, PSA
Renal (papillary, chromophobe)	PAX8, PAX2, Racemase (AMACR), CD10, KIT
Clear Cell Renal cell CA	PAX8, PAX2, Racemase (AMACR), RCC-Ag, CD10
Salivary gland	GATA3, S100, SOX10, BRST2/GCDFP15, AR, HER2
Squamous Cell Carcinoma	p40, p63, CK5/6, p16 (if HPV expected)
Thyroid	CK7, PAX8, TTF1, TROP2, thyroglobulin
Upper Gastrointestinal	CK7, CK20 -, SATB2 +/-

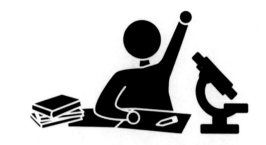

ACE MY PATH
Come Ace With Us!

CHAPTER 12: CUTANEOUS
LYMPHOPROLIFERATIVE DISORDERS

CHRISTINE AHN, MD
CASSANDRA DREW, MD

CUTANEOUS LYMPHOPROLIFERATIVE DISORDERS

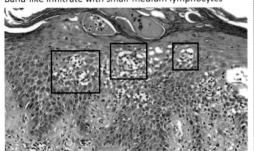
Band-like infiltrate with small-medium lymphocytes

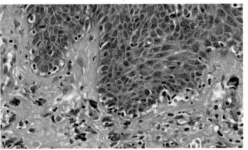
"Pautrier collections" of neoplastic lymphocytes

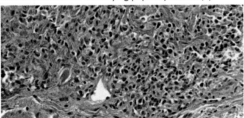
Lining of neoplastic lymphocytes along basal layer with halo and fibrosis of underlying papillary dermis (*)

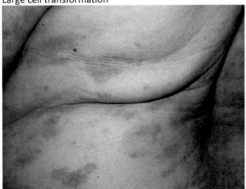
Large cell transformation

MYCOSIS FUNGOIDES (MF)

CLINICAL FEATURES
- Cutaneous T cell lymphoma (CTCL)
- Most common type of cutaneous lymphoma (~50%)
- Classic variant: patch, plaque, tumor stages
- Patch stage with thin scaly plaques on non-sun-exposed sites (buttocks, trunk, proximal extremities)
- Plaque stage with thicker plaques
- Tumor stage with non-specific indurated tumors
- Many clinical variants (discussed below)
- Can be observed in association with other hematologic disease (Hodgkin lymphoma, lymphomatoid papulosis, anaplastic large cell lymphoma)
- Extracutaneous involvement most often involves lymph nodes, spleen, liver

HISTOLOGIC FEATURES
- Early lesions with lichenoid patchy or band-like infiltrate in fibrotic papillary dermis with coarse collagen bundles
- Proliferation of small- to medium-sized pleomorphic "cerebriform" lymphocytes
- Collections of lymphocytes within the epidermis – "Pautrier collections"
- Neoplastic lymphocytes within the epidermis – "epidermotropism", may align along the basal layer, surrounded by clear halo
- Tumor stage with diffuse sheets of small, medium, and large, atypical lymphocytes in dermis, with little or no epidermotropism. Eosinophils may be present in tumor stage, not typical of patch and plaque stage
- In advanced stages, large cell transformation defined as large cells (immunoblasts, large pleomorphic cells, or large anaplastic cells) > 25% of infiltrate

IMMUNOHISTOCHEMISTRY
- Characterized by α/β T-cell phenotype: CD3+, CD4+, CD5+, βF1+, CLA +, CCR4 +,TCRδ-, TCRγ- Increased CD4:CD8 ratio, usually >10. Relative loss of CD5 and CD7 expression seen frequently
- Minority of cases exhibit T-cytotoxic or γ/δ T-cell phenotype: CD3+, CD4-, CD5+, CD8+, βF1-, TCRδ+, TCRγ+
- Tumor stage may show admixed B cells and high Ki-67 index
- Large cell transformation: CD30+/-, high Ki-67 and p53+

OTHER HIGH YIELD POINTS
- Monoclonal rearrangement of TCR commonly seen in plaque and tumor stage MF – must be interpreted with caution as benign dermatoses may also harbor monoclonal population of T lymphocytes
- Matching clones at 2 different skin sites or between skin or blood can be helpful
- Lymph node biopsy done for staging purposes
- Early-stage MF may show false negative results

DIFFERENTIAL DIAGNOSIS
- Spongiotic dermatitis – may be impossible to differentiate on histologic features alone
- Pseudolymphoma – presence of mixed T and B infiltrate
- Secondary syphilis – presence of plasma cells, demonstration of spirochetes
- Pityriasis lichenoides – infiltrate made of small, uniform lymphocytes

Path Presenter

Path Presenter

Path Presenter

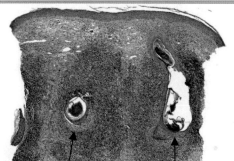
Inflammation around follicles with destruction of follicles, cystic dilation

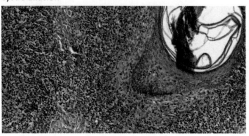
Small-medium neoplastic lymphocytes

Path Presenter

FOLLICULOTROPIC MYCOSIS FUNGOIDES

CLINICAL FEATURES
- Prominent involvement of hair follicles, erythematous, infiltrated plaques on hair-bearing sites
- May cause patchy alopecia
- Severely pruritic, secondary prurigo-like changes frequently observed
- May have a worse prognosis than classic MF

HISTOLOGIC FEATURES
- Dense infiltrates of small-medium neoplastic lymphocytes around hair follicles, with pleiotropic lymphocytes within hair follicles
- Granulomatous reaction, presence of eosinophils may be observed
- Mucin deposition restricted to hair follicle can be present, disrupts or destroys follicle
- On trunk and extremities, cystic dilation of hair follicles and less dense and superficial infiltrates are more characteristic

IMMUNOHISTOCHEMISTRY
- Predominantly CD4+ T lymphocytes

DIFFERENTIAL DIAGNOSIS
- Idiopathic follicular mucinosis – mucin deposition within follicle without a T-cell lymphoma, however, may progress to MF, clinical monitoring is recommended

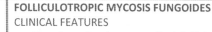
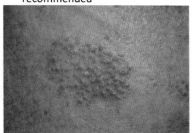
Erythematous plaque with pronounced follicles

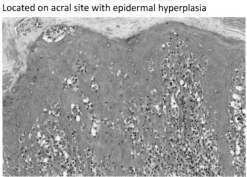
Located on acral site with epidermal hyperplasia

Epidermotropic lymphocytes with pagetoid spread

LOCALIZED PAGETOID RETICULOSIS

CLINICAL FEATURES
- Woringer-Kolopp type
- Localized psoriasiform, scaly erythematous patches or plaques
- Typically on extremities or acral sites

HISTOLOGIC FEATURES
- Marked epidermal hyperplasia with epidermotropic lymphocytes demonstrating "pagetoid" spread within epidermis and adnexal structures

IMMUNOHISTOCHEMISTRY
- CD8 +, cytotoxic T-cell phenotype
- Less frequently, helper phenotype or CD4-/CD8- phenotypes reported

OTHER HIGH YIELD POINTS
- Excellent prognosis

DIFFERENTIAL DIAGNOSIS
- Lymphomatoid papulosis, type D – may only be distinguishable by clinical course

Path Presenter

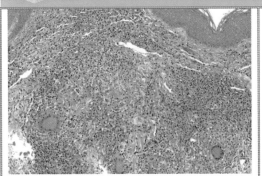

Diffuse infiltrate, multinucleated histiocytes, lack of epidermal involvement

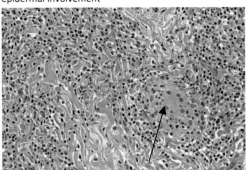

Emperipolesis with phagocytosis

GRANULOMATOUS SLACK SKIN

CLINICAL FEATURES

- Pendulous skin folds in flexural areas
- Seen in adults and elderly patients, rare cases in children

HISTOLOGIC FEATURES

- Diffuse granulomatous infiltrate with multinucleated histiocytes, lymphocytes, filling entire dermis and extending to subcutaneous tissue
- Emperipolesis with phagocytosis
- Loss of elastic fibers, fragments within cytoplasm of multinucleated histiocytes – "elastophagocytosis"
- Prominent epidermotropism or Pautrier collections notably absent

IMMUNOHISTOCHEMISTRY

- Similar immunophenotype to conventional MF

DIFFERENTIAL DIAGNOSIS

- Granulomatous MF – similar features histologically but usually more patchy, dermal granulomatous infiltrate, distinction may require clinicopathologic correlation

Path Presenter

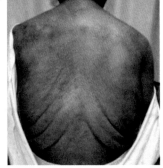

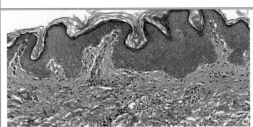

Sparse perivascular superficial infiltrate of atypical lymphocytes in hypopigmented MF

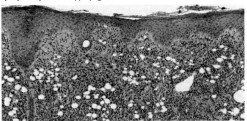

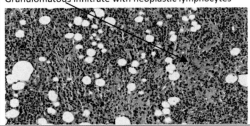

Granulomatous infiltrate with neoplastic lymphocytes

MYCOSIS FUNGOIDES – OTHER VARIANTS

Syringotropic

- Infiltrated plaques, single or multiple, frequently on palms and soles
- Dense lymphoid infiltrates around hyperplastic eccrine glands and coils, syringometaplasia common, may involve follicles

Hypopigmented

- Hypopigmented patches and plaques, more frequently in darker skin types and more frequently in children
- Predominant CD8+ phenotype more common than CD4+ phenotype

Poikilodermatous

- Atrophic red-brown macules and patches with telangiectasias, frequently on breast, buttocks, or generalized
- Atrophic epidermis, loss of rete ridges, band-like infiltrate of lymphocytes with epidermotropism, dilated capillaries within papillary dermis

Granulomatous

- Indurated papules and plaques
- Granulomatous infiltrate with neoplastic T-cells, epidermotropism is helpful clue to diagnosis
- Worse prognosis with higher association with secondary lymphoma

Path Presenter   Path Presenter

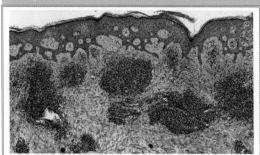
Infiltrate of lymphocytes with minimal epidermotropism

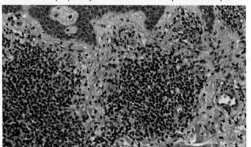
Small- and medium-sized pleomorphic lymphocytes

SÉZARY SYNDROME

CLINICAL FEATURES
- Triad of erythroderma, generalized lymphadenopathy, and circulating malignant T-cell (Sezary cells) (>1000 cell per microliter)
- Affects elderly, more often in men
- Pruritic erythroderma with hyperkeratosis, alopecia, onychodystrophy

HISTOLOGIC FEATURES
- Mild or absent epidermotropism
- Band-like infiltrate of lymphocytes with small- or medium-sized pleomorphic lymphocytes – "Sézary cells"-show abnormally shaped deeply grooved nuclei and nuclear convolutions
- Early or prodromal phase can be perivascular or nonspecific
- Other histopathologic variants include granulomatous reaction, follicular mucinosis, and large cell transformation

IMMUNOHISTOCHEMISTRY
- T-cells: CD3+, CD4+, CD7-, C8-
- Frequent loss of CD2, CD5, CD7 and/or CD26
- PD1 +, TOX +, CD25 +, CXCL13 +

DIFFERENTIAL DIAGNOSIS
- MF – histologic features and immunophenotype
- Inflammatory erythroderma – no atypical lymphocytes

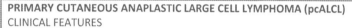

Path Presenter

Erythroderma and lymphadenopathy

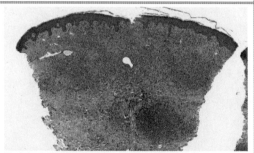
Nodular infiltrate throughout the dermis

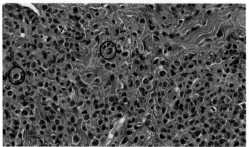
Large cells with irregular nuclei, Reed-Sternberg-like cells (circle), frequent mitoses (asterix)

Path Presenter

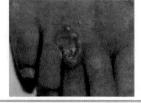

PRIMARY CUTANEOUS ANAPLASTIC LARGE CELL LYMPHOMA (pcALCL)

CLINICAL FEATURES
- Large, solitary ulcerated plaques or tumors
- Can occur on head/neck, extremities, mucosal regions
- Rapid growth with only partial regression

HISTOLOGIC FEATURES
- Sheets of large, atypical CD30+ cells in diffuse or nodular growth pattern
- Infiltrate in dermis and upper subcutis
- Additional features include epidermotropism, infiltration of adnexal structures, epidermal hyperplasia, reactive inflammation with neutrophils, lymphocytes, eosinophils
- Large cells with large, irregularly shaped nuclei and prominent nucleoli, giant Reed-Sternberg-like cells, and immunoblast-like cells
- Neutrophilic rich (pyogenic) and eosinophilic rich variants have been described

IMMUNOHISTOCHEMISTRY
- CD30+ in ≥75% neoplastic cells
- Usually CD3+, CD4+, CD8- although variability in immunophenotype observed
- Cytotoxic proteins (TIA, perforin, Granzyme) +
- ALK- and EMA- in majority of pcALCL in contrast to secondary skin lesions of nodal ALK+ ALCL
- MUM-1+, GATA3-

OTHER HIGH YIELD POINTS
- *IRF4* gene rearrangements (*DUSP22-IRF4*)
- Activating mutations of *JAK1*, *STAT3*
- Monoclonal TCR rearrangement (large CD30+ cells monoclonal)

DIFFERENTIAL DIAGNOSIS
- CD30+ MF with large cell transformation – nearly identical but GATA3 usually positive in this entity

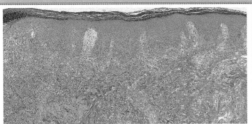
LyP type A with infiltrate of atypical large lymphocytes

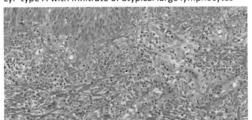
LyP type A with admixed reactive cells (eosinophils, lymphocytes, histiocytes)

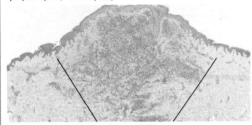
LyP type B with wedge-shaped infiltrate

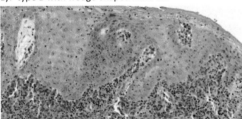
LyP type D with epidermotropism, dense underling infiltrate of large cells

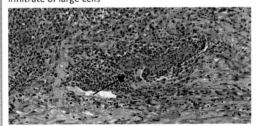
LyP type E with evidence of angiocentric tumor

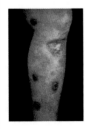
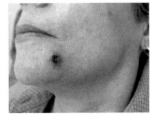

LYMPHOMATOID PAPULOSIS (LyP)

CLINICAL FEATURES

- Chronic, recurrent, self-healing papules and nodules
- Red-brown papules or nodules on trunk, extremities
- Rarely, larger tumors with spontaneous resolution with residual scarring
- Affects any age but usually young adults

HISTOLOGIC FEATURES

- 6 main histologic subtypes: A, B, C, D, E, LyP with 6p253 rearrangement – more than one can be observed within the same patient
- Type A (conventional or histiocytic type): most common, wedge-shaped infiltrate of large, atypical anaplastic cells (resembling histiocytes) mixed with small lymphocytes, histiocytes, neutrophils, and eosinophils, variable epidermotropism and necrosis, Reed-Sternberg-like cells can be present; CD4+, CD8-, CD30 +
- Type B (mycosis fungoides-like): band-like infiltrate of CD4+ small or medium pleomorphic cells with epidermotropism, Pautrier collections; CD4+, CD8-, CD30+/-
- Type C (anaplastic large cell lymphoma-like): nodular infiltrate with sheets of large monotonous atypical cells with few small lymphocytes, neutrophils, eosinophils; CD4+, CD8-, CD30+
- Type D (cutaneous aggressive epidermotropic CD8+ cytotoxic T-cell lymphoma-like): superficial, band-like, or wedge-shaped lymphoid infiltrate, prominent epidermotropism, CD4+,CD8+, CD30+
- Type E (angiocentric/angiodestructive): prominent angiotropism with angiodestruction (in contrast to focal angiotropism/angiodestruction in other types), CD4-, CD8+, CD30+
- LyP with 6p253 rearrangement: biphasic pattern with epidermotropism and wedge-shaped dermal infiltrate CD4+, CD8+ or CD4:CD8 double negative, CD30+
- Other rare variants include folliculotropic, syringotropic and granulomatous

IMMUNOHISTOCHEMISTRY

- Hallmark is CD30+ in neoplastic cells
- Usually T-helper lymphocytes (CD3+, CD4+), some cases T-cytotoxic (CD3+, CD8+, TIA-1-)

OTHER HIGH YIELD POINTS

- Monoclonal in 20-80% of cases
- 10-20% preceded by other lymphoma (Hodgkin lymphoma, MF, ALCL)
- *IRF4* translocation can be observed in LyP (less than ALCL)
- *DUSP22-IRF4* seen in subset of LyP

DIFFERENTIAL DIAGNOSIS

- Mycosis fungoides – with type B, only distinguishable by clinicopathologic correlation
- Anaplastic large cell lymphoma – with type C, only distinguishable by clinicopathologic correlation
- Cutaneous aggressive epidermotropic CD8+ cytotoxic T-cell lymphoma – with type D, demonstration of CD30+ prerequisite of diagnosis
- Hodgkin lymphoma – presence of Reed-Sternberg-like cells
- Extranodal NK/T-cell lymphoma, nasal type – with Type E, in situ hybridization demonstrating EBV- can differentiate

Path Presenter   Path Presenter   Path Presenter   Path Presenter   Path Presenter

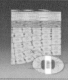

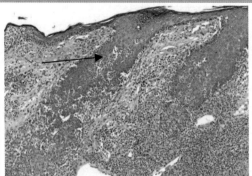

Pagetoid epidermotropism and dense infiltrate of lymphocytes

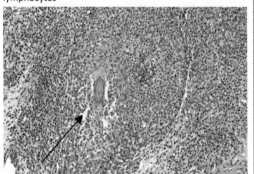

Destruction of follicle with proliferation of neoplastic cells

PRIMARY CUTANEOUS AGGRESSIVE EPIDERMOTROPIC CD8+ CYTOTOXIC T-CELL LYMPHOMA

CLINICAL FEATURES
- Generalized patches, plaques, tumors, often ulcerated; acral sites common
- Aggressive clinical course, seen usually in adults

HISTOLOGIC FEATURES
- Epidermotropism can be pagetoid or subtle
- Dense proliferation of lymphocytes, commonly invade and destroy adnexal skin structures, angiodestruction uncommon
- Variable cytomorphology (ranges small to large) with pleomorphic cells and indented nuclei
- Associated spongiosis and vesiculation
- Dermal involvement can be extensive; sometimes also involve subcutaneous fat with rimming of adipocytes

IMMUNOHISTOCHEMISTRY
- βF1+, CD3+, CD4-, CD7+, CD8+, CCR4-, EBV- , Ki-67 >75%
- Cytotoxic proteins positive: TIA-1, granzyme B, perforin
- CD30 usually negative

OTHER HIGH YIELD POINTS
- Monoclonal TCR rearrangement

DIFFERENTIAL DIAGNOSIS
- LyP, type D – usually CD30+

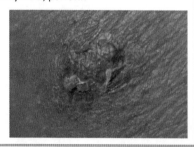

Path Presenter

Interface dermatitis-like changes, epidermotropism

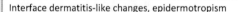

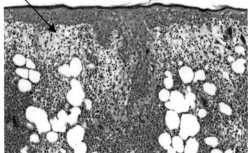

Angiocentricity with associated hemorrhage, panniculitis-like distribution

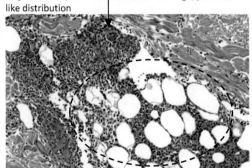

Angiocentricity

PRIMARY CUTANEOUS δ/γ T-CELL LYMPHOMA

CLINICAL FEATURES
- Localized or generalized plaques, tumors, often ulcerated
- Can involve mucosal regions
- Typically seen in adults
- Frequently associated with fever, night sweats and weight loss

HISTOLOGIC FEATURES
- Dense proliferation of lymphocytes with subcutaneous and dermal involvement
- Panniculitis-like distribution
- Variable epidermotropism
- Angiodestruction or angiocentricity frequently seen
- Interface dermatitis-like features, pronounced hemorrhage, necrosis

IMMUNOHISTOCHEMISTRY
- βF1-, CD3+, CD4-, CD8+/-, CD56+, TCR-γ+, TCR-δ+
- TIA-1+, granzyme B+, perforin+
- Ki-67 high (50-100%)

OTHER HIGH YIELD POINTS
- Monoclonal TCR rearrangement with overexpression of genes of NK-cell-associated molecules (killer cell immunoglobulin-like receptor genes – KIR, killer cell lectin-like receptor genes - KLR)

DIFFERENTIAL DIAGNOSIS
- Primary cutaneous aggressive epidermotropic CD8+ cytotoxic T-cell lymphoma – less involvement of subcutaneous fat, angiotropism less frequent

Path Presenter

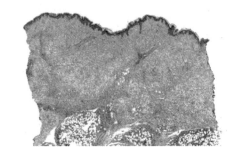

Patchy infiltrate extending into subcutaneous fat

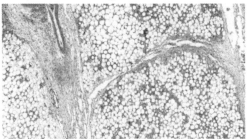

Lobular panniculitis-like architecture

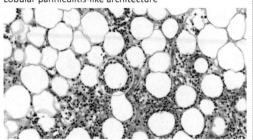

Rimming of adipocytes with neoplastic lymphocytes

SUBCUTANEOUS PANNICULITIS-LIKE T-CELL LYMPHOMA
CLINICAL FEATURES
- Solitary or multiple infiltrated plaques, most frequently on extremities
- Can sometimes mimic rheumatologic disease with malaise, fatigue, weight loss, and even positivity for antinuclear antibodies

HISTOLOGIC FEATURES
- Dense, nodular, or diffuse infiltrates of small and medium lymphocytes resembling lobular panniculitis
- Neoplastic lymphocytes line up around adipocytes – "rimming" of adipocytes
- Necrotic lymphocytes or "ghost cells" present

IMMUNOHISTOCHEMISTRY
- α/β T-cytotoxic phenotype: βF1+, CD3+, CD4-, CD8+, TCRγ-, TCRδ-
- TIA-1+, granzyme B+, perforin+ (cytotoxic proteins), CD56-, CD30-, EBV-
- Ki-67 highlights increased staining in clusters around adipocytes

OTHER HIGH YIELD POINTS
- History of autoimmune disorder in up to 20% of patients
- Association with hemophagocytic syndrome
- Majority of cases have monoclonal rearrangement

DIFFERENTIAL DIAGNOSIS
- Mycosis fungoides – usually CD4+ phenotype
- Subcutaneous anaplastic large cell lymphoma – large pleomorphic or anaplastic cells, CD4+, CD30+
- Extranodal NK/T-cell lymphoma – NK-cell phenotype, CD56+, EBER-1+, lack TCR rearrangement
- Lupus panniculitis – lack cellular atypia, should have mix of B lymphocytes, CD4+ cells present, clusters of CD123 plasmacytoid dendritic cells

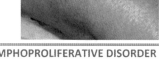

Path Presenter

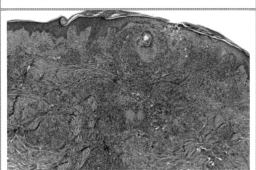

Nodular lymphoid infiltrate within the dermis

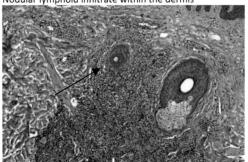

Infiltrate around follicle with follicular destruction

CUTANEOUS CD4+ SMALL/MEDIUM T-CELL LYMPHOPROLIFERATIVE DISORDER
CLINICAL FEATURES
- Affects adults and elderly, benign behavior
- Usually solitary tumor, head/neck most frequently involved

HISTOLOGIC FEATURES
- Nodular or diffuse lymphoid infiltrate within the dermis composed of small- and medium-sized T cells admixed with reactive cells, no lymphoid follicles
- Less frequently, a subepidermal band like infiltrate in superficial dermis in association with periadnexal involvement has been described
- Involvement of hair follicles with follicular destruction is characteristic
- Large cells rare (<40 %), epidermotropism not prominent

IMMUNOHISTOCHEMISTRY
- CD3+, CD4+, CD8-, CD30+/-; a small portion of the admixed reactive lymphocytes positive for CD8 and CD30
- Proportion of cells positive for PD-1, Bcl-6, ICOS, CXCL13+, Ki-67 <20%
- Variable reactive infiltrate of B lymphocytes

OTHER HIGH YIELD POINTS
- Monoclonal TCR rearrangement present in three-fourth of cases

DIFFERENTIAL DIAGNOSIS
- Mycosis fungoides – characterized by small- and medium-T helper cells, but immunostains can help distinguish

Path Presenter

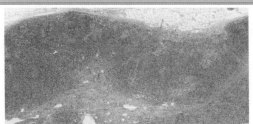

Nodular collections in the subcutaneous tissue

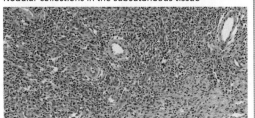

Proliferation of venules as seen here

Path Presenter

ANGIOIMMUNOBLASTIC T-CELL LYMPHOMA

CLINICAL FEATURES
- Affects elderly adults
- Erythematous papules, plaques, tumor
- Primarily a lymph node disease, involves skin in 50% of cases

HISTOLOGIC FEATURES
- Moderately dense perivascular and/or periadnexal collections of pleomorphic lymphocytes admixed with reactive cells (plasma cells, histiocytes and eosinophils)
- Proliferation of venules with prominent endothelial lining

IMMUNOHISTOCHEMISTRY
- T follicular helper lymphocyte phenotype: CD3+, CD4+, CD8-, CD10+, Bcl-6+, PD-1+, CXCL13+, ICOS+

OTHER HIGH YIELD POINTS
- Monoclonal TCR rearrangement present

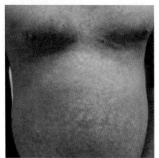

DIFFERENTIAL DIAGNOSIS
- Pseudolymphoma – reactive infiltrate but lacks atypia and monoclonal populations of T lymphocytes
- Infection, inflammatory dermatoses – can appear similar, usually less dense, lack of atypia and monoclonal population of T lymphocytes

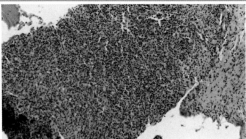

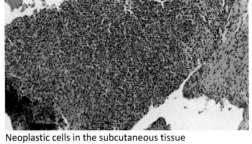

Neoplastic cells in the subcutaneous tissue

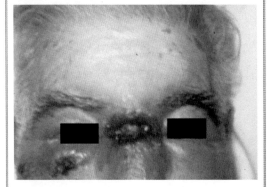

Path Presenter

EXTRANODAL NK/T-CELL LYMPHOMA

CLINICAL FEATURES
- Cytotoxic lymphoma of the nasal cavity and upper respiratory tract
- Majority associated with EBV infection
- Affects adults, more common in men, more common in Asia and South America
- Midline facial destructive, ulcerated plaques - "lethal midline granuloma"
- Persistent facial swelling
- Infiltrated erythematous or violaceous plaques on the trunk, frequent involvement of oral cavity and upper respiratory tract

HISTOLOGIC FEATURES
- Neoplastic lymphocytes diffusely throughout dermis and subcutaneous tissue; can present as perivascular pattern
- Epidermotropism and interface changes variable
- Angiotropism/angiodestruction focal if present
- Increased mitosis

IMMUNOHISTOCHEMISTRY
- NK cell phenotype: CD2+, CD3+, CD56+
- Usually CD4-, CD5-, CD8-
- TIA-1+, granzyme B+, perforin+
- CD30 can be positive
- EBER-1+ (helpful in CD56- cases)

OTHER HIGH YIELD POINTS
- Neoplastic cells overexpress EBV-induced genes, including oncogene *C-MYC*
- JAK/STAT signaling pathway affected through recurrent mutations

DIFFERENTIAL DIAGNOSIS
- Cutaneous γ/δ T-cell lymphoma – NK phenotype and EBER-1+ helps differentiate from other lymphomas

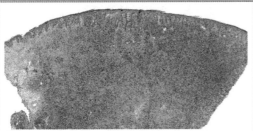
Diffuse nodular infiltrate filling the dermis

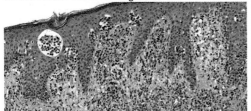
Prominent epidermotropism with neoplastic lymphocytes

Path Presenter

CUTANEOUS ADULT T-CELL LEUKEMIA/LYMPHOMA

CLINICAL FEATURES
- Associated with HTLV-1, endemic to Japan, Caribbean, Central Africa
- Affects adults or elderly
- Non-specific papules or plaques and tumor, erythroderma
- Leukemia and bone marrow involvement seen in >50%

HISTOLOGIC FEATURES
- Pleomorphic lymphocytes with prominent epidermotropism and dermal perivascular infiltrate
- Admixed eosinophils may be noted
- Polylobated flower cells may be seen in blood and tissue

IMMUNOHISTOCHEMISTRY
- CD3+, CD4+, CD8-, CD25+, PD-1+, CD103+, FOX-P3+/-
- Some cases may be CD4-/CD8+ or CD4+/CD8+

OTHER HIGH YIELD POINTS
- Monoclonal TCR rearrangement
- Monoclonal integration of HTLV-1

DIFFERENTIAL DIAGNOSIS
- Mycosis fungoides – other features may be identical but presence of monoclonal integration of HTLV-1 distinguishes the two entities

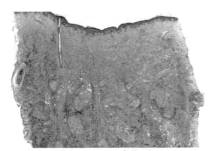
Nodular infiltrates demonstrating follicular pattern, no involvement of epidermis

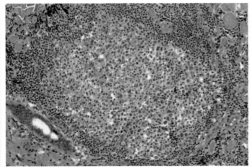
Neoplastic follicle without mantle zone

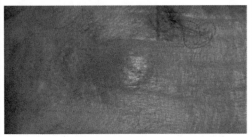

PRIMARY CUTANEOUS FOLLICLE CENTER LYMPHOMA

CLINICAL FEATURES
- Erythematous papules, plaques, tumors on head, neck, and trunk
- Expand centrifugally, often with surrounding erythema

HISTOLOGIC FEATURES
- Can show follicular, follicular and diffuse or diffuse growth pattern
- Nodular infiltrates with follicular pattern, spares epidermis and involves dermis and subcutaneous tissue
- Neoplastic follicles are ill-defined and do not demonstrate mantle zones, tingible body macrophages, and lack demarcation of dark and light areas
- Can show abnormal reversal of light area at periphery (neoplastic cells) around dark areas (reactive lymphocytes)
- Small and large centrocytes mixed with centroblasts admixed with reactive small lymphocytes
- Disrupted meshwork of CD21+/CD35+ follicular dendritic cells in atypical follicles
- Prominent stromal fibroblastic or fibro-histiocytic component present
- Diffuse growth pattern shows lack of follicles and monotonous population of large centrocytes mixed with centroblasts and reactive small lymphocytes

IMMUNOHISTOCHEMISTRY
- CD20+, CD79a+, Bcl-6+
- Bcl-2-, CD5-, CD43-
- CD10 + in follicular growth pattern; negative in diffuse growth pattern
- MUM-1 can be positive in minority of cells
- KI67 can be high

OTHER HIGH YIELD POINTS
- Monoclonal rearrangement of Ig genes

DIFFERENTIAL DIAGNOSIS
- Primary cutaneous diffuse large B-cell lymphoma, leg type – usually positive for Bcl-2, MUM-1, cytoplasmic IgM, MYC, FOX-P1

Path Presenter

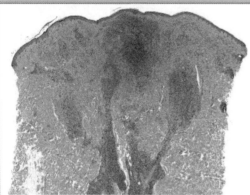
Nodular infiltrate forming lymphoid follicles

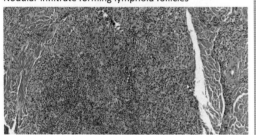
Neoplastic cells surrounded by reactive lymphocytes and inflammatory cells

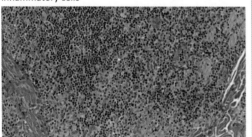
Lymphoplasmacytoid cells with admixed reactive lymphocytes

Path Presenter

PRIMARY CUTANEOUS MARGINAL ZONE LYMPHOMA

CLINICAL FEATURES
- Low-grade malignant B-cell lymphoma
- Associated with *B. burgdorferi* in some areas
- Observed in young adults, men more frequent
- Red-brown papules, plaques, or nodules with predilection for upper extremities and trunk

HISTOLOGIC FEATURES
- Patchy, nodular, or diffuse dermal infiltrate forming lymphoid follicles
- In conventional variant, reactive germinal centers are surrounded by neoplastic population of marginal zone cells, lymphoplasmacytoid lymphocytes and plasma cells
- Infiltrate heavily admixed with reactive lymphocytes and other inflammatory cells
- Reactive germinal centers show positive Bcl-6 +, Bcl-2 – cells in a meshwork of CD21 dendritic cells
- In **lymphoplasmacytic variant**: predominant lymphoplasmacytoid cells, PAS-positive intranuclear inclusions (Dutcher bodies), lack reactive lymphoid follicles and germinal centers, surrounding reactive infiltrate sparse
- In **plasmacytic variant**: predominant mature plasma cells, some blastoid cells, intracytoplasmic Ig inclusions (Russell bodies) can be seen, reactive germinal centers rare
- In **blastoid variant**: blastoid cells comprise majority of infiltrate, lack Dutcher and Russell bodies, few small reactive germinal centers
Two subtypes have been described:
- Heavy chain class-switched subtype shows expression of IgG, IgA, IgE and high number of T cells
- IgM positive non-class switched subtype is IgM positive and shows sheets of B cells with few T cells

IMMUNOHISTOCHEMISTRY
- CD20+, CD79a+, Bcl-2+, Bcl-6-, CD10-, cyclin-D1-, CD5-
- IRTA-1+
- Kappa or lambda light chain restriction
- In plasmacytoid variant: CD20-, CD38+, CD138+
- In blastoid variant: MUM-1+, Bcl-6-, CD10-, CD20+/-, CD79+/-, CD138+/-, CD5+, CD23+

OTHER HIGH YIELD POINTS
- Monoclonal rearrangement of Ig genes in 50-60%

DIFFERENTIAL DIAGNOSIS
- Cutaneous follicle center lymphoma – presence of follicular B lymphocytes in both entities, but Bcl-6+ and CD10+ help differentiate

PRIMARY CUTANEOUS DIFFUSE LARGE B-CELL LYMPHOMA, LEG TYPE

CLINICAL FEATURES
- Observed in elderly patients, most common on the leg
- Non-specific infiltrative plaque, nodule, or ulcer

HISTOLOGIC FEATURES
- Dense infiltrate within dermis and subcutaneous fat comprised of immunoblasts and centroblasts (large cells with round nuclei)
- Absence of follicular dendritic cell meshwork
- Early lesions can show mild perivascular lymphoid infiltrates
- Few small reactive lymphocytes, numerous mitoses

IMMUNOHISTOCHEMISTRY
- CD20+, CD79a+, PAX5+ (partial loss possible)
- Bcl-2+, MUM-1+, FOX-P1+, Bcl-6+
- CD10- (usually), CD138-

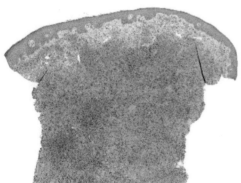
Dense sheets of neoplastic cells in the dermis

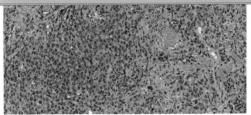

Immunoblasts and centroblasts with numerous apparent mitoses

Path Presenter

- Ki67 high (>40 %)

OTHER HIGH YIELD POINTS
- Monoclonal rearrangement of Ig genes
- Loss of *CDKN2A*, *CDKN2B* – associated with worse prognosis
- Activation of NF-κB pathway

DIFFERENTIAL DIAGNOSIS
- Cutaneous follicle center lymphoma – usually Bcl-2-
- Primary cutaneous diffuse large B-cell lymphoma, NOS- when criteria do not meet for either Primary cutaneous diffuse large B cell lymphoma, leg type or Follicle center cell lymphoma, diffuse pattern

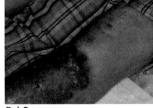

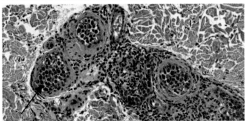

Perivascular infiltrate within the dermis

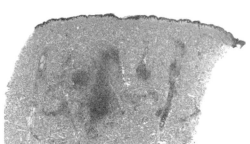

Intravascular large B lymphocytes seen in neurovascular bundles

Path Presenter

INTRAVASCULAR B-CELL LYMPHOMA

CLINICAL FEATURES
- Indurated, erythematous or violaceous patches and plaques with telangiectasias
- Favor trunk and thighs
- Can be associated with hemophagocytosis

HISTOLOGIC FEATURES
- Large B lymphocytes within dilated vessels in the dermis and subcutaneous tissue
- Perivascular infiltrate may be present
- Tumors can colonize hemangiomas

IMMUNOHISTOCHEMISTRY
- CD20+, CD79a+
- Aberrant CD5+
- Bcl-2+, MUM-1+ (usually)
- Bcl-6-, CD10- (usually)
- Cyclin D1-

OTHER HIGH YIELD POINTS
- High prevalence of *MYD88* and *CD79B* mutations

DIFFERENTIAL DIAGNOSIS
- Intralymphatic anaplastic large cell lymphoma – neoplastic cells of T cell lineage
- Intravascular large NK/T-cell lymphoma – neoplastic cells of NK lineage
- Reactive angioendotheliomatosis – intravascular proliferation of endothelial cells
- Intralymphatic histiocytosis – clusters of intralymphatic histiocytes
- Benign intralymphatic proliferation of T-cell lymphoid blasts

---

Nodular infiltrate in perivascular and periadnexal distribution

LYMPHOMATOID GRANULOMATOSIS

CLINICAL FEATURES
- B-cell lymphoproliferative disorder, associated with EBV infection
- Lungs are most frequently affected organ, followed by skin and CNS
- Erythematous papules, plaques, tumors on trunk and extremities – can precede lung lesions in minority of cases

HISTOLOGIC FEATURES
- Angiocentric/angiodestructive infiltrate with large B cells and admixed plasma cells and histiocytes
- Early lesions can show non-specific perivascular and periadnexal infiltrates

IMMUNOHISTOCHEMISTRY
- EBER-1+ (can be minimally positive or absent in grade 1 lesions)
- CD20+ in large B lymphocytes

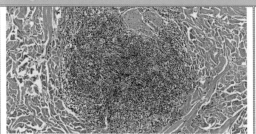
Angiocentric infiltrate with large B-cells and surrounding granulomatous inflammation

- Variably positive for CD30, CD15-
- Reactive lymphocytes typically CD3+, CD4+

OTHER HIGH YIELD POINTS

- Monoclonal rearrangement of Ig genes

Path Presenter

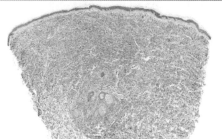
Diffuse infiltrate filling entirety of dermis with neoplastic cells

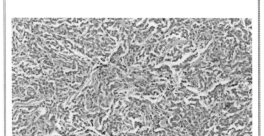
Single filing of neoplastic cell dissecting between collagen bundles

LEUKEMIA CUTIS

CLINICAL FEATURES

- Cutaneous involvement of myelogenous leukemia
- Multiple localized or generalized red-brown or violaceous papules or nodules
- May involve mucosa with gingival hypertrophy

HISTOLOGIC FEATURES

- Dermal infiltrate of neoplastic cells, may be perivascular or periadnexal
- Medium sized cells with distinct indented, bilobular, or kidney-shaped nuclei
- Single cells may line up between collagen bundles
- Neoplastic cells layer around lymphovascular and adnexal structures
- Angiocentric patterns may be seen

IMMUNOHISTOCHEMISTRY

- Depends on type of myelogenous leukemia
- Typically positive for lysozyme+, MPO+, CD13+, CD14+, CD15+, CD33+, CD43+, CD45+, CD68+ (ranges from expression of few to all markers)
- CD34+, CD117+ in more immature forms

OTHER HIGH YIELD POINTS

- Management is treatment of underlying leukemia

Path Presenter

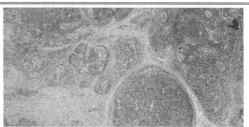
Nodular proliferation in deep dermis/subcutaneous tissue of epithelial islands

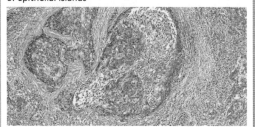
Central island of epithelial cells surrounded by lymphocytes

LYMPHOEPITHELIOMA-LIKE CARCINOMA

CLINICAL FEATURES

- Variant of cutaneous squamous cell carcinoma with prominent lymphoid infiltrate
- Papule or nodule, usually on face or scalp

HISTOLOGIC FEATURES

- Islands of epithelial cells surrounded by dense infiltrate of lymphocytes and plasmacytoid cells

IMMUNOHISTOCHEMISTRY

- Epithelial cells express cytokeratin and EMA

DIFFERENTIAL DIAGNOSIS

- Cutaneous lymphoma – with prominent lymphoid infiltrate, however negative for epithelial cells
- Merkel cell carcinoma – small neuroendocrine cells, lack admixture of lymphocytes

Path Presenter

CHAPTER 12: CUTANEOUS LYMPHOPROLIFERATIVE DISORDERS

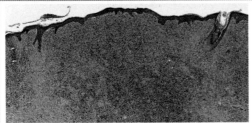

Dense infiltrate with mix of non-neoplastic lymphocytes, histiocytes, eosinophils, and plasma cells

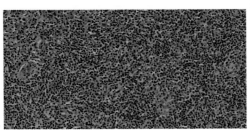

Uniform small lymphocytes with surrounding mixed inflammatory infiltrate

Path Presenter

PSEUDOLYMPHOMA

CLINICAL FEATURES

- Heterogenous group of disorders that mimic malignant cutaneous lymphoma
- Includes cutaneous hyperplasia simulating B-cell lymphoma, lymphomatoid drug reactions, pseudolymphomatous folliculitis, reactions resembling CD30+ lymphoproliferative disorders, cutaneous CD8+ T-cell infiltrates in HIV/AIDS, acral pseudolymphomatous angiokeratoma

HISTOLOGIC FEATURES

- Lymphoid hyperplasia with infiltrates of non-neoplastic, reactive lymphocytes, varying based on the entity
- Cutaneous hyperplasia simulating B-cell lymphoma demonstrates top-heavy infiltrate with lymphoid follicles in most cases, occasionally with mantle zones
- Lymphomatoid drug reactions with band-like dermal infiltrate with lymphocytes, histiocytes, few eosinophils and plasma cells
- Pseudolymphomatous folliculitis with perifollicular infiltrate of lymphocytes, rarely lymphoid follicles

IMMUNOHISTOCHEMISTRY

- Mixed infiltrate with B and T cell populations identified by conventional markers

OTHER HIGH YIELD POINTS

- Usually show polyclonal infiltrate

DIFFERENTIAL DIAGNOSIS

- Includes most entities spanning the B and T cell cutaneous lymphomas – clinicopathologic correlation, immunophenotype, and clonality studies can help differentiate

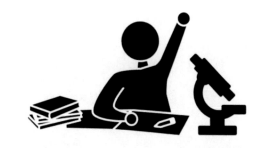

ACE MY PATH
Come Ace With Us!

CHAPTER 13: HISTIOCYTIC,
XANTHOMATOUS, AND MAST CELL
DISORDERS

CHRISTINE AHN, MD

HISTIOCYTIC, XANTHOMATOUS, AND MAST CELL DISORDERS

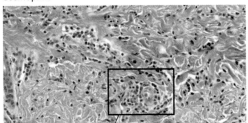

Dense infiltrate of cells in the papillary and mid dermis

Sheets of Langerhans cells with scattered lymphocytes and eosinophils

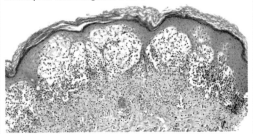

Eosinophils with Langerhans cells with reniform nuclei

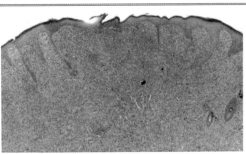

Collections of Langerhans cells in dermal papillae with associated spongiosis

LANGERHANS CELL HISTIOCYTOSIS (LCH)

CLINICAL FEATURES

- Spectrum of diseases with clonal proliferation of Langerhans cells, includes 4 distinct overlapping entities
- **Letterer-Siwe disease**: acute diffuse form, pink papules, pustules, vesicles with scale on the scalp, fissures of flexures of neck, axilla, and perineum, develops within first 2 years of life
- **Hand-Schüller-Christian disease**: triad of diabetes insipidus, bone lesion, exophthalmos, only 30% develop skin lesions like Letterer-Siwe disease, develops between ages 2-6 years
- **Eosinophilic granuloma**: localized variant, usually single lesion of bone and skin involvement rare, affects older children
- **Congenital self-healing reticulohistiocytosis (Hashimoto-Pritzker disease)**: widespread eruption of red to purple-brown papules and nodules, limited to skin and rapidly self-healing, presents within first few days of life

HISTOLOGIC FEATURES

- Clusters or sheets of Langerhans cells in the papillary dermis
- Langerhans cell characterized by reniform nuclei, abundant eosinophilic cytoplasm
- Surrounding admixed inflammation with eosinophils, neutrophils, lymphocytes, plasma cells, and mast cells
- Lipidized/xanthomatous changes seen in Hand-Schüller-Christian variant

IMMUNOHISTOCHEMISTRY

- Positive for Langerhans cell markers: S100, CD1a, Langerin (CD207), fascin (not seen in normal epidermal Langerhans cells)
- Negative for Factor XIIIa and other macrophage/monocyte markers: CD68, CD163, HAM56

OTHER HIGH YIELD POINTS

- Oncogenic *BRAFV600E* mutation seen in up to 60% of LCH specimens
- Cytoplasmic Birbeck granules on electron microscopy (tennis-racket shape and a zipper-like appearance)

DIFFERENTIAL DIAGNOSIS

- Spongiotic dermatitis – Langerhans cell hyperplasia can be seen secondary to other processes including contact dermatitis, scabies
- Juvenile xanthogranuloma – well-formed Touton giant cells, lack reniform nuclei
- Mycosis fungoides – epidermotropism seen in both, but characterized by atypical lymphocytes, presence of T cell markers will differentiate

Path Presenter

JUVENILE XANTHOGRANULOMA

CLINICAL FEATURES

- Most common non-LCH
- Affects infants and young children
- Pink to red-brown dome-shaped papule or nodule, most common on head and neck, followed by upper trunk, extremities

HISTOLOGIC FEATURES

- Well-demarcated, dense infiltrate of histiocytes within the superficial to deep dermis
- Early lesions with polygonal or spindle-shaped and plump monomorphous histiocytes

Dense infiltrate of histiocytes

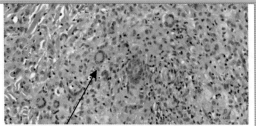

Numerous Touton giant cells and foam cells

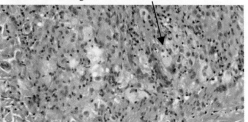

Path Presenter

- Mature lesions with Touton giant cells, foam cells, and scattered lymphocytes, eosinophils, and plasma cells
- *Spindle cell* and *scalloped cell* variants reported

IMMUNOHISTOCHEMISTRY
- Histiocytes positive for non-LCH markers: HAM56, CD68, Factor XIIIa

OTHER HIGH YIELD POINTS
- Extracutaneous lesions: eye most common, followed by lung
- Associations between JXG and café-au-lait macules; JXG and juvenile myelomonocytic leukemia; triple association between JXG, JMML, and neurofibromatosis 1 (NF1)

DIFFERENTIAL DIAGNOSIS
- Langerhans cell histiocytosis – histiocytes with reniform nuclei, epidermal infiltration
- ALK-positive Histiocytosis-Foamy or spindled histiocytes with abundant eosinophilic cytoplasm and irregularly folded nuclei, may show emperipolesis. Admixed Touton giant cells may be seen. Histiocytes show ALK positivity

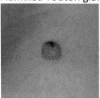 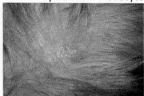

Yellowish papules and nodules typical of JXG

NECROBIOTIC XANTHOGRANULOMA

CLINICAL FEATURES
- Rare, progressive, multisystem histiocytic disease affecting adults
- Indurated plaque or nodule, violaceous to red with yellowish hue, central atrophy, ulceration and telangiectasia may be present
- Most commonly on periorbital region, followed by trunk, face, extremities

HISTOLOGIC FEATURES
- Palisading xanthogranulomatous infiltrate in the mid dermis to subcutaneous tissue
- Histiocytes, foam cells, lymphoid follicles, plasma cells, Touton giant cells and foreign body giant cells, large zones of necrobiosis with cholesterol clefts

IMMUNOHISTOCHEMISTRY
- Histiocytes positive for non-LCH markers: lysozyme, CD68, CD11b

OTHER HIGH YIELD POINTS
- Up to 70% cases associated with paraproteinemia - IgG monoclonal gammopathy

DIFFERENTIAL DIAGNOSIS
- Necrobiosis lipoidica – rarely have cholesterol clefts, less cellular, less foreign body giant cells and Touton-type giant cells

Path Presenter

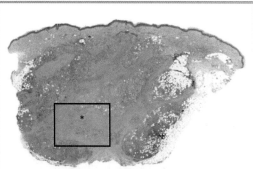

Zones of necrosis (*) in the dermis and subcutis surrounded by palisading infiltrate

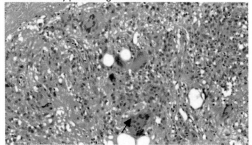

Infiltrate with histiocytes, giant cells, foam cells

Path Presenter

RETICULOHISTIOCYTOSIS

CLINICAL FEATURES
- Group of non-LCH histiocytosis
- Solitary reticulohistiocytoma, giant cell reticulohistiocytoma: single yellow-red nodule at any cutaneous site, no systemic associations
- Multicentric reticulohistiocytosis: severe arthropathy, cutaneous and mucous membrane papules and nodules on the face, distal extremities, "coral bead" appearance when small papules arranged along nailfolds

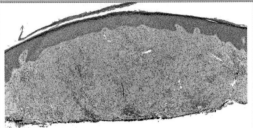

Dermal infiltrate of histiocytes

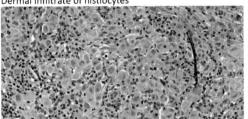

Histiocytes with "ground glass" cytoplasm, scattered lymphocytes, plasma cells, eosinophils

HISTOLOGIC FEATURES

- Well-circumscribed dermal infiltrate of mononuclear and multinucleate histiocytes with eosinophilic, finely granular "ground glass" cytoplasm
- Lymphocytes, occasional plasma cells and eosinophils

SPECIAL STAINS / IMMUNOHISTOCHEMISTRY

- PAS and Sudan black highlight material within multinucleate histiocytes
- Histiocytes positive for CD68, HAM56
- Negative for S100, CD34, CD1a

DIFFERENTIAL DIAGNOSIS

- Juvenile xanthogranuloma – lipidized cells and Touton giant cells
- Langerhans cell histiocytosis – reniform nuclei, S100

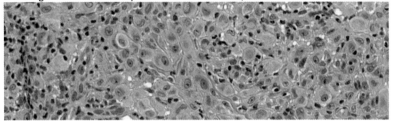

ROSAI-DORFMAN DISEASE

CLINICAL FEATURES

- Histiocytic proliferative disorder also known as sinus histiocytosis with massive lymphadenopathy
- Bilateral painless cervical lymphadenopathy with extranodal involvement, fever, anemia, neutrophilia, polyclonal hypergammaglobulinemia
- Cutaneous lesions in 10% of RDD in systemic form, usually multiple red-brown or xanthomatous macules, papules, nodules, or plaques
- Skin-limited form can present as single nodule or plaque, panniculitis

HISTOLOGIC FEATURES

- Dense dermal and/or subcutaneous infiltrate of histiocytes with large, vesicular nuclei, abundant foamy eosinophilic cytoplasm
- Emperipolesis – inflammatory cells (usually lymphocytes) within cytoplasm of histiocytes
- Scattered multinucleate cells, Touton cells, plasma cells (usually perivascular, can contain Russell bodies), lymphocytes (can form lymphoid aggregates)

IMMUNOHISTOCHEMISTRY

- Histiocytes are positive for S100, CD68, fascin, lysozyme
- Negative for CD1a, Langerin

DIFFERENTIAL DIAGNOSIS

- Juvenile xanthogranuloma – Touton giant cells, lack other inflammatory components and emperipolesis in most cases
- Langerhans cell histiocytosis – reniform nuclei, will express CD1a and Langerin
- Erdheim-Chester Disease- Foamy histiocytes with single small nuclei, admixed Touton giant cells, neutrophils, plasma cells, lymphocytes, BRAF positive

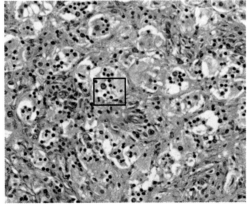

Dense infiltrate of histiocytes and lymphocytes in the dermis and subcutis

Emperipolesis (lymphocytes within histiocyte cytoplasm)

Path Presenter

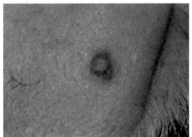

Solitary reddish brown nodule on the face

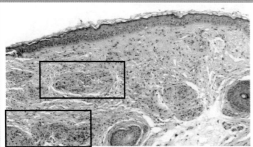
Aggregates of foam cells in the upper dermis

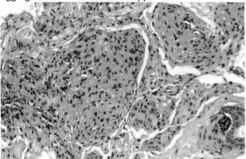
Foam cells with few inflammatory cells

XANTHELASMA

CLINICAL FEATURES
- Yellow to orange flat-topped papules on the face, particularly in periocular distribution

HISTOLOGIC FEATURES
- Aggregates of foam cells in upper dermis with minimal associated fibrosis or inflammatory cells

DIFFERENTIAL DIAGNOSIS
- Granuloma annulare – overlapping features with early lesions of xanthelasma without prominent foam cell change
- Dermatofibroma, xanthomatous variant – lipidized xanthomatous cells between hyalinized collagen bundles, peripheral collagen trapping, epidermal changes typical of dermatofibroma

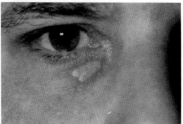
Flat yellowish plaque in periorbital region

Path Presenter

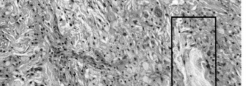
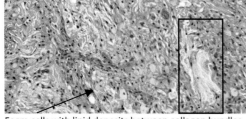
Foam cells with lipid deposits between collagen bundles in tuberous xanthoma

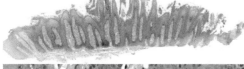

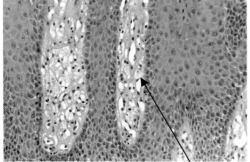
Verruciform acanthotic epidermis with foam cells within dermal papillae

Path Presenter

XANTHOMA (ERUPTIVE, TUBEROUS, VERRUCIFORM)

CLINICAL FEATURES
- Group of entities with **foam cells** (lipid-rich macrophages)
- Yellow or yellow-brown papules, nodules, or plaques
- Often associated with disorders of lipoprotein metabolism
- **Eruptive xanthoma**: multiple small red-yellow papules in crops, located on buttocks, thighs, extensor extremities
- **Tuberous xanthoma**: yellowish nodules on the elbows, knees, buttocks, most characteristic of familial hyperlipoproteinemia (type III)
- **Verruciform xanthoma**: warty papules or plaques most often on oral cavity, also genital and extragenital skin

HISTOLOGIC FEATURES
- Infiltrate of foam cells in the dermis with extravascular lipid deposits dissecting between collagen bundles
- Neutrophils and lymphocytes accompany histiocytic infiltrate in early lesions
- Tuberous xanthoma with larger nodular sheet of foam cells within the dermis
- Verruciform xanthoma with hyperkeratosis, parakeratosis, verrucous acanthosis, papillary dermis filled with large xanthoma cells

IMMUNOFLUORESCENCE/IMMUNOHISTOCHEMISTRY
- Foam cells positive for CD68, negative for S100

DIFFERENTIAL DIAGNOSIS
- Granuloma annulare – [see xanthelasma]
- Dermatofibroma, xanthomatous variant – [see xanthelasma]

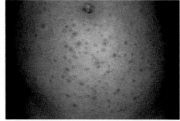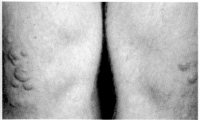
Eruptive xanthomas and tuberous xanthomas with red-yellowish hue

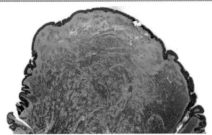

Dense infiltrate of mast cells within dermis in mastocytoma

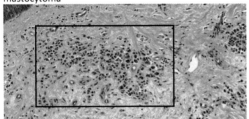

Aggregates of mast cells

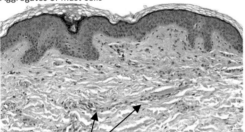

Subtle increased mast cells around superficial blood vessels in TMEP

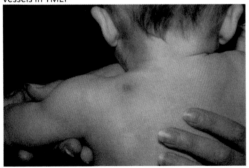

Hyperpigmented tan-brown papule with positive Darier sign after rubbing

MASTOCYTOSIS (URTICARIA PIGMENTOSA, MASTOCYTOMA, TMEP)

CLINICAL FEATURES

- Spectrum of related diseases with increased mast cells
- **Urticaria pigmentosa**: most common clinical variant (80%), generalized eruption of red-brown macules and papules on the trunk, extremities, and head, onset within 4 years of life
- **Mastocytoma**: solitary or few red-brown lesions, favor trunk and wrists, rarely associated with pruritus, flushing, headaches, gastrointestinal symptoms
- **Telangiectasia macularis eruptiva perstans (TMEP)**: mostly adult form of cutaneous mastocytosis, erythema and telangiectasia seen on subtle, hyperpigmented macules on trunk and extremities

HISTOLOGIC FEATURES

- Similar features across all clinical types of mastocytosis
- Urticaria pigmentosa features infiltrate of perivascular mast cells in the upper dermis with scattered eosinophils, dermal edema, basal hyperpigmentation
- Mastocytoma features dense sheets of mast cells filling the dermis
- TMEP shows subtle increase in mast cells, less cuboidal and more fusiform and loosely arranged around dilated vessels
- Variable features include papillary edema, basal hyperpigmentation, usually no eosinophils

SPECIAL STAINS / IMMUNOHISTOCHEMISTRY

- Special stains to highlight mast cells: toluidine blue, astra blue, Giemsa, chloroacetate esterase
- IHC: CD117 (KIT), tryptase

OTHER HIGH YIELD POINTS

- Mutation in *KIT* proto-oncogene
- **Darier sign**: firm stroking or rubbing of lesion leads to urticaria-like wheal

DIFFERENTIAL DIAGNOSIS

- Langerhans cell histiocytosis – similar cytologic features but reniform nuclei and lacks cytoplasmic granules of mast cells
- Melanocytic nevi – arranged in nests, aggregated in nests or cords in the dermis
- Juvenile xanthogranuloma – in cases without lipidized cells or Touton giant cells, can appear similar but express CD68 and Factor XIIIa
- Inflammatory dermatoses – can be difficult to distinguish from a mastocytosis with sparse infiltrate as mast cells can be part of inflammation of other disorders including lichen planus, spongiotic dermatitis, erythema multiforme

Path Presenter

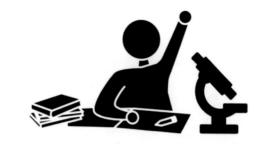

SECTION 2: NON - NEOPLASTIC
DERMATOPATHOLOGY

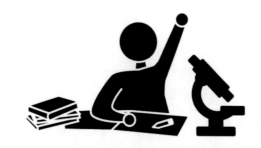

ACE MY PATH
Come Ace With Us!

CHAPTER 14: SPONGIOTIC
REACTION PATTERN
GEORGE TINOTENDA MUKOSERA, PhD

CHAPTER 14: SPONGIOTIC REACTION PATTERN

SPONGIOTIC DERMATITIS

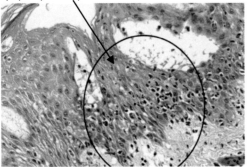
Intraepidermal vesicle / Spongiosis

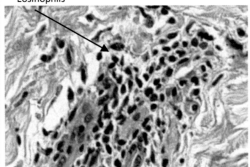
Lymphocytic exocytosis

Eosinophils

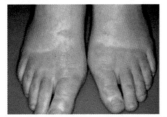

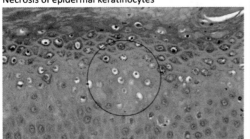
Path Presenter

ALLERGIC CONTACT DERMATITIS
CLINICAL FEATURES

- Allergic Contact Dermatitis (ACD) is a delayed **type IV hypersensitivity** reaction seen in individuals who have been previously sensitized
- This well delineated eruption **develops in 1-2 days** at the site of the allergen exposure as erythematous papules, vesicles, and weeping patches/plaques
- Vesicles may develop in the acute reaction, while chronic lesions are characterized by lichenified plaques
- ACD can occur in all ages, affecting both genders equally
- Top ten allergens as identified by the North American Contact Dermatitis group: **Nickel sulfate**, Neomycin Sulfate, Balsam of Peru, Fragrance mix, Thimerosal, Sodium gold thiosulfate, Formaldehyde, Quaternium-15, Cobalt chloride, Bacitracin

HISTOLOGIC FEATURES

- Histopathologic findings subdivided into acute, subacute, and chronic spongiotic stages
- **Acute** stage shows **spongiosis** with/without **vesiculation**
- **Focal parakeratosis with or without crust**
- Lymphocytic exocytosis common, Superficial perivascular lymphocytic infiltrate, often with eosinophils
- In the **subacute phase**, **spongiotic changes** are readily apparent but somewhat less pronounced
- A **moderate degree of acanthosis** is present, and there may be parakeratosis and a surface crust containing some neutrophils
- **Late** stages associated with **psoriasiform hyper**plasia and dermal fibroplasia **Spongiosis** is often **inconspicuous**

DIFFERENTIAL DIAGNOSIS
SEBORRHEIC DERMATITIS

- Psoriasiform and spongiotic dermatitis with overlying hyperkeratosis and parakeratosis
- Perifollicular parakeratosis (shoulder parakeratosis)
- Neutrophils in the stratum corneum with exocytosis and variable superficial mixed inflammatory infiltrate

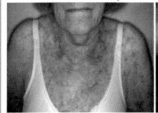
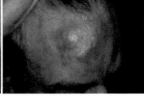

Necrosis of epidermal keratinocytes

IRRITANT CONTACT DERMATITIS
CLINICAL FEATURES

- This occurs at the site of contact with the irritant and varies from erythema to eczema to vesiculobullous lesions
- Lichenification +/- fissures and cracking in more chronic disease

HISTOLOGIC FEATURES

- Spongiotic epidermis with vesiculation, ballooning changes within keratinocytes often with focal necrosis
- Superficial perivascular infiltrate composed of lymphocytes and neutrophils

Superficial perivascular lymphocytic infiltrate

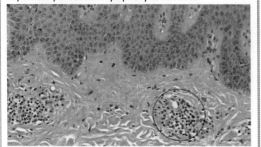

- Similar to allergic contact dermatitis but no/rare eosinophils

DIFFERENTIAL DIAGNOSIS

ALLERGIC CONTACT DERMATITIS

- Lymphocytic exocytosis common, Superficial perivascular lymphocytic infiltrate, often with eosinophils

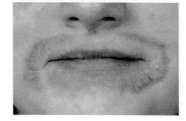

Path Presenter

Dense, wedge-shaped superficial and deep perivascular and interstitial inflammation

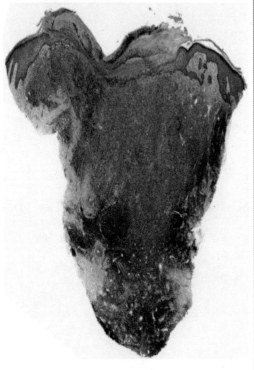

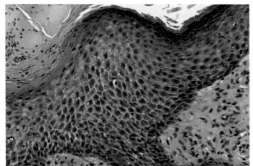

Path Presenter

ARTHROPOD BITE REACTION

CLINICAL FEATURES

- Clinical features of arthropod bite reactions are variable, ranging from small erythematous papules to vesicles to indurated nodules
- Erosion or ulceration may be seen
- A solitary punctum may be found at the site where insect mouth parts contact the skin
- Causative organisms include mosquitoes, fleas, ticks, bed bugs and spiders
- Some organisms are known for biting in a pattern. For example, bed bugs commonly bite in a linear configuration which has created the adage "breakfast, lunch and dinner" representing three arthropod bite "blood meals" linearly arranged
- Clinical presentation can mimic skin cancer (e.g., lymphoma or ulcerated carcinoma)

HISTOLOGIC FEATURES

- Histological findings in arthropod bite reaction are highly variable
- Classically, a dense, **wedge-shaped superficial and deep perivascular and interstitial inflammatory infiltrate** is present
- **Eosinophils are a prominent finding**, and are a useful clue when seen away from the vessels (interspersed between collagen bundles) and in the deeper dermis
- The **epidermis is variably spongiotic**; this is typically more prominent at the center where the arthropod mouth parts interrupt the skin
- **Mouth parts** may be present at the center of the lesion which aids in diagnosis Less often, secondary vasculitis and atypical lymphocytes can be identified
- Excoriated lesions may have prominent parakeratosis with scale crust formation, epidermal erosion or overt ulceration

DIFFERENTIAL DIAGNOSIS

PRODROMAL BULLOUS PEMPHIGOID

- The prodromal phase of bullous pemphigoid presents histologically with superficial and deep perivascular lymphocytic infiltrate admixed with eosinophils
- While the epidermis does not yet display the classic subepidermal split, spongiosis and eosinophilic exocytosis (eosinophilic spongiosis) may be identified
- **Eosinophils** are classically seen lining up along the dermo-epidermal junction

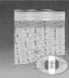

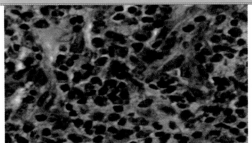

Eosinophils

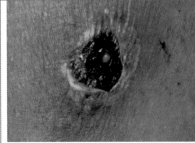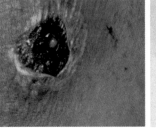

| Spider Bite | Tick Bite |

Superficial perivascular inflammation with eosinophils near the DEJ

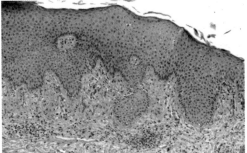

Eosinophilic spongiosis with exocytosis

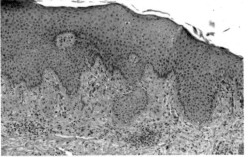

BULLOUS PRECURSORS (PEMPHIGUS AND PEMPHIGOID)

CLINICAL FEATURES

- Bullous pemphigoid (BP) can present with pruritus and erythematous patches or wheals prior to forming overt tense blisters
- Pemphigus vulgaris (PV) often involves mucosal sites +/- cutaneous blisters

HISTOLOGIC FEATURES

- Similar for both prodromal BP and PV
- Superficial and deep perivascular lymphocytic infiltrate with admixed eosinophils
- Eosinophilic **spongiosis** (epidermal) may be present
- **Eosinophils lining up along the dermal epidermal junction** (DEJ)

IMMUNOFLUORESCENCE/IMMUNOHISTOCHEMISTRY

- Perilesional skin in BP: **linear staining** along the DEJ with **IgG**
- Perilesional skin in PV: **intercellular IgG and C3, "chicken-wire pattern"**

DIFFERENTIAL DIAGNOSIS

- Arthropod reaction – usually without the lining of eosinophils along the DEJ, negative DIF
- Drug eruption – usually without the lining of eosinophils along the DEJ, negative DIF

Path Presenter   Path Presenter

Early prodromal plaque of BP

Hyperkeratosis and parakeratosis overlying spongiosis

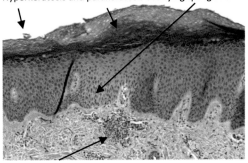

Perivascular inflammatory infiltrate with eosinophils

Path Presenter

SPONGIOTIC DRUG ERUPTION

CLINICAL FEATURES

- Similar to eczema, presents as generalized papules and eczematous plaques
- Most common implicated drugs include **ACE inhibitors, calcium channel blockers, thiazides,** and **atenolol**

HISTOLOGIC FEATURES

- **Spongiosis** with overlying **hyperkeratosis** and **parakeratosis**
- Perivascular inflammation in dermis, often extending deep with admixed **eosinophils**

DIFFERENTIAL DIAGNOSIS

- Allergic contact dermatitis - clinical drug history will help differentiate
- Atopic dermatitis - clinical drug history will help differentiate

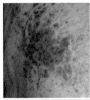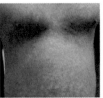

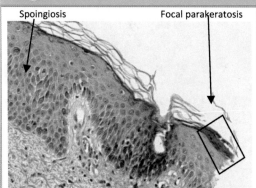

Spoingiosis   Focal parakeratosis

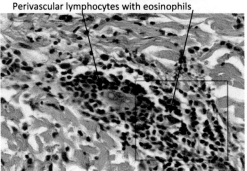

Perivascular lymphocytes with eosinophils

Path Presenter

PRURITIC URTICARIAL PAPULES AND PLAQUES OF PREGNANCY

CLINICAL FEATURES

- Clinical features highly suggest the diagnosis
- **Primigravida**, especially those having **twins**, can develop this pruritic eruption beginning in the **late third trimester** and **resolving with delivery**
- The erythematous papules begin in the **abdominal striae** and spread over the abdomen, buttocks, and thighs

HISTOLOGIC FEATURES

- Focal parakeratosis and spongiosis
- Perivascular lymphocytes with **interstitial eosinophils**
- **DIF-negative**

DIFFERENTIAL DIAGNOSIS

HERPES GESTATIONIS

- On H&E, lesional skin of herpes gestationis reveals a **subepidermal bullae with eosinophils**
- The epidermis may display spongiosis and eosinophilic spongiosis
- In the dermis, there is a superficial and mid perivascular lymphocytic infiltrate with eosinophils and papillary dermal edema
- Skin biopsy for H&E evaluation and demonstration of negative direct immunofluorescence helps to confirm the diagnosis and to rule out other dermatoses of pregnancy, such as herpes gestationis

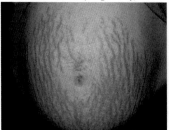 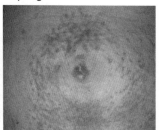

Erythematous papules on abdominal striae

Eosinophilic spongiosis progressing to vesiculation

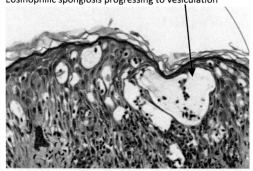

Dyskeratotic keratinocytes

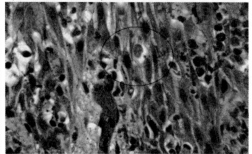

INCONTINENTIA PIGMENTI

CLINICAL FEATURES

- Also known as Bloch-Sulzberger syndrome
- Genetically transmitted: **X-linked dominant**
- Associated with **NEMO mutation**
- Affected females can have involvement of the hair, teeth, nails, eyes, skeleton, and central nervous system
- Lesions classically appear in **four stages: vesicular, verrucous, hyperpigmented and hypopigmentation**
- At birth, there is **linear** erythema and **vesicles** on the trunk and/or extremity
- With time this can evolve to a verrucous hyperkeratotic stage Hyper and hypopigmented stages also occur

HISTOLOGIC FEATURES

- **Vesiculobullous** stage: **Eosinophilic spongiosis** progressing to **vesiculation**
- Scattered **dyskeratotic keratinocytes**

DIFFERENTIAL DIAGNOSIS

ERYTHEMA TOXICUM NEONATORUM

- Spongiosis and subcorneal vesiculation, usually follicular based
- Numerous eosinophils in subcorneum, within spongiotic epidermis
- Rarely neutrophils can also be identified but are far outnumbered by eosinophils

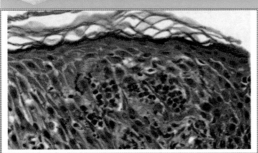

Subcorneal neutrophilic abscess   Hypogranulosis

Subcorneal neutrophils

Path Presenter

Subcorneal neutrophilic pustules

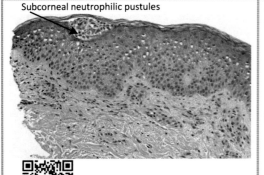

Path Presenter

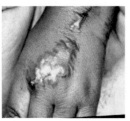

Erythematous linear patch   Hypopigmented linear patch

PUSTULAR PSORIASIS

CLINICAL FEATURES

- This can be a localized event within prior plaques of psoriasis or can be seen in acral psoriasis. Generalized pustular psoriasis can present suddenly with fever and generalized erythema in patients who are withdrawn from systemic corticosteroids
- Other triggers: pregnancy, hypocalcemia, infection, topical irritants

HISTOLOGIC FEATURES

Psoriasiform hyperplasia with neutrophilic abscesses, both in subcorneal and

- intraepidermal locations and associated spongiosis restricted to pustules
- Hypogranulosis under parakeratotic foci common
- Superficial perivascular infiltrate of lymphocytes and neutrophils
- Eosinophils may be sometimes seen

DIFFERENTIAL DIAGNOSIS

ACUTE GENERALIZED EXANTHEMATOUS PUSTULOSIS (AGEP)

- Can look histologically similar. Typically AGEP with more eosinophils but not always. Clinical history of drug exposure more indicative of DRESS

SUBCORNEAL PUSTULAR DERMATOSIS

- Can look histologically similar. Clinical correlation needed

IGA PEMPHIGUS

- IgA pemphigus shows a + DIF

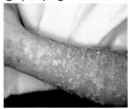
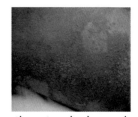

Numerous pustules studded on erythematous background

ACUTE GENERALIZED EXANTHEMATOUS PUSTULOSIS

CLINICAL FEATURES

- The majority of cases occur suddenly with fever a **few days after a new drug** is started (especially **beta-lactam antibiotics**)
- Starts as a diffuse macular erythema that rapidly develops **small non-follicular based pustules**
- Blood neutrophilia is usually seen

HISTOLOGIC FEATURES

- Parafollicular subcorneal or superficial intraepidermal neutrophilic and eosinophilic pustules with admixed few acantholytic keratinocytes
- Background of spongiosis with neutrophilic exocytosis and scattered dyskeratotic cells
- Papillary dermal edema

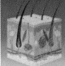
Spongiosis with neutrophilic exocytosis

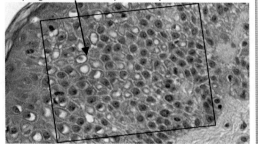

Perivascular mixed infiltrate with eosinophils

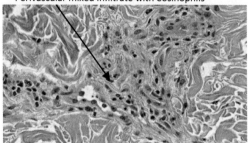

- Perivascular mixed inflammatory infiltrate of lymphocytes, neutrophils, and eosinophils
- Vasculitis may be seen in dermis

DIFFERENTIAL DIAGNOSIS

SUBCORNEAL PUSTULAR DERMATOSIS

- Can look histologically similar. Drug exposure not present and fewer eosinophils

IGA PEMPHIGUS

- IgA pemphigus shows a + DIF

DERMATOPHYTOSIS

- Hyphae may be apparent on H&E and are usually highlighted with PAS or GMS staining
- Varying degrees of spongiosis may be seen
- +/- Neutrophils, sometimes admixed in the parakeratotic horn

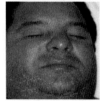 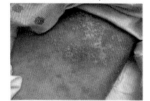

Numerous pustules studded on erythematous background

Intraepidermal spongiotic vesiculation

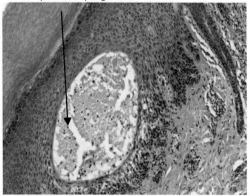

Parakeratosis

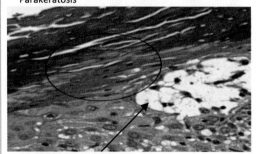

Intraepidermal vesicle

Path Presenter

DYSHIDROTIC ECZEMA

CLINICAL FEATURES

- A recurrent deep seated **vesicular**, pruritic eruption involving the **palms, soles**, and **sides of the fingers**

HISTOLOGIC FEATURES

- Parakeratosis and serum in the stratum corneum may be seen
- **Intraepidermal spongiotic vesiculation** with surrounding spongiosis
- Variable superficial perivascular infiltrate with/without eosinophils

DIFFERENTIAL DIAGNOSIS

ALLERGIC CONTACT DERMATITIS

- Clinical history helpful

DERMATOPHYTOSIS

- Hyphae present in stratum corneum with PAS or GMS

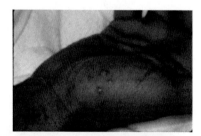

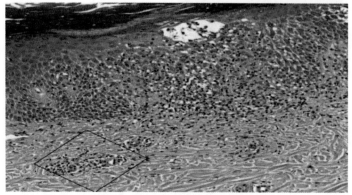

Superficial perivascular lymphocytic infiltrate

Hyperkeratosis   Psoriasiform hyperplasia

Superficial perivascular inflammation

Path Presenter

Parakeratosis   Spongiosis

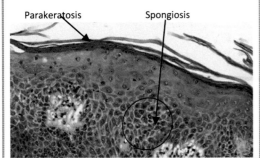

NUMMULAR ECZEMA

CLINICAL FEATURES

- Classically presents as pruritic **coin-shaped erythematous plaques** with scale on the lower legs, dorsal hands and extensor arms

HISTOLOGIC FEATURES

- Hyperkeratosis and parakeratosis with focal scale crust
- **Spongiotic** and psoriasiform hyperplasia
- Superficial perivascular mixed inflammatory infiltrate

DIFFERENTIAL DIAGNOSIS

ALLERGIC CONTACT DERMATITIS

- Can have overlapping histology Langerhans cell micro-abscesses and eosinophils more indicative of allergic contact dermatitis

DERMATOPHYTOSIS

- Hyphae present in the stratum corneum with PAS or GMS staining

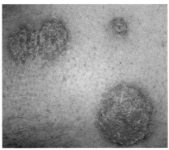
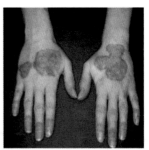

Pruritic coin-shaped erythematous patches

Shoulder parakeratosis

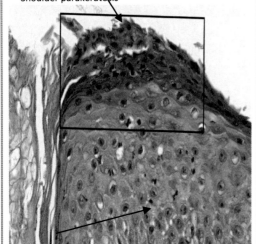

Spongiosis

Path Presenter

SEBORRHEIC DERMATITIS

CLINICAL FEATURES

- Greasy scale on an erythematous background Involves most commonly the scalp, ears, eyebrows, nasolabial folds, and chest

HISTOLOGIC FEATURES

- **Psoriasiform and spongiotic dermatitis** with overlying hyperkeratosis and parakeratosis
- Perifollicular parakeratosis (**shoulder parakeratosis**)
- Neutrophilic exocytosis and variable superficial inflammation

DIFFERENTIAL DIAGNOSIS

PSORIASIS

- Regular acanthosis, hypogranulosis, dilated dermal papillary blood vessels
- Neutrophils are also seen in the stratum corneum in the absence of significant serum crusting

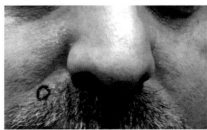
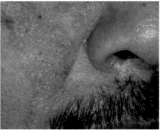

Greasy scale on an erythematous background

Lobular collection of blood vessels in the papillary dermis

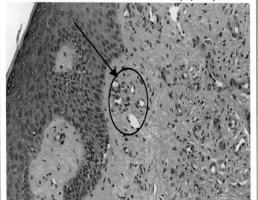

Dermal hemosiderin deposition

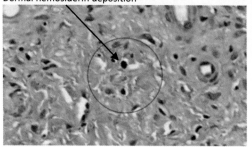

STASIS DERMATITIS
CLINICAL FEATURES
- Affects middle-aged and elderly patients, rarely occurring before the fifth decade of life
- This is most common on the **medial lower legs** presenting as pruritic, erythematous to tan scaly patches in patients with history of swollen legs
- More advanced cases encircle the lower leg and extend below the knee

HISTOLOGIC FEATURES
- **Lobular proliferation of thick-walled vessels** in superficial dermis with red cell extravasation, perivascular lymphocytic infiltrate and surrounding dermal fibrosis
- Overlying epidermis may show acute to chronic **spongiotic changes** with associated vacuolar changes at DEJ
- **Chronic lesions** show **epidermal acanthosis with hyperkeratosis** along with deep dermal aggregates of siderophages due to uptake of **hemosiderin** from degraded erythrocytes
- Dermal capillaries are frequently dilated with intimal thickening of small arterioles and venules along with dermal fibrosis

DIFFERENTIAL DIAGNOSIS
PIGMENTED PURPURIC DERMATOSIS
- Superficial perivascular lymphohistiocytic inflammation with extravasated red blood cells and siderophages. Typically more inflammatory than stasis dermatitis

Path Presenter

Spongiosis   Focal parakeratotic mounds

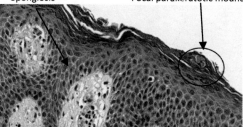

Superficial perivascular lymphocytic infiltrate

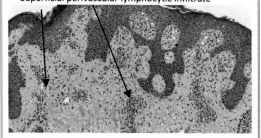

Path Presenter

PITYRIASIS ROSEA (PR)
CLINICAL FEATURES
- Most common on the trunk and upper extremities of teens and young adults starting with a single large, oval salmon pink, finely scaly patch (**herald patch**) that is joined by similar smaller lesions with the long axis along the lines of cleavage forming a **"Christmas tree" pattern**

HISTOLOGIC FEATURES
- **Mild spongiosis** and **focal parakeratotic mounds**
- Superficial perivascular lymphocytic infiltrate with **extravasated red blood cells**, sometimes admixed eosinophils

DIFFERENTIAL DIAGNOSIS
- Allergic contact dermatitis, **guttate psoriasis**, dermatophytosis

DERMATOPHYTOSIS
- Hyphae present in the stratum corneum with PAS or GMS staining

GUTTATE PSORIASIS
- Parakeratotic mounds and mild spongiosis often present. The presence of neutrophils in the stratum corneum and absence of red blood cell extravasation differentiates from pityriasis rosea

SEBORRHEIC DERMATITIS
- Parakeratotic mounds and mild spongiosis often present. The presence of neutrophils in the stratum corneum, shoulder parakeratosis, and the absence of red blood cell extravasation differentiates from pityriasis rosea

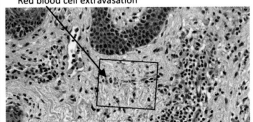

Red blood cell extravasation

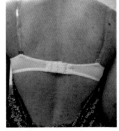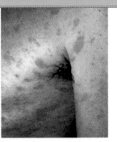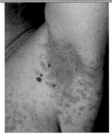

"Christmas tree" pattern of round to oval slightly scaly erythematous plaques

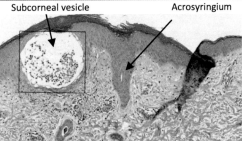

Subcorneal vesicle   Acrosyringium

Numerous 1-2mm vesicles on the trunk

MILIARIA CRYSTALLINA

CLINICAL FEATURES

- Numerous 1-2 mm clear vesicles without erythema
- This presents in neonates on the head, neck and upper trunk
- Also occurs in febrile adults and in tropical climates on the trunk

HISTOLOGIC FEATURES

- **Subcorneal vesicle** with few neutrophils in **association with the acrosyringium**

DIFFERENTIAL DIAGNOSIS

SUBCORNEAL PUSTULAR DERMATOSIS

- Subcorneal neutrophilic abscesses **+/-** acantholytic keratinocytes

DYSHIDROTIC ECZEMA

- Histologic overlap with intraepidermal vesicles but dyshidrotic eczema on classically acral sites

Path Presenter

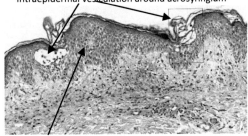

Intraepidermal vesiculation around acrosyringium

Spongiosis

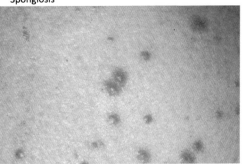

1-2mm erythematous papulo-vesicles

MILIARIA RUBRA

CLINICAL FEATURES

- Commonly referred to as "prickly heat," this presents as **papules and vesicles on an erythematous background**, involving the trunk and intertriginous areas of infants or adults, especially in hot, humid climates

HISTOLOGIC FEATURES

- **Spongiosis and intraepidermal vesiculation around acrosyringium** with accompanying lymphohistiocytic inflammation

DIFFERENTIAL DIAGNOSIS

INFUNDIBULOFOLLICULITIS

- Follicular spongiosis (hallmark of disseminated infundibulofolliculitis)
- It occurs in the setting of variable follicular plugging and overlying parakeratosis
- +/- perifollicular lymphocytic infiltrate

FOX-FORDYCE DISEASE

- Spongiosis and vesiculation of the follicular infundibulum where the apocrine gland joins the follicle
- In later stages, para-follicular xanthoma is seen
- Follicular plugging with variable parakeratosis and acanthosis
- Variable chronic inflammatory infiltrate within the surrounding dermis

Path Presenter

Vesiculation

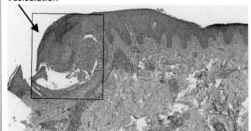

Lymphohistiocytic inflammation

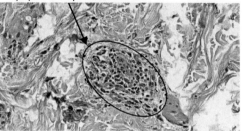

Path Presenter

MILIARIA PROFUNDUS

CLINICAL FEATURES

- Due to the deep obstruction of the sweat duct, small papules are seen, mostly on the trunk in tropical climates

HISTOLOGIC FEATURES

- **Spongiosis around acrosyringium** with accompanying **subepidermal edema and vesiculation**
- Associated with lymphohistiocytic inflammation

DIFFERENTIAL DIAGNOSIS

FOX-FORDYCE DISEASE

- Spongiosis and vesiculation of the follicular infundibulum where the apocrine gland joins the follicle
- In later stages, para-follicular xanthoma is seen
- Follicular plugging with variable parakeratosis and acanthosis
- Variable chronic inflammatory infiltrate within the surrounding dermis

INFUNDIBULOFOLLICULITIS

- Follicular spongiosis (hallmark of disseminated infundibulofolliculitis)
- It occurs in the setting of variable follicular plugging and overlying parakeratosis
- +/- perifollicular lymphocytic infiltrate

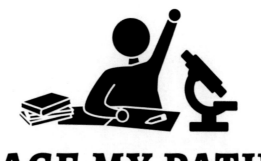

ACE MY PATH

Come Ace With Us!

CHAPTER 15: PSORIASIFORM
REACTION PATTERN

NATHAN BOWERS, MD, PhD
JESUS ALBERTO CARDENAS-DE LA GARZA, MD

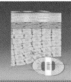
PSORIASIFORM REACTION PATTERN

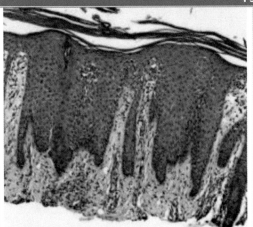

Regular acanthosis with thinning of and suprapapillary plate

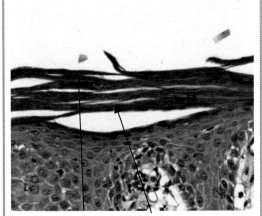

Alternating neutrophils with parakeratosis "shoulder sign"

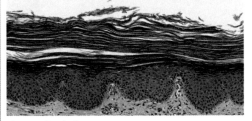

Guttate Psoriasis

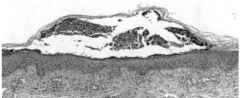

Pustular Psoriasis

PSORIASIS

CLINICAL FEATURES

- Sharply demarcated erythematous plaques and patches. Predilection for extensor surfaces of elbows, knees, scalp, trunk, nails, and buttocks
- Mean age at presentation is 25-35 years old
- Patients may develop seronegative arthritis
- Auspitz's sign: Pinpoint bleeding occurs when scale is removed

HISTOLOGIC FEATURES

- **Confluent parakeratosis** with admixed neutrophilic microabscesses in the stratum corneum
- **Neutrophilic microabscesses** may be seen in in epidermis
- **Loss of granular layer** below **parakeratosis**
- **Regular epidermal acanthosis with clubbed rete ridges, thinning of the suprapapillary plates** and **tortuous blood vessels** in the dermal papillae
- **Mild perivascular inflammation in superficial dermis**

VARIANTS

GUTTATE PSORIASIS:

- Acute onset of numerous drop-like psoriasiform papules. Often preceded by *S pyogenes* infection and commonly affects individuals less than 30 years of age. Histologically characterized by less prominent epidermal hyperplasia with mild spongiosis and focal areas of parakeratosis with neutrophils

PUSTULAR PSORIASIS:

- Presents with individual and/or confluent yellow/white pustules with underlying erythema/edema. May be generalized with fever and malaise, localized annular, or seen during pregnancy. Histologically characterized by regular epidermal hyperplasia with neutrophils in the stratum corneum, and subcorneal neutrophilic dermatosis

OTHER HIGH YIELD POINTS

- **HLA-Cw6** strongly associated with psoriasis and predicts earlier disease onset
- Differential diagnosis for collections of **neutrophils in the stratum corneum**: Psoriasis, tinea, impetigo, *Candida*, seborrheic dermatitis, and syphilis **(PTICSS)**

DIFFERENTIAL DIAGNOSIS

LICHEN SIMPLEX CHRONICUS

- Irregular acanthosis, hypergranulosis, and superficial dermal fibrosis with vertically oriented vessels in papillary dermis, no neutrophils in stratum corneum

PITYRIASIS RUBRA PILARIS

- Alternating parakeratosis and orthokeratosis in checkerboard pattern
- No loss of granular layer, follicular keratin plugs common

SUPERFICIAL FUNGAL INFECTION

- PAS highlighting fungal organisms

Path Presenter

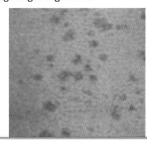

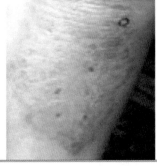

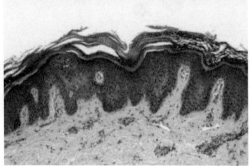

Acanthosis, hypergranulosis, and thickened suprapapillary plates

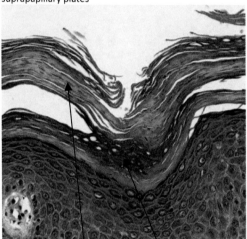

Alternating parakeratosis and orthokeratosis "checkerboard sign"

Follicular plugging

PITYRIASIS RUBRA PILARIS (PRP)

CLINICAL FEATURES

- Papulosquamous eruption of unknown etiology
- Presents as characteristic papules with follicular accentuation, perifollicular erythema, and **islands of sparing**
- May affect children or adults and be associated with infections (like HIV), drugs, and vaccines
- **Palms and soles** can present orange-yellowish hyperkeratosis (keratoderma)

HISTOLOGIC FEATURES

- Characteristically presents alternating **vertical and horizontal orthokeratosis and parakeratosis** similar to a **checkerboard**
- **Irregular epidermal acanthosis** is present with **hypergranulosis** and thickened suprapapillary plates
- **Follicular plugging** with parakeratosis adjacent to the hair follicles **(shoulder parakeratosis)**
- **Occasional focal acantholysis**
- Perivascular and perifollicular lymphocytic infiltrate

OTHER HIGH YIELD POINTS

- Five distinct subtypes:
  ➢ Type 1: most common form, rapid onset of classic PRP features, good prognosis (80% resolve within 3 yrs.)
  ➢ Type 2: slow onset, ichthyosiform leg lesions + keratoderma +/– alopecia; chronic course
  ➢ Type 3: same presentation/course as type 1; peaks in adolescence
  ➢ Type 4: most common form in **children**; only **localized** form of PRP; p/w follicular papules and erythema on **elbows and knees**; variable course
  ➢ Type 5: first few years of life, PRP +, sclerodermoid changes of hands/feet; chronic
- Psoriasis is the main pathological differential diagnosis
- High number of plasma cells must raise the possibility of syphilis

DIFFERENTIAL DIAGNOSIS

PSORIASIS

- Regular acanthosis, thinning of suprapapillary plates with tortuous blood vessels, alternating neutrophils with parakeratosis, and neutrophilic spongiform pustules

LICHEN SIMPLEX CHRONICUS

- Irregular acanthosis, hypergranulosis, and superficial dermal fibrosis with vertical oriented vessels in papillary dermis

PSORIASIS

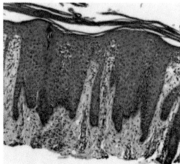

LICHEN SIMPLEX CHRONICUS

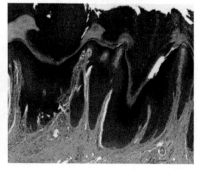

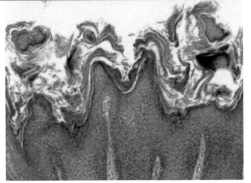

Papillomatosis

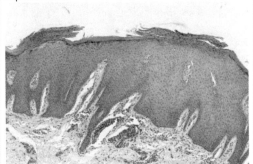

Psoriasiform hyperplasia

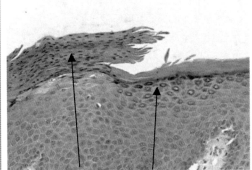

Alternating parakeratosis and orthokeratosis

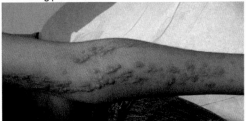

Inflammatory Linear Verrucous Epidermal Nevus

Path Presenter

INLFLAMMATORY LINEAR VERRUCOUS EPIDERMAL NEVUS (ILVEN)

CLINICAL FEATURES

- Epidermal nevus usually appears before age 5
- Rare cases of adult onset have been reported
- Presents as a linear psoriasiform plaque following **Blaschko's lines**
- Legs, thighs, and buttocks most frequently affected
- Associated intense pruritus

HISTOLOGIC FEATURES

- **Psoriasiform hyperplasia** and **papillomatosis**
- Characteristically, there are **columns of orthokeratosis** with underlying hypergranulosis **alternating** with **columns of parakeratosis** with underlying hypogranulosis
- Neutrophils may be present in the stratum corneum (Munro's microabscesses)
- Superficial mixed dermal infiltrate

OTHER HIGH YIELD POINTS

- Clinical history is important to differentiate from similar conditions
- Psoriasis lacks alternating hypergranulosis with orthokeratosis and hypogranulosis with parakeratosis

DIFFERENTIAL DIAGNOSIS

LINEAR PSORIASIS

- Regular acanthosis, thinning of suprapapillary plates with tortuous blood vessels, alternating neutrophils with parakeratosis, and neutrophilic spongiform pustules

BLASCHKITIS/LICHEN STRIATUS

- Spongiosis with lichenoid inflammatory infiltrate Lymphocytes surrounding sweat glands Clinically not pruritic

EPIDERMAL NEVUS

- Papillomatosis with orthokeratosis, lacks alternating orthokeratosis and parakeratosis. Resembles seborrheic keratosis histologically

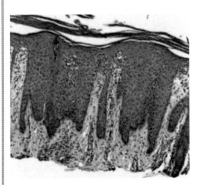

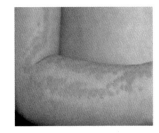

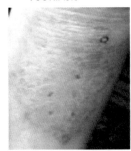

PSORIASIS

BLASCHKITIS/LICHEN STRIATUS

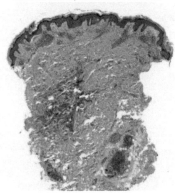

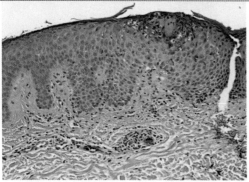

Psoriasifrom hyperplasia with absent thinning of suprapapillary plates and tortuous papillary vessels

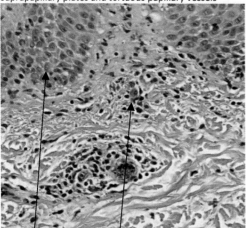

Spongiosis and dermal eosinophil

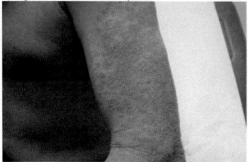

Psoriasifrom papules and plaques on sun exposed skin

PSORIASIFORM DRUG ERUPTION

CLINICAL FEATURES

- Medication may induce or exacerbate psoriasis
- Presentation of drug-induced psoriasis is similar to plaque or guttate psoriasis
- Time to onset is variable (usually 1-3 months)
- Frequent drugs include **beta-blockers**, **anti-TNF alpha**, lithium, hydroxychloroquine, and immune checkpoint inhibitors

HISTOLOGIC FEATURES

- Histology may be identical to psoriasis
- Suprapapillary thinning and tortuous papillary vessels may be absent
- Munro's microabscesses are rare
- There can be variable hypogranulosis or spongiosis
- **Eosinophils** may be present in the **superficial dermis**

OTHER HIGH YIELD POINTS

- Medication history is important to differentiate from psoriasis
- Eosinophils are a useful clue that favors drug eruption
- Acute generalized exanthematous pustulosis (AGEP) has similar histology to pustular psoriasis and many consider both diseases as a spectrum. AGEP has eosinophils in dermis and is usually associated with NSAID use

DIFFERENTIAL DIAGNOSIS

PSORIASIS

- Can look identical histologically Regular acanthosis, thinning of suprapapillary plates with tortuous blood vessels, alternating neutrophils with parakeratosis, and neutrophilic spongiform pustules

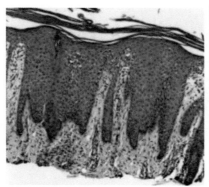

Path Presenter

PSORIASIS

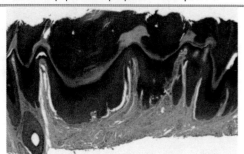

Orthokeratosis, hypergranulosis and irregular acanthosis

PRURIGO NODULARIS/LICHEN SIMPLEX CHRONICUS

CLINICAL FEATURES

- Prurigo nodularis and lichen simplex chronicus present identical histological features, but the clinical presentation is distinct
- Prurigo nodularis presents as very pruritic firm nodules usually on the trunk or extremities
- Lichen simplex chronicus presents as thick, scaly plaques usually on the shins, scalp, neck or genital area
- Both are secondary to chronic scratching or rubbing
- Usually associated with conditions causing chronic pruritus like atopic or contact dermatitis

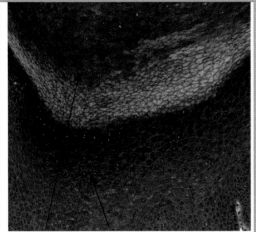

Othokeratosis and hypergranulosis

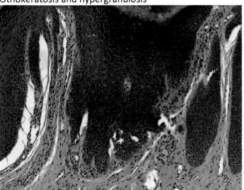

Vertical-oriented collagen bundles and blood vessels

Path Presenter

HISTOLOGIC FEATURES

- **Compact orthokeratosis** with **hypergranulosis** and focal areas of parakeratosis in the setting of **irregular acanthosis**
- Spongiosis and lymphohistiocytic perivascular infiltrate may be present
- Vertically oriented collagen bundles and blood vessels in the papillary dermis

OTHER HIGH YIELD POINTS

- Pseudoepitheliomatous hyperplasia in prurigo nodularis may be confused with squamous cell carcinoma
- Absence of neutrophils in the stratum corneum, hypergranulosis, and irregular acanthosis may help differentiate from psoriasis

DIFFERENTIAL DIAGNOSIS

PSORIASIS

- Regular acanthosis, thinning of suprapapillary plates with tortuous blood vessels, alternating neutrophils with parakeratosis, hypogranulosis, and neutrophilic spongiform pustules

SQUAMOUS CELL CARCINOMA (KERATOACANTHOMA TYPE)

- Exoendophytic crateriform and infiltrative growth pattern
- Well-differentiated, 'glassy' keratinocytes

HYPERTROPHIC LICHEN PLANUS

- Hyperplastic epidermis with wedge-shaped hypergranulosis and lichenoid inflammation

PERFORATING DERMATOSES

- Regular to irregular acanthosis with trans-epidermal elimination of amorphous debris

LICHEN SIMPLEX CHRONICUS

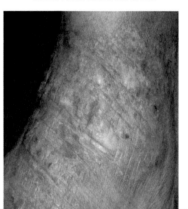

PRURIGO NODULARIS

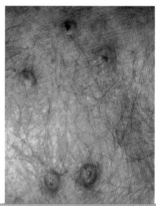

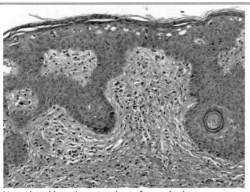

Vacuolated keratinocytes, loss of granular layer, dyskeratosis, and superficial dermal mixed infiltrate

NECROLYTIC MIGRATORY ERYTHEMA (GLUCAGONOMA SYNDROME)

CLINICAL FEATURES

- **Glucagonoma** (neuroendocrine tumor of the alpha cells of the pancreas) syndrome presents with weight loss, glucose intolerance/diabetes mellitus, and necrolytic migratory erythema (NME)
- NME presents as scaly erythematous patches and plaques with necrosis, central bullae, and erosions
- Most common topography includes intertriginous areas, perioral, and distant extremities
- May be associated with **multiple endocrine neoplasia type 1**
- Rarely, NME has been associated with other disorders including hepatitis C and Crohn's disease

HISTOLOGIC FEATURES

- **Superficial necrosis** of the **upper spinous layer** of the epidermis with **vacuolated keratinocytes**

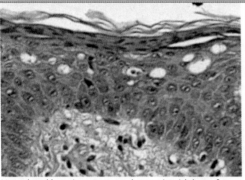

Vacuolated keratinocytes, parakeratosis with loss of granular layer, and dyskeratosis

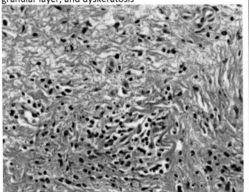

Superficial mixed dermal infiltrate with pallor
Path Presenter

- **Pallor** of the **mid and upper epidermis**
- Parakeratosis and **irregular acanthosis**
- **Loss of granular layer**
- Dyskeratosis
- Superficial dermal mixed infiltrate
- Dilated blood vessels in the dermal papillae

OTHER HIGH YIELD POINTS

- Histological features of NME also appear in **niacin and zinc deficiency**, and **necrolytic acral erythema**

DIFFERENTIAL DIAGNOSIS

PSORIASIS

- Regular acanthosis, thinning of suprapapillary plates with tortuous blood vessels, alternating neutrophils with parakeratosis, and neutrophilic spongiform pustules

NUTRITIONAL DEFICIENCY DERMATOSIS

- Can look identical histologically Psoriasiform hyperplasia with focal or confluent parakeratosis, loss of granular layer, and pallor of the epidermis

PSORIASIS   NUTRITIONAL DEFICIENCY DERMATOSIS

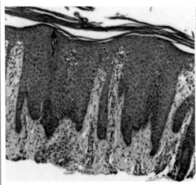 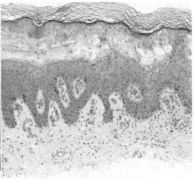

ACRODERMATITIS ENTEROPATHICA (ZINC DEFICIENCY-ASSOCIATED DERMATITIS)

CLINICAL FEATURES

- Secondary to **zinc deficiency** due to an **inherited autosomal recessive** zinc transporter deficiency **or acquired** usually associated with prolonged exclusive **breastfeeding, restrictive diets, or inflammatory bowel disease**
- Classic **triad** of **dermatitis, alopecia, and diarrhea**
- Dermatitis is **periorificial and acral initially** with vesiculobullous plaques that evolve to a desquamative and psoriasiform appearance

HISTOLOGIC FEATURES

- **Psoriasiform hyperplasia** with focal or confluent **parakeratosis**
- Loss of granular layer
- Pallor of the superficial epidermis
- Ballooning degeneration and dyskeratosis
- Mild superficial perivascular lymphocytic infiltrate

OTHER HIGH YIELD POINTS

- Acrodermatitis enteropathica shares the same histological features as pellagra and necrolytic migratory erythema associated with glucagonoma

DIFFERENTIAL DIAGNOSIS

PSORIASIS

- Regular acanthosis, thinning of suprapapillary plates with tortuous blood vessels

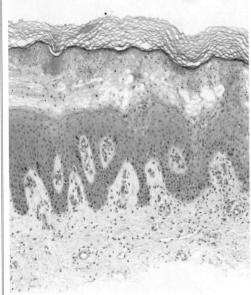

Psoriasiform hyperplasia with focal or confluent parakeratosis, loss of granular layer, and pallor of the epidermis

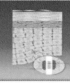

- Alternating neutrophils with parakeratosis, and neutrophilic spongiform pustules
- Typically no pallor in upper epidermis

NECROLYTIC MIGRATORY ERYTHEMA

- Can look identical histologically Need to distinguish clinically
- Vacuolated keratinocytes, loss of granular layer, dyskeratosis, and superficial dermal mixed infiltrate

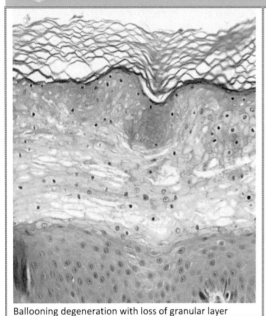

Ballooning degeneration with loss of granular layer

Path Presenter

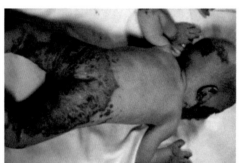

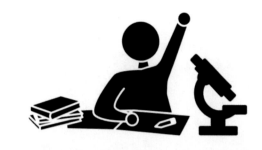

ACE MY PATH
Come Ace With Us!

CHAPTER 16: INTERFACE REACTION
PATTERN

AAYUSHMA REGMI, MBBS

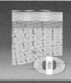

INTERFACE REACTION PATTERNS

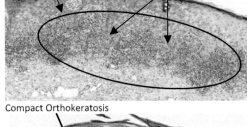

Lichenoid inflammation   Saw-toothed rete ridges

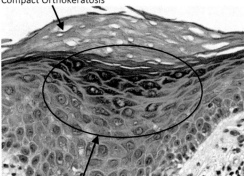

Compact Orthokeratosis

Wedge shaped hypergranulosis
Apoptotic bodies (Civatte bodies)

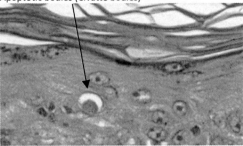

Basement membrane vacuolar changes

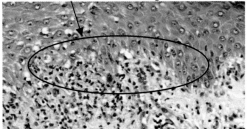

Subepidermal clefting

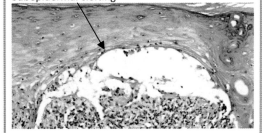

LICHEN PLANUS

CLINICAL FEATURES

- Clinically the **"6 Ps"**: **purple, pruritic, planar (flat), polygonal, papules, and plaques**
- Distribution: **Flexural wrists, forearms, dorsal hands**, **shins, ankle**, presacral area, mucous membranes (oral mucosa, genitalia, rarely esophagus), hair, nails
- **Wickham's striae** (fine white lines on the surface of lesions corresponding to areas of hypergranulosis) or **Koebner phenomenon** (new lesions at trauma sites, e.g., scratching) may be present in some cases
- Typically **resolves spontaneously**, though some patients experience a relapsing and remitting course
- Variant morphologies: Atrophic, hypertrophic, linear, annular, actinic, follicular, bullous, ulcerative, and pigmented (lichen planus pigmentosus)
- Nail matrix involvement leads to nail plate thinning, onychorrhexis, dorsal pterygium formation, and trachyonychia

HISTOLOGIC FEATURES

- **Compact hyperorthokeratosis** (no parakeratosis)
- **Irregular acanthosis** with **saw-tooth rete ridges**
- **Wedge-shaped hypergranulosis**
- **Lichenoid band-like lymphohistiocytic infiltrate** within the superficial dermis
- Apoptotic bodies (Civatte / cytoid bodies), more frequent near BM or lower layers of epidermis
- **Basement membrane vacuolar change** with basal cell squamatization (flattening of cells)
- Occasionally subepidermal clefting ("**Max Joseph space**"- artifactual cleft formation between the epidermis and the papillary dermis)
- Melanophages in dermis signifying pigment incontinence
- Plasma cells and eosinophils generally absent

IMMUNOFLUORESCENCE/IMMUNOHISTOCHEMISTRY

- Direct immunofluorescence – **Fibrillar band of fibrin** along dermo-epidermal junction Civatte bodies highlighted with IgM, IgA and C3

DIFFERENTIAL DIAGNOSIS

BENIGN LICHENOID KERATOSIS

- Clinically a solitary lesion
- Orthokeratosis, usually with parakeratosis, variable epidermal acanthosis, and Civatte bodies with extensive band-like lichenoid inflammation in DEJ

LICHENOID DRUG REACTION

- Lichenoid lymphocytic inflammation at the DEJ, often with admixed eosinophils

SECONDARY SYPHILIS

- Combined psoriasiform epidermal hyperplasia with hyperkeratosis and parakeratosis with long thin rete ridges
- Superficial and deep perivascular and periadnexal lymphocytic infiltrate with admixed plasma cells, sometimes in a lichenoid distribution

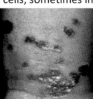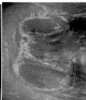

Path Presenter

Subepidermal bullae

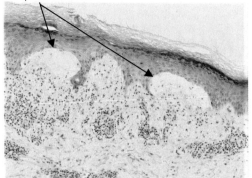

Interface changes with sawtooth rete ridges

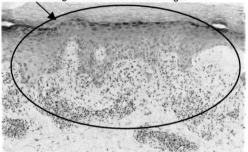

Robust interface reaction

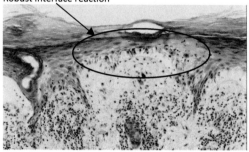

Path Presenter

BULLOUS LICHEN PLANUS

CLINICAL FEATURES

- **Similar to the typical lichen planus (LP) eruption** (pruritic, polygonal, planar, purple, papules, and plaques)
- Tense vesicles or bullae **arising within existing lichen planus lesion**
- No autoantibody mediated blistering

HISTOLOGIC FEATURES

- Similar features of LP with associated **subepidermal bullae arising within existing lichen planus lesions**
- **Robust interface dermatitis** that disrupts basement membrane zone integrity
- Plasma cells and eosinophils generally absent

OTHER HIGH YIELD POINTS

- It is important to **exclude lichen planus pemphigoides**, which can have similar morphology. In lichen planus pemphigoides, **the vesicles or bullae arise in previously uninvolved skin** (i.e., not within preexisting lichen planus lesions)
- Negative Immunofluorescence

DIFFERENTIAL DIAGNOSIS

LICHEN PLANUS PEMPHIGOIDES

- Subepidermal bullae arising in uninvolved skin (not within preexisting LP)
- Sparse to moderate superficial perivascular and interstitial lymphocytic infiltrate with eosinophils and neutrophils
- DIF: Linear IgG along basement membrane

PARANEOPLASTIC PEMPHIGUS

- An overt interface or lichenoid infiltrate associated with necrotic keratinocytes at all levels of the epidermis (epidermal suprabasal acantholysis)

TOXIC EPIDERMAL NECROLYSIS

- Subepidermal bulla with confluent full thickness necrosis of epidermis
- Sparse perivascular lymphocytic infiltrate with eosinophils

BULLOUS LUPUS ERYTHEMATOSUS

- Subepidermal bulla with interface changes and neutrophils along DEJ
- Perivascular and periadnexal infiltrate with increased mucin

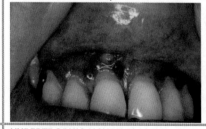 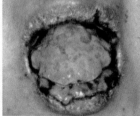

Hyperkeratosis with pronounced epidermal hyperplasia

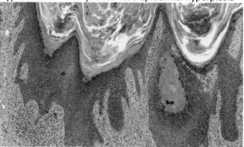

HYPERTROPHIC LICHEN PLANUS

CLINICAL FEATURES

- Also called **lichen planus verrucous or lichen planus hypertrophicus**
- Usually presents as **symmetric lesions, more common in African American patients**
- **Red, yellow-gray, violaceous, or hyperpigmented hypertrophic papules and plaques**
- Lesions are **more firm/thick** and often have a **verrucous of hyperkeratotic surface**
- Often **extremely pruritic** and **more chronic in nature** than classic lichen planus

Prominent epidermal hyperplasia

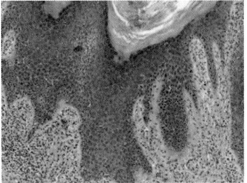

Horizontally-oriented collagen bundles

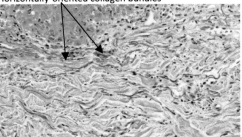

Band like lichenoid inflammation

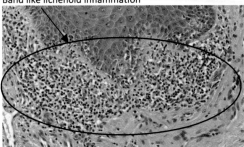

Interface changes

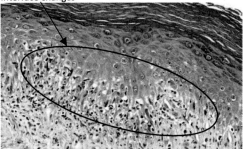

Epidermal atrophy with lichenoid inflammation

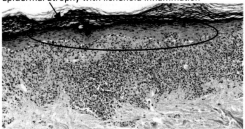

- Similar distribution pattern to classic lichen planus, but lesions more commonly found on the pretibial lower leg and/or ankles
- Often has superimposed features of lichen simplex chronicus from chronic scratching/rubbing

HISTOLOGIC FEATURES

- Similar features of LP with more **prominent epidermal hyperplasia with enlarged rete ridges**
- **Horizontally oriented, thickened collagen bundles** in the papillary dermis
- **Eosinophils** may be seen compared to other variants
- Variable subepidermal clefting ("Max Joseph space")
- Sometimes inflammation less dense than LP and often **concentrated at tips of rete ridges**

OTHER HIGH YIELD POINTS

- Squamous cell carcinoma (SCC) can occur in this variant

DIFFERENTIAL DIAGNOSIS

LICHEN SIMPLEX CHRONICUS

- Compact orthokeratosis with focal parakeratosis with overlying irregular acanthosis and curvilinear, blunt rete ridges
- Papillary dermal fibrosis, with vertically oriented collagen bundle
- Perivascular lymphocytic infiltrate

SQUAMOUS CELL CARCINOMA

- Single lesion
- Proliferation of atypical keratinocytes with prominent intercellular bridging
- Variable pleomorphism, nuclear atypia and mitotic figures with keratinization

HYPERTROPHIC LUPUS ERYTHEMATOSUS

- Hyperkeratosis, marked acanthosis and papillomatosis with lichenoid dermatitis
- Basement membrane thickening and follicular plugging
- Superficial and deep inflammatory cell infiltrate
- Increased dermal mucin deposition

PRURIGO NODULARIS

- Hyperorthokeratosis, psoriasiform epidermal hyperplasia, and pseudoepitheliomatous hyperplasia
- Focal parakeratosis
- Collagen bundles in papillary dermis run perpendicular to the surface
- Admixed vessels and chronic inflammation

LICHEN AMYLOIDOSIS

- Amyloid (eosinophilic globules) deposits in the papillary dermis, usually at the tips of the dermal papillae
- Hyperkeratosis and epidermal acanthosis
- Vacuolar alteration, colloid bodies and pigmentary incontinence maybe seen

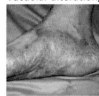 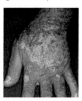

Path Presenter

Orthokeratosis Hypergranulosis

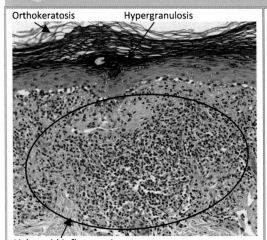

Lichenoid inflammation

Path Presenter

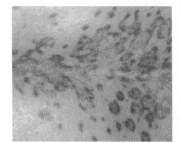

ATROPHIC LICHEN PLANUS
CLINICAL FEATURES

- **Well-demarcated, shiny, violaceous, flat, or atrophic macules and patches**
- Variably pruritic and lesions may koebnerize
- It may occur in areas previously affected by annular or ulcerative lichen planus
- Similar distribution to typical lichen planus. Common sites include the **lower extremities, trunk, axillae, penis**
- Typically **resolves spontaneously**, though some patients experience a relapsing and remitting course
- Patients may also have pseudopelade (form of cicatricial alopecia)

HISTOLOGIC FEATURES

- Features similar to typical lichen planus but with **more pronounced epidermal atrophy**
- Scattered Civatte bodies may be seen
- Some cases may have associated porokeratosis

DIFFERENTIAL DIAGNOSIS
LUPUS ERYTHEMATOSUS

- Hyperkeratosis, epidermal atrophy or hypertrophy, attenuation of rete ridges, basement membrane thickening, and follicular keratotic plugging
- Vacuolar interface changes with keratinocyte apoptosis in the basilar layer
- Dense superficial and deep lymphocytic infiltrate

LICHENOID DRUG REACTION

- Compact orthokeratosis with parakeratosis, wedge shaped hypergranulosis, and irregular acanthosis
- Lichenoid lymphocytic inflammation at the DEJ, often with admixed eosinophils

ERYTHEMA DYSCHROMICUM PERSTANS

- Hyperkeratosis with variable epidermal atrophy
- Focal lichenoid lymphocytic infiltrate with vacuolar degeneration of the basal layer and pigment incontinence

Hyperkeratosis

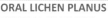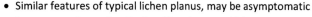

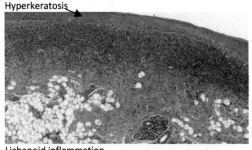

Lichenoid inflammation

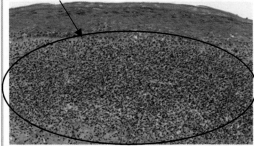

ORAL LICHEN PLANUS
CLINICAL FEATURES

- Similar features of typical lichen planus, may be asymptomatic
- Large percentage of patients with cutaneous LP have mucous membrane involvement and primarily affects women ages 40 - 60 years
- Lesions consists of **lacy, netlike, white plaques with a violaceous base** on the tongue or buccal mucosa
- Painful erosions and ulcers may also be seen, as well as atrophic, bullous, pigmented, reticular and papular forms
- Some studies associate oral LP with chronic liver disease (especially hepatitis C)

HISTOLOGIC FEATURES

- Features **similar to typical lichen planus**, usually hyperparakeratosis but may have orthokeratosis
- Epithelium may be atrophic, acanthotic
- May contain plasma cells in addition to lymphocytes
- No epithelial dysplasia or verrucous architectural change

Path Presenter
Interface changes

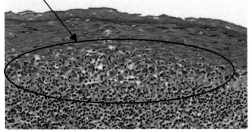

Subepidermal clefting

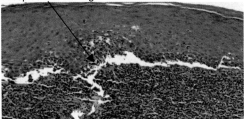

DIFFERENTIAL DIAGNOSIS

LUPUS ERYTHEMATOSUS

- Epidermal atrophy or hypertrophy, attenuation of rete ridges, and basement membrane thickening
- Vacuolar interface changes with keratinocyte apoptosis in the basilar layer
- Lamina propria is edematous and inflammation varies from sparse to lymphocyte rich
- Both superficial and deep inflammatory (perivascular) infiltrates

ORAL LICHENOID DRUG REACTION

- May have a higher number of apoptotic keratinocytes
- The inflammation may be more diffuse rather than band-like and contain plasma cells and eosinophils

MUCOUS MEMBRANE PEMPHIGOID

- Subepithelial clefting with detachment from the lamina propria
- No hydropic degeneration of the basal cells or colloid bodies
- Inflammation often patchy, variable and contains lymphocytes, plasma cells and possibly eosinophils

CHRONIC ULCERATIVE STOMATITIS

- Ulcerated mucosa with mixed inflammatory infiltrate

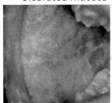 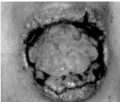 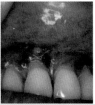

Mild interface inflammation

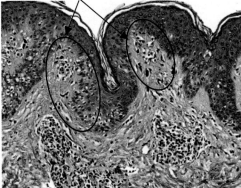

Pigment incontinence

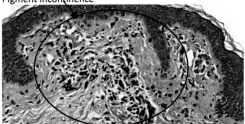

Perivascular inflammation

ERYTHEMA DYSCHROMICUM PERSTANS

CLINICAL FEATURES

- Also known as **Ashy dermatosis (of Ramirez)**, that describes its **gray macules**
- It is a form of **acquired dermal macular hyperpigmentation**
- **Well-circumscribed round to oval or irregular patches** on the **face, neck, and trunk**, most commonly **symmetrically distributed**
- There may be a transient inflammatory erythematous border that extends peripherally
- Most often affects **darker-skinned people** (Fitzpatrick skin types III-V) and has a preference for Latin American and Asian females in their 30s

HISTOLOGIC FEATURES

- **Lichenoid interface dermatitis** in the acute phase
- **Melanin incontinence** in the papillary dermis
- More typically presents with mild perivascular and lichenoid lymphocytic infiltrate (absent in late lesions)

DIFFERENTIAL DIAGNOSIS

LICHEN PLANUS

- Compact hyperorthokeratosis, irregular acanthosis and saw-tooth rete ridges with wedge-shaped hypergranulosis
- Lichenoid band-like lymphohistiocytic infiltrate within the superficial dermis
- Apoptotic bodies (Civatte /cytoid bodies)
- Basement membrane vacuolar change with basal cell squamatization (flattening of cells)

POST INFLAMMATORY PIGMENT ALTERATION

- Focal reduction of melanin pigmentation in the basal layer of the epidermis with normal number of melanocytes, pigment incontinence in dermis

Path Presenter

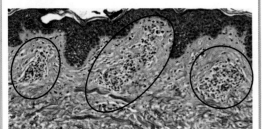

Hyperkertosis   Mild interface inflammtion

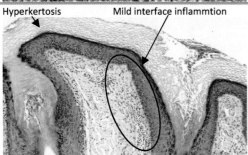

Infundibulum and upper isthamus with lymphocytic inflammation

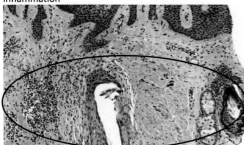

Wedge shaped scar

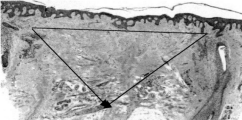

Inflammation around hair follicles

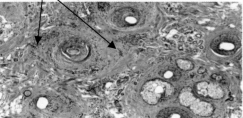

ATROPHIC ACTINIC KERATOSIS

- Thin epidermis with atypia of basal keratinocytes with loss of polarization, crowding and overlapping
- Focal parakeratosis

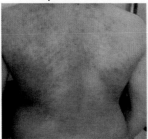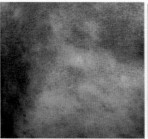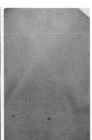

LICHEN PLANOPILARIS

CLINICAL FEATURES

- Also known as **follicular lichen planus (LP), lichen follicularis, or lichen planus acuminatus**
- Characterized by **perifollicular erythema and scale** that can progress to **cicatricial (scarring) alopecia with "lonely hairs"** over time, often associated with burning pain or pruritus
- **Scalp** is the most common location (typically with patchy involvement of vertex and parietal scalp), but it can affect the axillae, pubic hair, face, and other sites
- Most commonly affects **middle-aged and post-menopausal women**
- Subdivided into three main clinical types:
  - A Classic LPP
  - B Frontal fibrosing alopecia (FFA)
  - C Graham–Little Syndrome
- **Classic LPP**
  - Presents with **follicular violaceous erythema** and **perifollicular fine scale**, interfollicular erythema may also be seen
  - The perifollicular erythema is usually seen at the periphery of patches of alopecia, which corresponds to active areas of disease
- **Frontal fibrosing alopecia (FFA)**
  - The **progressive recession of frontal hairline** and development of scarring alopecia with **"lonely hairs"** within the hypopigmented scar
  - Typically seen in **postmenopausal women**
  - **Eyebrows** commonly affected
- **Graham-Little Syndrome**
  - **Triad** of scalp LPP, non-cicatricial pubic/axillary alopecia, and keratosis pilaris

HISTOLOGIC FEATURES

- **Early Disease**:
  - **Lichenoid lymphocytic inflammation, dyskeratotic keratinocytes, and Civatte bodies** within affected **infundibula and upper isthmus**
  - **Minimal interfollicular lichenoid** interface dermatitis
  - Loss/reduction of sebaceous gland is noted
  - Artifactual cleft may be seen between the follicular epithelium and perifollicular stroma
  - The infiltrate of LPP is mostly CD3+ T-lymphocytes with a normal CD4: CD8 ratio
  - Concentric, lamellar perifollicular **mucinous fibroplasia** with **hourglass-like narrowing** at the level of the follicular infundibulum

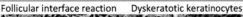
Follicular interface reaction   Dyskeratotic keratinocytes

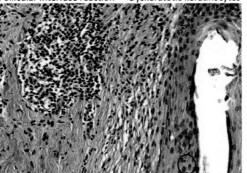
Peri-follicular inflammation and artifactual clefting

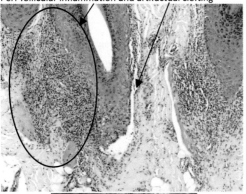

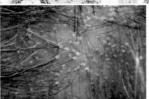

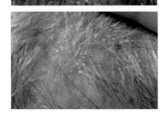

- Deep perivascular and peri eccrine inflammation and interstitial mucin are absent
- **Late / Chronic Stage**:
  - **Wedge-shaped** superficial follicular scar with **follicular drop-out** with minimal scar affecting the intervening epidermis
  - **Peri-follicular fibrosis** most prominent at the level of the infundibulum
  - **Polytrichia** with a fusion of 2-3 follicular units
  - Loss of sebaceous glands with entrapped arrector pili muscles

OTHER HIGH YIELD POINTS
- **Alcian blue and colloidal iron** stains demonstrate a **normal amount of dermal mucin** in the surrounding normal dermis in contrast to lupus
- **Loss of peri-follicular fibers** at the level of the infundibulum is highlighted by **Movat or elastic stain**

DIFFERENTIAL DIAGNOSIS
LUPUS ASSOCIATED ALOPECIA
- Vacuolar interface or lichenoid inflammation within the follicular epithelium and intervening epidermis
- Presence of deeper inflammation prominent within the isthmus and epidermal involvement distinguishes LE from LPP
- Thickening of the basement membrane with underlying pigment incontinence
- Concentric fibrosis and mucinous degeneration of fibrous tracts with loss of sebaceous glands of follicles
- Superficial and deep perivascular and periadnexal lymphoplasmacytic inflammation
- DIF: "Full house" with deposition of granular IgG, IgM, IgA and C3 at the BMZ

SYPHILITIC ALOPECIA
- Psoriasiform and lichenoid/vacuolar dermatitis with perifollicular lymphohistiocytic infiltrate with admixed plasma cells
- Can have many miniaturized hairs
- Telangiectasia with endothelial cell swelling

ALOPECIA AREATA
- Normal total number of hairs with increased miniaturized hairs
- Increased number of terminal catagen and telogen hairs
- Characteristic "swarm of bees" peribulbar mononuclear cell inflammation affecting terminal anagen and catagen hairs

Path Presenter

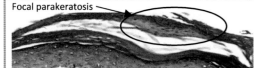
Focal parakeratosis

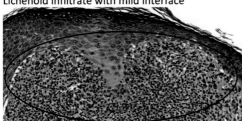
Lichenoid infiltrate with mild interface

LICHEN NITIDUS
CLINICAL FEATURES
- Clusters of numerous **monomorphic, pinpoint-sized flat-topped papules** that are **skin-colored**, hypo-, or hyperpigmented
- May have a disseminated or localized, linear distribution, commonly on the **ventral arms, chest, abdomen, and/or genitalia.** Oral involvement invariably absent
- Nail involvement may include pitting, splitting, or ridging
- Predominately seen in **children and young adults**, but can affect any age with no apparent gender or race predilection
- Usually asymptomatic, but may be pruritic and lesions may koebnerize
- Often resolves spontaneously without residual atrophy or pigmentary changes

HISTOLOGIC FEATURES

Ball in claw appearance

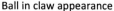

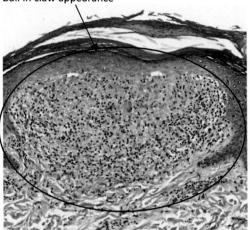

Lymphohistiocytic infiltrate

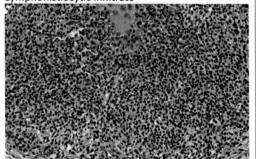

Path Presenter

- **Epidermal atrophy** with **overlying parakeratosis**
- Well-circumscribed dense aggregate of lichenoid lymphohistiocytic infiltrate
- Lichenoid infiltrate is **limited to 1 or 2 rete ridges** (or 1 - 4 dermal papillae) surrounded by a collarette formed by rete ridges - **'ball in claw' appearance**
- Mild interface change with few cytoid bodies may be present
- Melanophages/pigment incontinence is common in richly pigmented individuals
- Occasional multinucleate giant cells and plasma cells are present

OTHER HIGH YIELD POINTS

- The shaft and glans of the penis are considered favored sites for lichen nitidus, which should be considered in the differential for penile papules

DIFFERENTIAL DIAGNOSIS

LICHEN PLANUS

- Compact hyperorthokeratosis, irregular acanthosis, wedge-shaped hypergranulosis with saw-tooth rete ridges
- Lichenoid band-like lymphohistiocytic infiltrate within the superficial dermis
- Basement membrane vacuolar change with apoptotic bodies

LICHEN PLANUS LIKE KERATOSIS

- Clinically a solitary lesion
- Orthokeratosis, usually with parakeratosis, variable epidermal acanthosis, and Civatte bodies with extensive band-like lichenoid inflammation in DEJ

LICHEN STRIATUS

- Hyperkeratosis with focal parakeratosis, mild spongiosis and acanthosis with dyskeratotic cells (Civatte bodies) at all levels of the epidermis
- Mild to dense band-like lichenoid lymphohistiocytic inflammation at DEJ
- Extension of inflammation into the deep dermis in a perivascular or perifollicular pattern. Peri eccrine inflammation is characteristically present

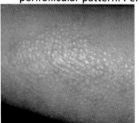

Focal parakeratosis

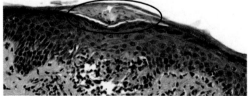

Lichenoid inflammation

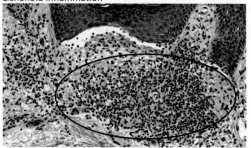

LICHEN STRIATUS

CLINICAL FEATURES

- Uncommon, **self-limited** dermatosis of **young children**
- Numerous **pinpoint (1-3mm) skin-colored to hyperpigmented or brownish scaly, flat-topped papules** coalescing into a curvilinear plaque
- Distributed along the **lines of Blaschko**, usually unilateral
- Can occur anywhere (including nails), however, most often on the **leg**
- Occasionally pruritic, but usually asymptomatic
- Resolution can result in hypo or hyperpigmentation

HISTOLOGIC FEATURES

- Hyperkeratosis with **focal parakeratosis**, mild spongiosis and acanthosis of the epidermis
- Dyskeratotic cells (Civatte bodies) at **all levels of the epidermis**
- Mild to dense band-like lichenoid lymphohistiocytic inflammation at DEJ
- Extension of inflammation into the **deep dermis** in a perivascular or perifollicular pattern
- **Peri eccrine inflammation** is characteristically present

Peri eccrine inflammation

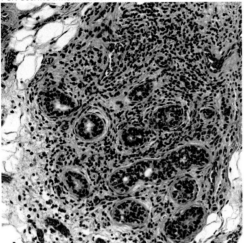

Path Presenter

Epidermal atrophy   Homogenization of collagen

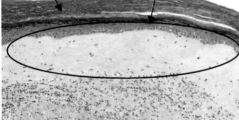

Dense lichenoid inflammation

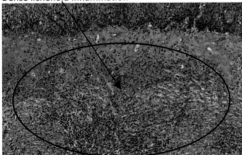

Path Presenter

- Papillary dermal edema and pigment incontinence may be present

DIFFERENTIAL DIAGNOSIS

LICHEN PLANUS

- Compact hyperorthokeratosis, irregular acanthosis, wedge-shaped hypergranulosis with saw-tooth rete ridges
- Lichenoid band-like lymphohistiocytic infiltrate within the superficial dermis
- Basement membrane vacuolar change with apoptotic bodies

SUBACUTE-CHRONIC ECZEMATOUS DERMATITIS

- Parakeratosis and scale crust overlying mildly acanthotic epidermis
- Spongiotic changes, sometimes with vesiculation
- Superficial perivascular lymphohistiocytic infiltrate with associated dermal fibroplasia

DRUG ERUPTION

- Superficial and deep perivascular lymphocytic infiltrate with admixed eosinophils
- Exocytosis and vacuolar change with rare apoptotic keratinocytes

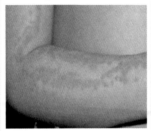
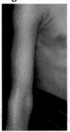
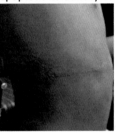

LICHEN SCLEROSUS

CLINICAL FEATURES

- Chronic condition that begins with a short inflammatory stage, followed by chronic scarring and atrophy
- Lesions evolve **from white to slightly erythematous macules or plaques** (often with a violaceous border) into **white, sclerotic, and atrophic patches or thin plaques** that have a shiny porcelain appearance
- Follicular plugs and telangiectasia may be observed
- Over 85% of lesions are found on **anogenital skin**, but lichen sclerosis can also occur in the extragenital regions (typically occurring on the trunk, buttocks, or thighs)
- Predominantly affects **females.** Female genital forms are typically distributed on the labia majora and/or the labia minora, clitoris, and anus
- Lesions have an **hourglass or figure of eight appearances.** Can be intensely pruritic
- If left untreated can evolve into complete loss of the labia minora and fusion of the clitoral hood and clitoris
- The male genital form typically occurs in **uncircumcised males** on the glans or prepuce and is also referred to as balanitis xerotica obliterans

HISTOLOGIC FEATURES

- **Early lesions** may only show **subtle changes** and may be confined to adnexal structures, which include luminal hyperkeratosis & hypergranulosis, psoriasiform epidermal hyperplasia, and basement membrane zone thickening
- Lymphohistiocytic infiltrate may be **sparse, dense, lichenoid, or interstitial**
- Lymphocytic exocytosis may be seen
- Later lesions are associated with epidermal atrophy, a broad zone of pallor in the papillary dermis, and a mild perivascular lymphocytic infiltrate

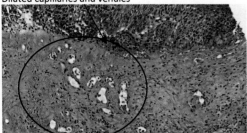
Dilated capillaries and venules

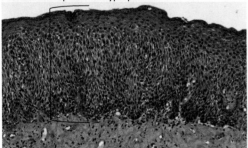
Psoriasiform epidermal hyperplasia

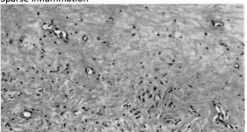
Sparse inflammation

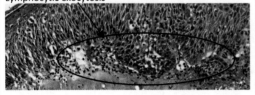
Lymphocytic exocytosis

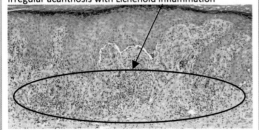
Irregular acanthosis with Lichenoid inflammation

Eosinophils mixed with lymphocytes

- **Homogenization of collagen** in the upper dermis with loss of spaces in between them, appearing like a pale eosinophilic sheet, mimicking edema
- This can result in subepidermal vesicle formation
- Plasma cells and eosinophils may be present
- Loss of elastic fibers in the sclerotic zone
- Dilated superficial capillaries and venules

OTHER HIGH YIELD POINTS

- Squamous cell carcinoma can develop in untreated genital lesions Biopsy is necessary if malignant transformation is suspected

DIFFERENTIAL DIAGNOSIS

MORPHEA

- Biopsy has a rectangular shape on low magnification
- Epidermis is normal or atrophic
- Superficial and deep perivascular, interstitial and perineural infiltrates of lymphocytes, sometimes admixed with plasma cells and eosinophils
- Collagen bundles in the reticular dermis are crowded, thickened, brightly eosinophilic
- The spaces in between are narrowed, but not obliterated
- Loss of periadnexal fat with atrophy of adnexal structures, especially the pilosebaceous units

RADIATION DERMATITIS

- Hyperkeratosis often with epidermal atrophy and acanthosis
- Sclerosis of upper dermis, sometimes involving the entire thickness and extending into subcutis
- Large bizarre, stellate radiation fibroblasts within sclerotic areas
- Ectatic blood vessels with fibrin

LICHEN PLANUS

- Compact hyperorthokeratosis with irregular acanthosis, wedge shaped hypergranulosis, and saw-tooth rete ridges
- Lichenoid band-like lymphohistiocytic infiltrate within the superficial dermis with no homogenization of collagen

 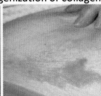 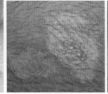 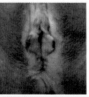

LICHENOID DRUG ERUPTION

CLINICAL FEATURES

- **Erythematous to violaceous small-scaling papules** coalescing into larger plaques. **Pruritus** is a common feature
- Distribution is often **symmetrical and widespread,** commonly involving the **trunk and extremities.** Oral lesions are sometimes seen
- Morphology resembles lichen planus; however, lichenoid drug lesions are **larger in size,** have secondary eczematization and significant post-inflammatory hyperpigmentation, often lack Wickham's striae, and less commonly involve the mucosa
- Latency period between the onset of the eruption and initiation of the implicated medication varies from weeks to months and even years
- More common in adults, with a female predominance
- Occasionally exacerbated by sun exposure
- Classic cutaneous lichenoid drug eruptions may be caused by **angiotensin-converting enzyme (ACE) inhibitors,** antimalarials, beta-blockers, gold, lithium, mercury amalgam, methyldopa, penicillamine, quinidine,

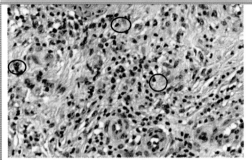
Hyperkeratosis and hypergranulosis

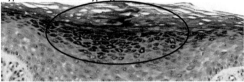
Civatte bodies

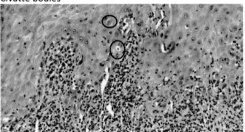
Wedge shaped hypergranulosis

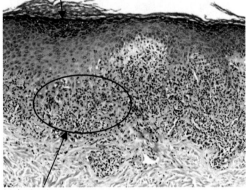
Melanin pigment

Basket-weave stratum corneum with interface reaction

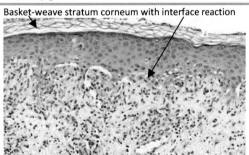
Dyskeratotic keratinocytes

sulfonylureas, thiazide diuretics, tumor necrosis factor (TNF)-α inhibitors, and tyrosine kinase inhibitors
- Typically, the eruption occurs 2-3 months after initiation of the culprit medication, although onset may be as short as a few weeks or as long as several years
- Resolution often takes months or up to a year after its discontinuation

HISTOLOGIC FEATURES
- **Compact orthokeratosis with parakeratosis**, **wedge-shaped hypergranulosis**, and **irregular acanthosis**
- **Lichenoid lymphocytic inflammation** at the DEJ, often with admixed **eosinophils**
- Civatte bodies are occasionally seen within the superficial epidermis
- Melanin pigment incontinence can be seen
- Plasma cells can be present

DIFFERENTIAL DIAGNOSIS

LICHEN PLANUS
- Compact hyperorthokeratosis, irregular acanthosis, wedge-shaped hypergranulosis with saw-tooth rete ridges
- Lichenoid band-like lymphohistiocytic infiltrate within the superficial dermis
- Basement membrane vacuolar change with apoptotic bodies
- Plasma cells and eosinophils are generally absent

BENIGN LICHENOID KERATOSIS
- Clinically a solitary lesion
- Orthokeratosis, usually with parakeratosis, variable epidermal acanthosis, and Civatte bodies
- Extensive band-like lichenoid inflammation at the DEJ with interface change

FIXED DRUG ERUPTION
- Basket-weave stratum corneum with necrotic/dyskeratotic keratinocytes
- Vacuolar interface dermatitis
- Prominent pigment incontinence around superficial vessels with overlying papillary dermal fibrosis

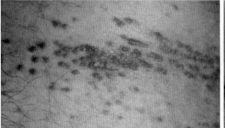
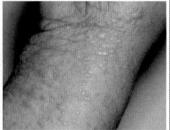

FIXED DRUG ERUPTION
CLINICAL FEATURES
- Cutaneous adverse drug reaction that recurs within minutes to hours at the **same body site** each time the individual is **re-exposed to the culprit drug**
- One to several sharply demarcated **annular, red, or violaceous plaques** (size varies from 05 to several centimeters). Overtime, lesions can become bullous due to severe DEJ damage
- Usually asymptomatic, although burning, pain, or pruritus may occur
- Common sites: **face (oral mucosa)**, hands, feet, and **genitalia**
- Etiology: common medications - **sulfonamides, NSAIDs, tetracyclines, barbiturates, carbamazepine, phenolphthalein (in laxatives)**
- The lesions classically resolve with **post-inflammatory hyperpigmentation.**
- Hypopigmented variant: pseudoephedrine

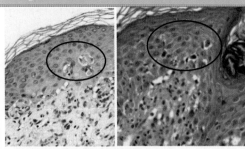
Vacuolar interface changes

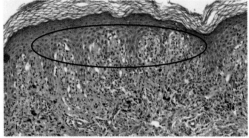
Pigment incontinence and interface changes

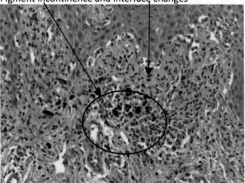

Path Presenter

Necrotic keratinocytes at all levels

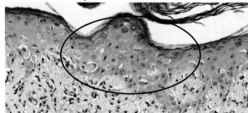
Interface vacuolar dermatitis

- If medication is continued, there is a risk for the development of generalized FDE
- Provocation by patch testing at a previously involved site can be useful in identifying the culprit drug

HISTOLOGIC FEATURES
- **Basket-weave stratum corneum** with **necrotic/dyskeratotic keratinocytes** and **vacuolar interface dermatitis**
- Prominent pigment incontinence around superficial vessels with overlying **papillary dermal fibrosis**
- Superficial perivascular mixed infiltrate with eosinophils may extend deep into dermis

DIFFERENTIAL DIAGNOSIS
ERYTHEMA MULTIFORME
- Preserved basket-weave stratum corneum with necrotic/dyskeratotic keratinocytes at all levels
- Interface vacuolar dermatitis
- Superficial perivascular lymphocytic infiltrate +/- eosinophils

ARTHROPOD BITE
- Highly variable histology
- Classically, a dense, wedge-shaped superficial and deep perivascular and interstitial inflammatory infiltrate
- Eosinophils are a prominent finding, and are a useful clue when seen away from the vessels (interposed between collagen bundles) and in the deeper dermis
- The epidermis is variably spongiotic and mouth parts may be present at the center of the lesion which aids in diagnosis

GRAFT VERSUS HOST DISEASE
- Apoptosis in epidermal basal layer or lower Malpighian layer or infundibulum/outer root sheath of hair follicle or acrosyringium/sweat ducts
- ± lichenoid inflammation, vacuolar change and lymphocytic satellitosis

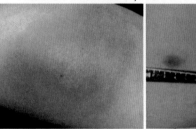
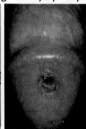
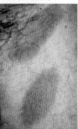

ERYTHEMA MULTIFORME (EM)
CLINICAL FEATURES
- Self-limited hypersensitivity reaction of the skin and mucous membranes
- Characterized by the **acute onset of fixed lesions** of concentric color change
- Two subtypes: **EM major and EM minor.** Major subtypes include mucosal involvement and systemic symptoms such as fever, arthralgias, and asthenias which are absent in minor
- Commonly affects **young adults**
- **Targetoid erythematous** thin plaques, predominantly on the acral extremities, occasionally with mucosal membrane involvement

HISTOLOGIC FEATURES
- **Preserved basket-weave** stratum corneum
- **Necrotic/dyskeratotic keratinocytes at all levels**
- **Interface vacuolar dermatitis**
- Superficial perivascular lymphocytic infiltrate +/- eosinophils

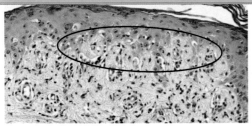

Basket-weve stratum corneum

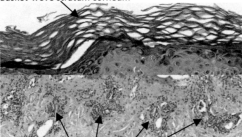

Superficial perivascular inflammation
Subepidermal bulla

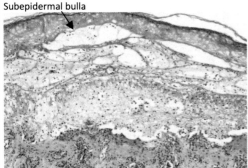

Path Presenter

Subepidermal split

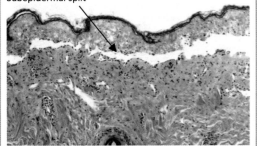

Full-thickness epidermal necrosis

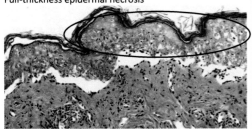

- **Subepidermal cleft/bullae** in erythema multiforme bullosa

OTHER HIGH YIELD POINTS

- Common triggers include **herpes simplex infection** (most common), M. pneumoniae, and drugs in <10% of cases
- Although a strong association exists between HSV and EM, a direct immunofluorescence test or viral culture for HSV will be negative in EM lesions

DIFFERENTIAL DIAGNOSIS

FIXED DRUG ERUPTION

- Basket-weave stratum corneum with necrotic/dyskeratotic keratinocytes and vacuolar interface dermatitis
- Prominent pigment incontinence around superficial vessels with overlying papillary dermal fibrosis
- Superficial perivascular mixed infiltrate with eosinophils may extend deep into dermis

TOXIC EPIDERMAL NECROLYSIS

- Subepidermal bulla with confluent full-thickness necrosis of epidermis
- Sparse perivascular lymphocytic infiltrate with eosinophils

GRAFT VERSUS HOST DISEASE

- Apoptosis in epidermal basal layer or lower Malpighian layer or infundibulum/outer root sheath of hair follicle or acrosyringium/sweat ducts
- ± lichenoid inflammation, vacuolar change and lymphocytic satellitosis

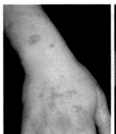
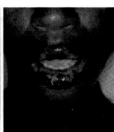

STEVENS- JOHNSON SYNDROME/TOXIC EPIDERMAL NECROLYSIS (SJS/TEN)

CLINICAL FEATURES

- Rare, **severe drug reactions** that are characterized by **mucosal erosions** (mucosa is involved in nearly 100% of cases) with **skin pain and detachment**, most commonly triggered by **medications**
- **SJS: <10% Body Surface Area (BSA)**
- **TEN: >30% BSA**
- **SJS-TEN overlap: 10-30% BSA**
- The primary medications most frequently implicated include **allopurinol, NSAIDs, antibiotics, and anticonvulsants.** Additional causes, albeit rare, include immunizations and infections
- SJS/TEN can affect all ages and races, with a slight preponderance seen in women (15:1) and an increasing incidence with age
- Onset: Occurs 1-3 weeks, and sometimes as long as 8 weeks, after the ingestion of the culprit medication
- It is typically preceded by **nonspecific prodromal symptoms** followed by characteristic **skin and mucosal lesions.** Prodromal symptoms may precede skin/mucosal findings by 1-3 days
- **Prodromal symptoms** include fevers, malaise, arthralgias/myalgias, ocular irritation, upper respiratory tract symptoms, and oropharyngeal pain

Necrotic keratinocytes at all levels of epidermis

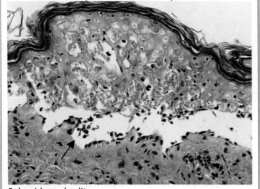

Subepidermal split
Full-thickness epidermal necrosis

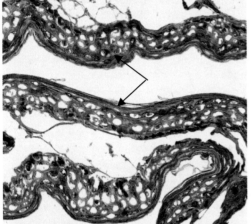

Epidermal necrosis-high power

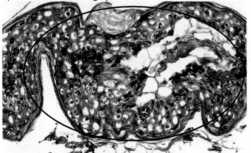

Minimal perivascular inflammation

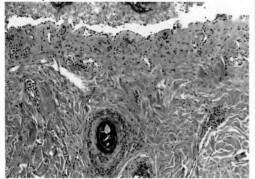

- **Cutaneous lesions** may begin as a typical exanthematous eruption evolving to dusky, irregular, ill-defined coalescing macules typically on the central trunk, palms, and soles and then spread to involve the face and proximal extremities. As the disease progresses, large areas of serous blistering and sloughing may occur
- **Mucosal lesions**: Oral mucosal sloughing and crusting are present in more than 90% of cases, and ocular involvement in more than 80%. Urogenital and, more rarely, respiratory and gastrointestinal (GI) mucosa may also be involved
- With severe involvement of the eyes, ulceration, scarring, visual impairment, and ultimately **blindness** may result
- **Nikolsky's sign**: tangential pressure-induced blister
- **Asboe-Hansen sign**: vertical pressure applied to bulla will result in an extension of the split to previously unaffected skin

HISTOLOGIC FEATURES

- **Subepidermal bulla** with confluent **full-thickness necrosis of the epidermis**
- **Necrotic cells** at **all levels of the epidermis**
- Minimal to mild perivascular lymphocytic infiltrate with neutrophils and/or eosinophils
- On frozen section, one may get a roll of necrotic epidermis completely sloughed off from dermis

OTHER HIGH YIELD POINTS

- Cutaneous pain or burning skin is a prominent early feature of SJS/TEN, and its presence could signify an ominous sign of impending necrolysis
- Worse prognosis: Extent of BSA involved, older age, malignancy, number of medications, leukopenia, and elevated serum urea, glucose, and creatinine levels
- **SCORTEN** is a prognostic scoring system for patients with epidermal necrolysis
- SJS carries a 1%-5% mortality risk, may or may not have systemic symptoms and involves the trunk and face with many isolated lesions
- TEN carries a 25%-35% mortality risk, invariably has systemic symptoms, and the lesions on the trunk and face are largely coalesced

DIFFERENTIAL DIAGNOSIS

ERYTHEMA MULTIFORME

- Preserved basket-weave stratum corneum with necrotic/dyskeratotic keratinocytes at all levels
- Interface vacuolar dermatitis
- Superficial perivascular lymphocytic infiltrate +/- eosinophils

GRAFT VERSUS HOST DISEASE

- Apoptosis in epidermal basal layer or lower malpighian layer or infundibulum/outer root sheath of hair follicle or acrosyringium/sweat ducts
- ± lichenoid inflammation
- ± vacuolar change
- ± lymphocytic satellitosis

STAPHYLOCOCCAL SCALDED SKIN SYNDROME

- Subcorneal split without much inflammation. On frozen section, one may get roll of stratum corneum only

Path Presenter

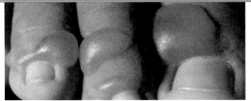
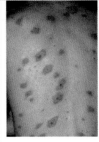
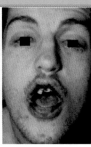
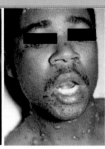
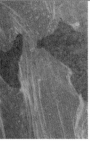

Epithelial damage and peri-follicular inflammation

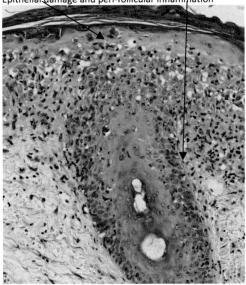

Hyperkeratosis and parakeratosis

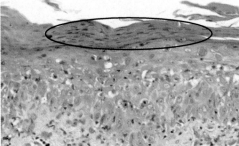

Dyskeratotic keratinocytes

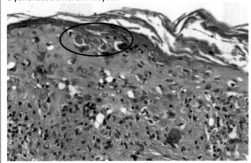

GRAFT VERSUS HOST DISEASE (GVHD)

CLINICAL FEATURES

- GVHD occurs in patients mostly with **allogeneic bone marrow transplants**, but it may occur in solid organ transplant and blood transfusion recipients
- **Acute GVHD** normally occurs **within 2-4 weeks** of stem cell infusion around the time of engraftment and typically presents as **a morbilliform eruption that may progress to erythroderma or, rarely, a TEN-like picture** often involving the palms and soles
- According to revised National Institute of Health (NIH) criteria, classic acute GVHD occurs within 100 days following hematopoietic stem cell transplantation and late-onset acute GVHD occurs after 100 days, and affects mainly the skin, gastrointestinal tract and liver
- **Chronic cutaneous GVHD** usually presents a mean of 4 months after transplantation (100 days after hematopoietic stem cell transplantation) with **mucocutaneous manifestations; sclerotic (sclerodermoid) and nonsclerotic (lichen planus-like/lichenoid) skin lesions** are most common

HISTOLOGIC FEATURES

Acute GVHD:
- Hypergranulosis
- Epithelial damage (**dyskeratotic keratinocytes**) initially occurs at the tips of rete ridges and within hair follicles. Dyskeratotic keratinocytes are often accompanied by two or more lymphocytes, a picture of **satellite cell necrosis** (lymphocyte-associated apoptosis)
- Vacuolar interface dermatitis
- Sparse superficial perivascular lymphocytic infiltrate

Chronic GVHD has 2 stages: lichenoid and sclerodermatous
- Lichenoid GVHD is similar to that of classic lichen planus: hyperkeratosis, hypergranulosis, acanthosis, and dyskeratotic keratinocytes with basal cell vacuolization
- Sclerodermatous GVHD resembles lichen sclerosus and morphea lesions

OTHER HIGH YIELD POINTS

- Clinical appearance and history of bone marrow transplant may be highly suggestive of the diagnosis
- Dyskeratotic keratinocytes involving the adnexal epithelium can differentiate between GVHD and drug eruption in difficult cases

DIFFERENTIAL DIAGNOSIS

SCLERODERMA
- Dermal sclerosis with thick closely packed hyalinized collagen bundles
- Loss of periadnexal fat and atrophy of adnexal structures, especially the pilosebaceous units
- Blood vessels appear narrowed with severe intimal fibrosis in small arteries and arterioles with sparse lymphoplasmacytic infiltrate

FIXED DRUG ERUPTION
- Basket-weave stratum corneum and necrotic/dyskeratotic keratinocytes
- Vacuolar interface dermatitis and papillary dermal fibrosis

Dermal sclerosis- Sclerodermatous GVHD

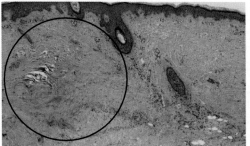

Path Presenter

Follicular plugging

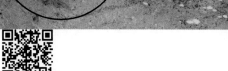

Pigment incontinence   Hyperkeratosis

Basement membrane thickening

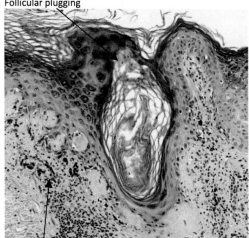

- Superficial perivascular mixed infiltrate with eosinophils, may extend deep into dermis

LUPUS ERYTHEMATOSUS

- Epidermal atrophy or hypertrophy with vacuolar interface reaction, basement membrane thickening and attenuation of rete ridges
- Follicular plugging and increased dermal mucin
- Superficial and deep perivascular and periadnexal inflammation

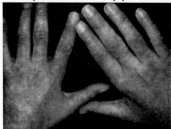 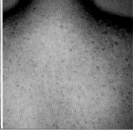 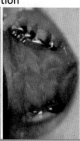

DISCOID LUPUS ERYTHEMATOSUS

CLINICAL FEATURES

- Most common in **women** in the **third to fifth decade** of life. Individuals of African and Hispanic descent are at increased risk, and there may be a positive family history of lupus or connective tissue disease
- **Sun-exposed areas** of the **head and neck** but can involve the non-exposed trunk and upper extremities. The **conchal bowl** is a characteristic site of involvement
- **Early plaques are red/erythematous** and scaly with **follicular plugging**
- Established lesions are **atrophic, hypopigmented, and scarred** with resultant **alopecia**

HISTOLOGIC FEATURES

- **Hyperkeratosis** with **follicular keratotic plugging**
- Epidermal atrophy or hypertrophy with attenuation of rete ridges
- Vacuolar interface dermatitis
- **Thickening of basement membrane**
- Pigment incontinence
- **Superficial and deep** perivascular and periadnexal lymphocytic infiltrate (CD123 positive lymphocytes)
- **Increased dermal mucin**

IMMUNOFLUORESCENCE/IMMUNOHISTOCHEMISTRY

- **Positive lupus band test**: IgM is most common, while **IgG** is most specific, and C3 may also be paired with IgM
- **Granular IgM** is continuous in sun-exposed skin and interrupted in sun-protected skin

OTHER HIGH YIELD POINTS

- **Most common** form of chronic cutaneous lupus erythematosus
- **Squamous cell carcinoma** may rarely develop in chronic DLE scars, especially in sun-exposed areas
- 20% of patients with SLE will manifest discoid lesions but only 5%-10% of patients with DLE demonstrate systemic involvement or will go on to develop SLE

DIFFERENTIAL DIAGNOSIS

LICHEN PLANUS

- Compact hyperorthokeratosis, irregular acanthosis, wedge-shaped hypergranulosis with saw-tooth rete ridges
- Lichenoid band-like lymphohistiocytic infiltrate within the superficial dermis
- Basement membrane vacuolar change with apoptotic bodies

Path Presenter

Vacuolar interface

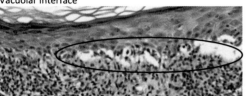

Deep peri-vascular and peri-adnexal inflammation

- Plasma cells and eosinophils are generally absent

SECONDARY SYPHILIS
- Combined psoriasiform epidermal hyperplasia with hyperkeratosis and parakeratosis with long thin rete ridges
- Superficial and deep perivascular and periadnexal lymphocytic infiltrate with admixed plasma cells, sometimes in a lichenoid

POLYMORPHOUS LIGHT ERUPTION
- Marked papillary dermal edema in association with an underlying superficial and deep tight perivascular lymphocytic infiltrate
- Commonly, the overlying epidermis may demonstrate varying degrees of spongiosis and dyskeratosis

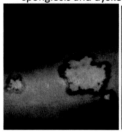
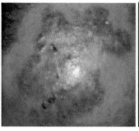
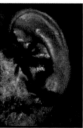
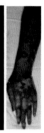

Unremarkable epidemis with minimal DEJ changes

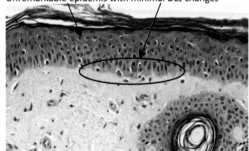

Perivascular inflammation

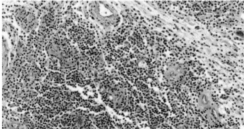

Increased dermal mucin

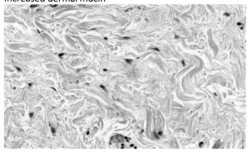

TUMID LUPUS ERYTHEMATOSUS (TLE)

CLINICAL FEATURES
- **Asymptomatic, edematous, red/erythematous papules and plaques** with **no surface changes**, most commonly on the **trunk, face, and neck**; sun-exposed areas
- Annular and gyrate configurations may also be seen
- **Photosensitivity** is a characteristic feature: lesions are often after ultraviolet (UV) light exposure. However, it may also be present on skin not exposed to the sun

HISTOLOGIC FEATURES
- Epidermal involvement is uncommon with normal appearing DEJ
- **Increased dermal mucin**, predominantly in the reticular dermis, and is often accompanied by subepidermal edema
- Some cases have only a **sparse superficial and deep** inflammatory cell infiltrate, whereas others have a **heavy superficial and deep**
- Predominance of CD4 T-cells over CD8 in immunohistochemical staining

IMMUNOFLUORESCENCE/IMMUNOHISTOCHEMISTRY
- Direct immunofluorescence is usually **negative**

OTHER HIGH YIELD POINTS
- Considered to be a relatively **uncommon subtype** of cutaneous lupus erythematosus (CLE), but unlike others, its association with SLE is rare
- Lack of atrophy, scarring, follicular plugging, and dyspigmentation are the salient features of TLE
- It has also been postulated that TLE is in the **same spectrum** as **lymphocytic infiltrate of Jessner** and reticular erythematous mucinosis (**REM**) due to similar findings on histology. The lesions of REM tend to have a **reticular appearance clinically**

DIFFERENTIAL DIAGNOSIS
RETICULAR ERYTHEMATOUS MUCINOSIS
- Superficial and deep perivascular mixed infiltrate (mostly lymphocytic)
- May have telangiectasias and hemorrhage in the upper dermis
- Mucin in between collagen bundles in the upper dermis and around the infiltrate and appendages

Periadnexal inflammation

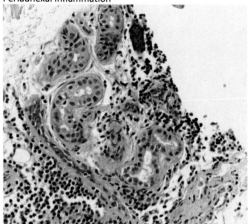

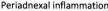
- Usually minimal to no epidermal changes

LUPUS ERYTHEMATOSUS

- Epidermal atrophy or hypertrophy with follicular plugging
- Vacuolar interface reaction, basement membrane thickening, and attenuation of rete ridges
- Increased dermal mucin
- Superficial and deep perivascular and periadnexal inflammation

CUTANEOUS FOCAL MUCINOSIS

- Localized deposition of mucin in the mid to upper dermis associated with an increased number of spindled cells and stellate fibroblasts
- Separated from the epidermis by a grenz zone
- The lesion may be flanked by an epidermal collarette

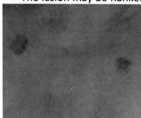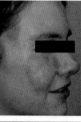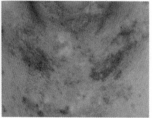

Hyperkeratosis   Mild DEJ changes

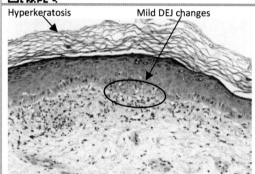

Periadnexal (perifollicular) inflammation

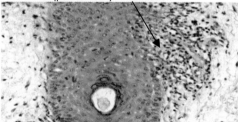

SUBACUTE LUPUS ERYTHEMATOSUS (SCLE)

CLINICAL FEATURES

- **Photosensitive, nonscarring, nonatrophic**-producing eruption on **sun-exposed areas**
- Two variants:
  a) **Erythematous annular variant**: raised pink-red borders and central clearing
  b) **Papulosquamous variant**: chronic psoriasiform or eczematous appearance
- Patient can have a mild systemic illness with musculoskeletal complaints and serological abnormalities
- Commonly resolves with **hypopigmentation**
- Drug-induced SCLE: **HCTZ, penicillamine**, glyburide, griseofulvin, piroxicam, spironolactone, diltiazem, ACE inhibitors, terbinafine

HISTOLOGIC FEATURES

- Variable vacuolar or lichenoid interface dermatitis and scattered cytoid bodies
- **Dyskeratotic keratinocytes** extending into **upper spinous layers** is a hallmark but rare finding of SCLE
- Acanthosis may be present in psoriasiform lesions
- Occasional focal hypergranulosis may be seen
- Mild, predominantly **superficial perivascular and periadnexal** lymphocytic infiltrate
- Increased dermal mucin
- **Drug-induced variants** are more commonly associated with **leukocytoclastic vasculitis** and have **less mucin deposition**

OTHER HIGH YIELD POINTS

- Approximately **50% of patients** with SCLE meet criteria for SLE
- Epidermal atrophy, follicular plugging, basement membrane thickening, dermal mucin, and pigment incontinence may be present but **less prominent** than in chronic lupus erythematosus
- **Concomitant Sjögren syndrome** may occur due to shared presence of anti-SSA/Ro antibodies

Increased dermal mucin

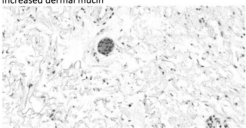

Perivascular inflammation

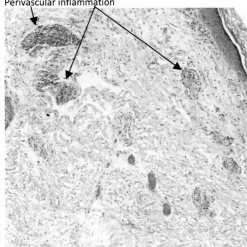

DIFFERENTIAL DIAGNOSIS

DERMATOMYOSITIS

- Hyperkeratosis, epidermal atrophy, flattened rete ridges, apoptotic keratinocytes
- Vacuolar interface dermatitis
- Pigment incontinence and a sparse to moderate perivascular and periadnexal infiltrate in the dermis
- Increased dermal mucin deposition

SECONDARY SYPHILIS

- Combined psoriasiform epidermal hyperplasia with hyperkeratosis and parakeratosis
- Interface/vacuolar change and long thin rete ridges
- Superficial and deep perivascular and periadnexal lymphocytic infiltrate with admixed plasma cells, sometimes in a lichenoid

LUPUS ERYTHEMATOSUS

- Hyperkeratosis, epidermal atrophy with follicular plugging
- Vacuolar interface dermatitis and thickening of basement membrane
- Pigment incontinence, increased dermal mucin
- Superficial and deep perivascular and periadnexal lymphocytic infiltrate

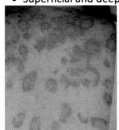 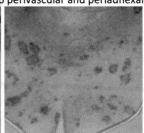 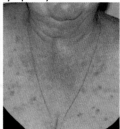

Hyperkeratosis and follicular plugging

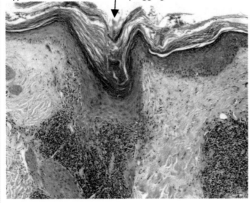

Vacuolar interface change

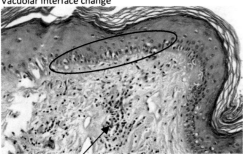

Superficial inflammation

SYSTEMIC LUPUS ERYTHEMATOSUS

CLINICAL FEATURES

- Classic "**butterfly**" malar rash (involving the cheeks and nose) developing after sun exposure
- Slightly **scaly erythematous** edematous eruption on the **sun-exposed area**
- **Photosensitivity**
- There are three main specific subtypes based on morphology and distribution, chronicity, association with SLE, and histologic features including location/depth of inflammatory infiltrate:

a) **Acute cutaneous lupus erythematosus (ACLE):**
- Transient cutaneous findings presenting as malar erythema without scarring
- Strongly associated with systemic findings
- Inflammatory infiltrate in the superficial dermis

b) **Subacute cutaneous lupus erythematosus (SCLE):**
- Photosensitive cutaneous eruption lasting longer than ACLE but without scarring
- Systemic findings are seen in 10%-15% of patients
- Inflammatory infiltrate in the upper dermis

c) **Chronic cutaneous lupus erythematosus (CCLE):**
- Includes most common variant Discoid lupus erythematosus (DLE) also with less common variants like lupus tumidus, lupus panniculitis, and chilblain lupus
- DLE and CCLE are often interchangeably used
- DLE presents with chronic discoid lesions with permanent disfiguring scars most often seen on the scalp, face, and ears
- Systemic findings are seen in 5%-15% of patients

Periadnexal inflammation

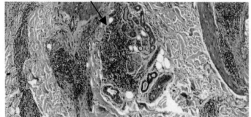

Perivascular inflammation

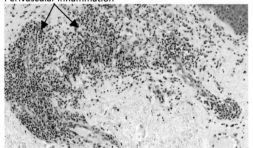

Increased dermal mucin

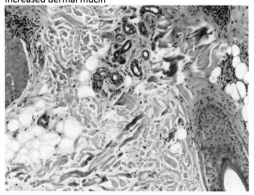

Path Presenter

- In DLE, significant inflammatory infiltrate seen in superficial and deep dermis as well as prominent involvement of the adnexa on biopsy

HISTOLOGIC FEATURES

- **Hyperkeratosis** and **follicular plugging**
- **Vacuolar interface changes**
- **Thickened basement membrane (highlighted by PAS)**
- Dense **superficial and deep** periadnexal and perivascular lymphocytic infiltrate
- Increased dermal mucin can often be seen
- Early lesion can show subtle and mild features

IMMUNOFLUORESCENCE/IMMUNOHISTOCHEMISTRY

- **Positive lupus band test**

DIFFERENTIAL DIAGNOSIS

DERMATOMYOSITIS

- Hyperkeratosis, epidermal atrophy, flattened rete ridges, apoptotic keratinocytes
- Vacuolar interface dermatitis
- Pigment incontinence, and a sparse to moderate perivascular and periadnexal infiltrate in the dermis

POLYMORPHOUS LIGHT ERUPTION (PMLE)

- Epidermal acanthosis, spongiosis, occasional dyskeratotic cells and lymphocytic exocytosis
- Mild DEJ change and papillary dermal edema
- Perivascular lymphohistiocytic infiltrate in superficial and sometimes deep dermis

GRAFT VERSUS HOST DISEASE

- Apoptosis in epidermal basal layer or lower Malpighian layer or infundibulum/outer root sheath of hair follicle or acrosyringium/sweat ducts
- ± lichenoid inflammation
- ± vacuolar change
- ± lymphocytic satellitosis

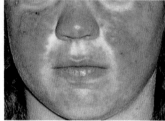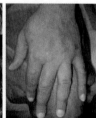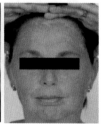

Epidermal atrophy

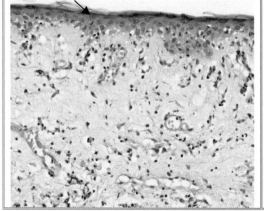

DERMATOMYOSITIS

CLINICAL FEATURES

Typical cutaneous manifestations of dermatomyositis most often include:

- **Violaceous to erythematous poikiloderma** (atrophic skin with changes in pigmentation and telangiectasia in photo-exposed or non-exposed areas)
- Violaceous to erythematous discoloration and swelling of the eyelids and periorbital skin **(Heliotrope rash)**
- Erythema in a shawl-like distribution on the upper chest and back, often photo distributed **(shawl sign)**
- Erythematous hyperkeratotic/atrophic dermal papules over the MCP, PIP, or DIP joints **(Gottron's papules)**
- Erythematous macules or patches over joints, especially knuckles, knees, and elbows **(Gottron's sign)**
- Erythema of lateral thighs **(Holster sign)**

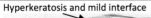
Hyperkeratosis and mild interface

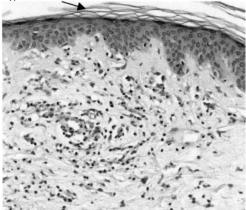

Hyperkeratosis and mild interface

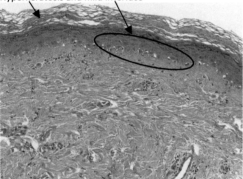

Pigment incontinence

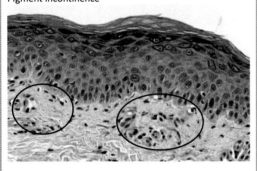

Perivascular inflammation

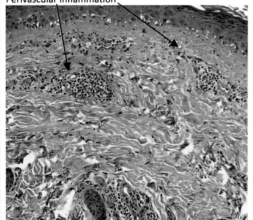

- Ill-defined erythematous macules involving the anterior aspect of the neck and the upper chest **(V sign)**
- Depending on the dermatomyositis subtype, proximal muscle weakness may be present
- Ragged cuticles **(Samitz sign)** with nail fold telangiectasia
- Diffuse alopecia with erythema and scale
- **Rarely**, dermatomyositis can present with **papulosquamous lesions** that can somewhat resemble psoriasis:
- **Well-demarcated pink plaques with scale**
- Can involve elbows
- Follicular accentuation may be present
  Other observed clinical features can include:
- **Raynaud** phenomenon
- **Calcinosis cutis** (more common in juvenile form)
- Calcifying panniculitis
- Hyperkeratotic, cracked horizontal lines on the palmar and lateral aspects of the fingers **(Mechanic's hands)**

HISTOLOGIC FEATURES

- **Chronic nonspecific dermatitis** or **interface dermatitis** resembling systemic lupus erythematosus
  Typical findings:
- **Hyperkeratosis, epidermal atrophy**, and flattened rete ridges with **apoptotic keratinocytes**
- **Vacuolar interface dermatitis,** often with thickened basement membrane zone
- Pigment incontinence
- Telangiectasia with sparse to moderate perivascular and periadnexal lymphocytic infiltrate in the dermis
- Increased **dermal mucin** deposition
- **Gottron's papules**: lichenoid infiltrate but with acanthosis rather than epidermal atrophy
- Muscles show myositis with **myofiber necrosis, fragmentation and phagocytosis**; late myofiber atrophy, fibrosis and fatty change
  When presented clinically as a **papulosquamous lesions**:
- **Parakeratosis**, may be confluent or centered above follicles
- **Acanthosis**
- Interface change, subtle or not present
- Dermal edema may be prominent
- Dermal mucin may be increased

OTHER HIGH YIELD POINTS

- Laboratory workup for **auto-antibodies** (anti-Mi2, anti-Jo1, anti-SRP, anti-KU etc.) should be done for prognosis and associated disorders
- Can be associated with **underlying malignancy**, especially of the breast, stomach, and ovary

DIFFERENTIAL DIAGNOSIS

GRAFT VERSUS HOST DISEASE

- Apoptosis in epidermal basal layer or lower Malpighian layer or infundibulum/outer root sheath of hair follicle or acrosyringium/sweat ducts
- ± lichenoid inflammation, ± vacuolar change, ± lymphocytic satellitosis

LUPUS ERYTHEMATOSUS

- Hyperkeratosis, epidermal atrophy with follicular plugging
- Vacuolar interface dermatitis and thickening of basement membrane
- Superficial and deep perivascular and periadnexal lymphocytic infiltrate

DRUG ERUPTION

Increased dermal mucin

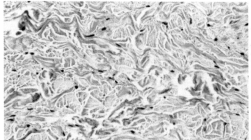

- Superficial and deep perivascular lymphocytic infiltrate with admixed eosinophils
- Exocytosis and vacuolar change with rare apoptotic keratinocytes

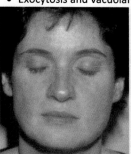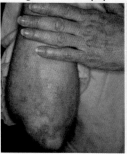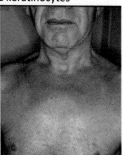

Hyperkeratosis   Parakeratosis

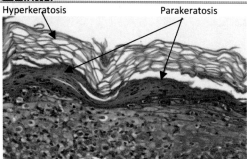

Wedhe shaped dermal inflammation

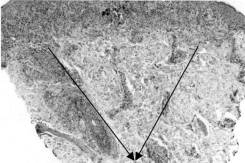

RBC extravasation

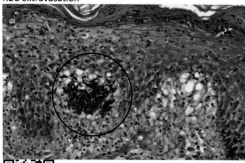

PITYRIASIS LICHENOIDES ET VARIOLIFORMIS ACUTA (PLEVA)
CLINICAL FEATURES

- **Acute onset** of asymptomatic to mildly pruritic **crops of red or brown**, 2- to 3-mm macules and papules
- Crops of papules that rapidly becomes **vesicular** and **hemorrhagic**, eventuating in **necrosis**
- **Ulcerated** and **crusted lesions** are common
- The crops usually recur over weeks to months before spontaneously resolving, often leaving **varioliform scars**
- Common in **males** in late childhood or early adulthood on the trunk
- Typically, various stages at the same time
- Most commonly scattered across the **trunk, buttocks, and proximal extremities**, but may also occur on the face, palms, soles, and scalp
- Occasionally associated with fever and systemic symptoms **(Mucha-Habermann disease)**

HISTOLOGIC FEATURES

- **Compact hyperkeratosis** and **focal parakeratosis** often with **neutrophilic** scale crust
- **Dyskeratotic cells** in epidermis
- Vacuolar interface dermatitis
- Dense **wedge-shaped** mixed infiltrate with lymphocytic exocytosis
- Lymphocytes are CD8>CD4 in dermis
- **Red cell extravasation** in the dermis
- Neutrophils within dermal vessels
- Eosinophils usually absent

DIFFERENTIAL DIAGNOSIS
PITYRIASIS ROSEA

- Focal mounds of parakeratosis overlying a spongiotic and slightly acanthotic epidermis
- In the dermis, there is a superficial perivascular lymphohistiocytic infiltrate
- Red blood cell (RBC) extravasation is a helpful diagnostic feature with RBCs found in the papillary dermis and occasionally in the epidermis

SECONDARY SYPHILIS

- Combined psoriasiform epidermal hyperplasia with hyperkeratosis and parakeratosis
- Interface/vacuolar change and long thin rete ridges
- Superficial and deep perivascular and periadnexal lymphocytic infiltrate with admixed plasma cells, sometimes in a lichenoid

Vacuolar interface changes

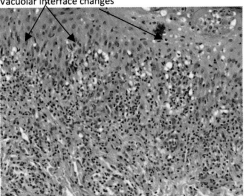

ERYTHEMA MULTIFORME

- Preserved basket-weave stratum corneum with necrotic/dyskeratotic keratinocytes at all levels
- Interface vacuolar dermatitis
- Superficial perivascular lymphocytic infiltrate +/- eosinophils

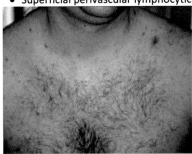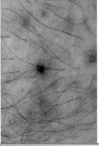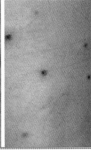

Parakeratotic scale

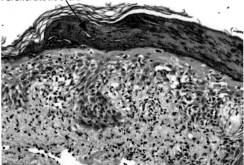

DEJ changes wiith dyskeratotic cells in epidermis

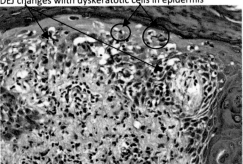

Dyskeratotic cells (high power)

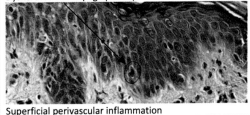

Superficial perivascular inflammation

PITYRIASIS LICHENOIDES CHRONICA

CLINICAL FEATURES

- Common in **males** in **late childhood or early adulthood** on the **trunk, extremities, and buttocks**
- Numerous **recurring crops of erythematous brown-red papules with central scale**
- There is seasonal variation to this condition, with onset more often occurring in the fall or winter

HISTOLOGIC FEATURES

- **Parakeratotic scale** with scattered **dyskeratotic cells** in epidermis
- **Upper dermal sparse inflammation**, mostly lymphocytes, sometimes with scattered melanophages
- Focal **vacuolar alteration** at DEJ and dermal fibrosis
- Red cell extravasation
- Neutrophils in vascular lumens in acute phase
- Superficial and deep inflammation in acute phase

OTHER HIGH YIELD POINTS

- A rare and more severe ulcerative variant of PLC with systemic symptoms is febrile ulceronecrotic **Mucha-Habermann disease,** which is a dermatologic emergency
- The relationship of PLC and lymphomatoid papulosis and whether PLC is a lymphoproliferative condition with malignant potential remains controversial

DIFFERENTIAL DIAGNOSIS

PITYRIASIS ROSEA

- Focal mounds of parakeratosis overlying a spongiotic and slightly acanthotic epidermis
- In the dermis, there is a superficial perivascular lymphohistiocytic infiltrate
- Red blood cell (RBC) extravasation is a helpful diagnostic feature with RBCs found in the papillary dermis and occasionally in the epidermis

SECONDARY SYPHILIS

- Combined psoriasiform epidermal hyperplasia with hyperkeratosis and parakeratosis
- Interface/vacuolar change and long thin rete ridges
- Superficial and deep perivascular and periadnexal lymphocytic infiltrate with admixed plasma cells, sometimes in a lichenoid

ERYTHEMA MULTIFORME

- Preserved basket-weave stratum corneum with necrotic/dyskeratotic keratinocytes at all levels
- Interface vacuolar dermatitis
- Superficial perivascular lymphocytic infiltrate +/- eosinophils

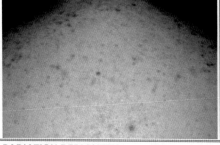
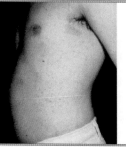

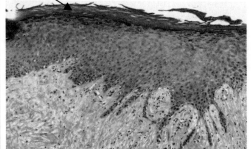

Hypekeratosis

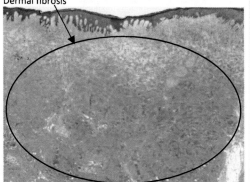

Dermal fibrosis

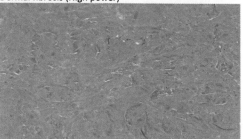

Dermal fibrosis (High power)

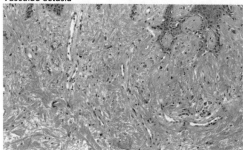

Vasculae ectasia

RADIATION DERMATITIS

CLINICAL FEATURES

- **Acute Radiation Dermatitis:**
  - Occurs within **90 days of exposure**
  - Lesions generally present in a **geometric configuration** at the irradiated site
  - Skin changes range from **faint erythema and dry desquamation to necrosis and ulceration**
  - **Classification of acute radiation dermatitis:**
  - Grade 0 – No change
  - Grade 1 – faint erythema or dry desquamation, epilation
  - Grade 2 – Moderate to brisk (bright) erythema or patchy, moist desquamation confined to skin folds and creases. Moderate edema
  - Grade 3 – Confluent, moist desquamation that is not confined to the skin folds. Pitting edema. Bleeding induced by minor trauma or abrasion
  - Grade 4 – Life-threatening consequences. Skin necrosis or ulceration of full thickness dermis. Hemorrhage or spontaneous bleeding from involved site. Skin graft indicated
- **Chronic Radiation Dermatitis**
  - Onset may occur from **15 days to decades** after the beginning of the procedure
  - More likely to occur in individuals with **unprotected sun exposure**, a larger dose per fraction delivered (> 4 Gy), larger total dose (> 55 Gy), and those who undergo radiation of large areas

HISTOLOGIC FEATURES

- **Acute Radiation Dermatitis:**
  - **Necrotic epidermis,** may be accompanied by both spongiosis and intracellular edema
  - **Vaculoar changes** at the basal layer of the epidermis, occasionally with subepidermal vesiculation
  - **Dermis is edematous** and may show fibrin deposition and dermal macrophages
  - Inflammatory response is often mixed with eosinophils, plasma cells and lymphocytes
  - In early stages, **vascular thrombosis can be seen**
- **Chronic radiation dermatitis:**
  - Epidermis is often **hyperkeratotic, acanthotic or atrophic with attenuation of ridge ridges**
  - May be associated with **epidermal spongiosis or basal vacuolar change**
  - **Dermal sclerosis** with **loss of appendages**, particularly hair follicles
  - **Elastosis** and **vascular ectasia** overlying an epidermis. Blood vessels have thickened wall with fibrointimal hyperplasia
  - Both the stroma **fibroblasts** and **endothelial** cells may show some **hyperchromasia, enlargement, and atypia (radiation fibroblasts)**
  - There is often a mixed inflammatory response

Loss of adnexal structures

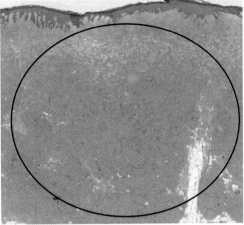

Atypical fibroblast and endothelial cells

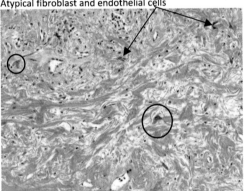

Path Presenter

- **Post UV-B radiation:**
  - Damaged keratinocytes, more in superficial epidermis **(sunburn cells)** with intercellular edema and exocytosis
  - **Endothelial cell swelling** and **perivenular edema** with a predominantly mononuclear intradermal chronic inflammatory cell infiltrate
  - Elastosis in fair skinned individuals
- **Post UV-A radiation:**
  - **Necrotic epidermis** and may be accompanied by both spongiosis and intracellular edema
  - **Keratinocyte swelling** and **vacuolation** accompanied by intercellular edema
  - **Diminished** number of Langerhans cells, but lacks sunburn cells
  - Dermis has mixed infiltrate of neutrophils, lymphocytes and occasionally basophils and eosinophils
  - Endothelial swelling may be seen

OTHER HIGH YIELD POINTS
- Certain diseases and syndromes increase the risk of radiation dermatitis (e.g., connective tissue diseases, HIV, Fanconi anemia, bloom syndrome etc.)

DIFFERENTIAL DIAGNOSIS

GRAFT VERSUS HOST DISEASE
- Apoptosis in epidermal basal layer or lower Malpighian layer or infundibulum/outer root sheath of hair follicle or acrosyringium/sweat ducts
- ± lichenoid inflammation, ± vacuolar change, ± lymphocytic satellitosis

MORPHEA/SCLERODERMA
- Biopsy has a rectangular shape on low magnification
- Epidermis is normal or atrophic
- Superficial and deep perivascular, interstitial and perineural infiltrates of lymphocytes, sometimes admixed with plasma cells and eosinophils
- Collagen bundles in the reticular dermis are crowded and thickened
- Loss of periadnexal fat with atrophy of adnexal structures, especially the pilosebaceous units

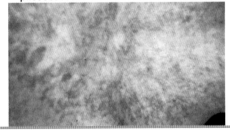

Epidermal spongiosis

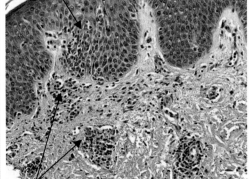

Superficial and deep inflammation

DRUG ERUPTION

CLINICAL FEATURES
- **Symmetric morbilliform or exanthematous** presentation
- **Red macules and papules** that often arise on the **trunk** and spread symmetrically to involve the **proximal extremities**
- In severe cases, lesions coalesce and may lead to erythroderma
- Palms, soles, and mucous membranes may also be involved
- Pruritus is a common feature
- Superficial desquamation and a dusky color may occur as the eruption resolves

HISTOLOGIC FEATURES
- Superficial and deep perivascular lymphocytic infiltrate with admixed eosinophils

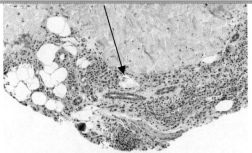
Lymphocytic infiltrate with eosinophils

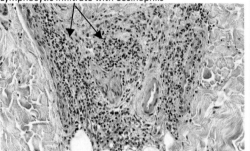
Eosiniphils (High power)

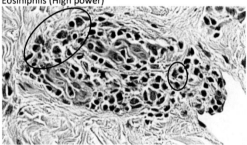

Path Presenter

- +/- Epidermal spongiosis with exocytosis and vacuolar change with rare apoptotic keratinocytes

OTHER HIGH YIELD POINTS

- Most commonly seen with the use of antibiotics (penicillin and sulfas), allopurinol, phenytoin, barbiturates, chlorpromazine, carbamazepine, gold, d-penicillamine, captopril, naproxen, piroxicam, etc.
- The eruption may occur even if the offending medication has already been discontinued
- Erythematous papules blanch with pressure, and thus can be differentiated from palpable purpura, which is indicative of vasculitis

DIFFERENTIAL DIAGNOSIS

LUPUS ERYTHEMATOSUS

- Hyperkeratosis, epidermal atrophy with follicular plugging
- Vacuolar interface dermatitis and thickening of basement membrane
- Superficial and deep perivascular and periadnexal lymphocytic infiltrate

PRODROMAL BULLOUS PEMPHIGOID

- Dermal inflammation with admixed eosinophils
- Eosinophilic exocytosis

ARTHROPOD BITE

- Classically, a dense, wedge-shaped superficial and deep perivascular and interstitial inflammatory infiltrate
- Eosinophils are a prominent finding, and are a useful clue when seen away from the vessels (interposed between collagen bundles) and in the deeper dermis
- The epidermis is variably spongiotic and mouth parts may be present at the center of the lesion which aids in diagnosis

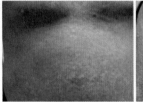 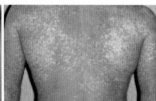 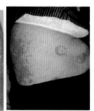

PHOTOTOXIC DERMATITIS

Path Presenter

CLINICAL FEATURES

- **Immediate/Mild** – Immediate onset of **erythema** occurring approximately **30 minutes** after UVL exposure. This reaction is associated with burning and pruritus but minimal edema It usually lasts for 1-2 days after stopping UVL exposure
- **Immediate/wheals** – Immediate onset of **transient wheals** associated with burning. This reaction can occur with room light (non-UVL) and resolves rapidly after light exposure is stopped
- **Delayed/Severe** – Onset is **8-24 hours** after UVL exposure and is associated with **dark erythema, edema, and hyperpigmentation. Blistering** may occur with severe reactions. It usually lasts 2-4 days after UVL exposure is stopped, but in some instances, it may persist for months

HISTOLOGIC FEATURES

- Prominent **dyskeratosis, more prominent in superficial epidermis**
- **Squamatization** of basal layer
- Papillary dermal edema

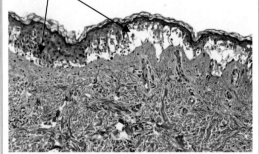
Prominent dyskeratosis

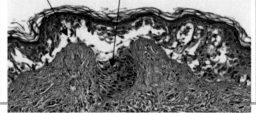
Dyskeratosis and squamatization

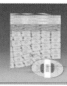

Mixed inflammatory infiltrate

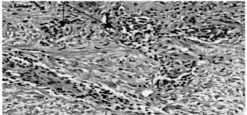

DEJ changes

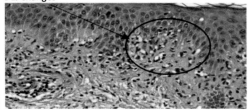

- Variable mixed perivascular infiltrate sometimes with admixed eosinophils

OTHER HIGH YIELD POINTS

- Implicated drugs include **tetracyclines, NSAIDs, sulfonamides**, thiazide diuretics, antiarrhythmics

DIFFERENTIAL DIAGNOSIS

SPONGIOTIC DRUG ERUPTION

- Parakeratosis overlying spongiosis
- A superficial and deep perivascular inflammatory infiltrate is commonly seen in the epidermis
- Eosinophils can be prominent within the dermal inflammatory infiltrate

IRRITANT CONTACT DERMATITIS

- Necrosis of epidermal keratinocytes: necrosis may be confluent or of individual keratinocytes
- Mild spongiosis
- Superficial perivascular infiltrate of lymphocytes

PITYRIASIS LICHENOIDES CHRONICA

- Parakeratotic scale, with scattered dyskeratotic cells in epidermis
- Upper dermal sparse inflammation, mostly lymphocytes, sometimes with scattered melanophages
- Focal vacuolar alteration at DEJ and dermal fibrosis
- Red cell extravasation

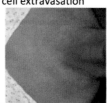
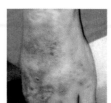
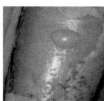

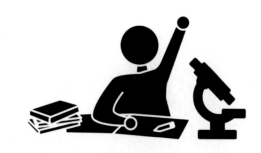

ACE MY PATH
Come Ace With Us!

CHAPTER 17: VESICULOBULLOUS
REACTION PATTERN

MICHAEL GREAS, MD

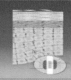
VESICULOBULLOUS DERMATOSES

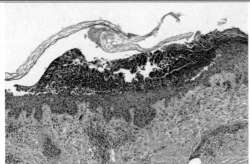
Subcorneal bulla with many neutrophils

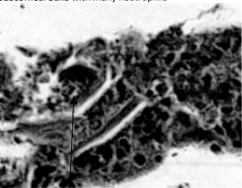
Gram positive cocci within the bulla

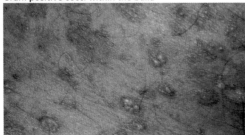
Pus filled bullae on erythematous background

BULLOUS IMPETIGO

CLINICAL FEATURES

- Common, highly **contagious** disease that affects infants, young children, and immunocompromised patients
- Commonly occurs on the face, flexures, and diaper area
- Presents as rapidly enlarging bullae that burst, leaving circinate, weepy **honey-colored** crusting
- Heals with no to minimal scarring

HISTOLOGIC FEATURES

- **Sub-corneal blister** with neutrophils and rare acantholytic cells
- **Gram positive cocci** usually seen within the bullae

IMMUNOFLUORESCENCE/IMMUNOHISTOCHEMISTRY

- Negative direct immunofluorescence (not required)

OTHER HIGH YIELD POINTS

- Culture is usually positive for S. aureus, phage group II type 71. The subcorneal split is due to exfoliative toxin A and B produced by S. aureus which result in cleavage of desmoglein-1

DIFFERENTIAL DIAGNOSIS

BULLOUS DERMATOPHYTOSIS

- Presence of fungal hyphae within the stratum corneum (PAS stain helps to visualize the fungal elements if not visible on H&E)

PEMPHIGUS FOLIACEUS

- Prominent acantholysis and an absence of bacterial cocci in the blister
- **DIF is positive for intercellular (net-like) staining for IgG and C3** predominately at the superficial layers of the epidermis

STAPHYLOCOCCAL SCALDED SKIN SYNDROME

- The subcorneal split is due to exfoliative toxin A and B produced by S. aureus which result in cleavage of desmoglein-1
- Pauci-inflammatory blister (absence of neutrophils unless secondary infected) without bacterial cocci in the blister
- Lack of epidermal necrosis and dyskeratotic cells with minimal dermal infiltrate

Path Presenter

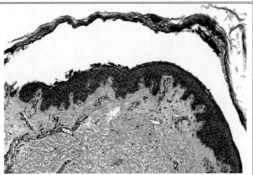
Subcorneal split with sparse dermal inflammation

STAPHYLOCOCCAL SCALDED SKIN SYNDROME (SSSS)

CLINICAL FEATURES

- Potentially life-threatening disorder and commonly affecting younger children
- Presents with acute fever, superficial erosions and peeling of skin that develops flaccid and easily ruptured bullae
- Mucous membrane spared except for conjunctivitis
- **Positive Nikolsky's sign**

HISTOLOGIC FEATURES

- Subcorneal split/bullae with rare acantholytic cells
- Sparse neutrophils can be seen within the bullae
- Sparse mixed dermal inflammation and perivascular edema

IMMUNOFLUORESCENCE/IMMUNOHISTOCHEMISTRY

- Negative direct immunofluorescence (not required)

OTHER HIGH YIELD POINTS

- The subcorneal split is due to **exfoliative toxin A and B produced by S. aureus** which result in **cleavage of desmoglein-1**

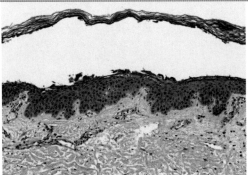
No significant acantholysis

DIFFERENTIAL DIAGNOSIS

BULLOUS DERMATOPHYTOSIS
- Presence of fungal hyphae within the stratum corneum (PAS stain helps to visualize the fungal elements if not visible on H&E)

PEMPHIGUS FOLIACEUS
- Prominent acantholysis and an absence of bacterial cocci in the blister
- **DIF is positive for intercellular (net-like) staining for IgG and C3** predominately at the superficial layers of the epidermis

BULLOUS IMPETIGO
- Subcorneal bulla with few neutrophils and rare acantholytic cells
- Gram positive cocci usually seen within the bullae

Path Presenter

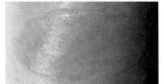
Superficial erosion and peeling of skin from flaccid and easily ruptured bullae

PEMPHIGUS FOLIACEUS (PF)

CLINICAL FEATURES
- Autoimmune blistering disorder that predominately affects the upper trunk, scalp and face. Widespread lesions presenting as exfoliative erythroderma can be also seen
- Blisters are superficial and fragile, rupturing easily and causing erosions and scale crust
- **No mucous membrane/oral involvement**

HISTOLOGIC FEATURES
- Subcorneal bullae and split with **acantholysis in the granular cell layer. Sometimes, the stratum corneum is completely sloughed off and not available in biopsy, leaving an erosion-epidermis present with missing cornified and granular layer and showing few acantholytic cells on surface**
- Variable acantholysis within the superficial epidermis
- Perivascular lymphocytic infiltrate with occasional eosinophils
- Early stage may show neutrophilic or eosinophilic spongiosis

IMMUNOFLUORESCENCE/IMMUNOHISTOCHEMISTRY
- **DIF is positive for intercellular (net-like) staining with IgG and C3** predominately at the **superficial** aspect of the epidermis
- Serum indirect immunofluorescence on **monkey esophagus** is positive for intercellular staining

OTHER HIGH YIELD POINTS
- Positive for serum **DSG1** and negative for serum DSG3
- **Associated with myasthenia gravis, thymoma, ACE inhibitors and penicillamine**

DIFFERENTIAL DIAGNOSIS

BULLOUS DERMATOPHYTOSIS
- Presence of fungal hyphae within the stratum corneum (PAS stain helps to visualize the fungal elements if not visible on H&E)

BULLOUS IMPETIGO
- Subcorneal bulla with few neutrophils and rare acantholytic cells
- Gram positive cocci usually seen within the bullae

STAPHYLOCOCCAL SCALDED SKIN SYNDROME
- The subcorneal split is due to exfoliative toxin A and B produced by S. aureus which result in cleavage of desmoglein-1

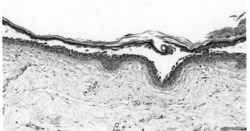
Subcorneal split with acantholysis in the granular cell layer

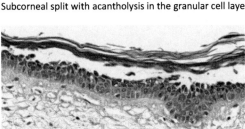
Variable acantholysis within the granular cell layer

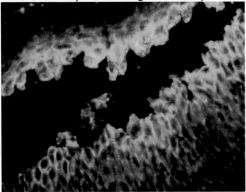
DIF is positive for intercellular (net-like) staining with IgG and C3 predominately in the superficial epidermis

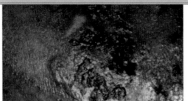

Blisters are superficial and fragile, causing erosions and scale crust

- Pauci-inflammatory blister (absence of neutrophils unless secondary infected) without bacterial cocci in the blister
- Lack of epidermal necrosis and dyskeratotic cells with minimal dermal infiltrate

Path Presenter

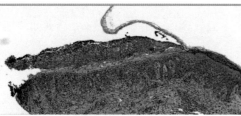

Subcorneal/mid-epidermal blister

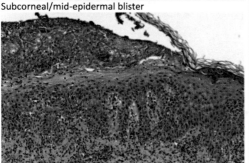

Blister cavity with many neutrophils and minimal acantholysis

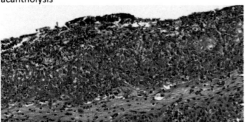

Path Presenter

PEMPHIGUS HERPETIFORMIS
CLINICAL FEATURES
- Clinical characteristics of dermatitis herpetiformis with the immunologic features of pemphigus (about 7% of pemphigus cases)
- Severe pruritic urticarial type plaques and vesicles in a herpetiform pattern with widespread distribution
- Uncommon mucous membrane involvement
HISTOLOGIC FEATURES
- Diffuse intraepidermal blister at the mid-epidermal level
- Blister cavity with many neutrophils and eosinophils
- Some acantholysis can be seen
IMMUNOFLUORESCENCE/IMMUNOHISTOCHEMISTRY
- DIF is positive for intercellular (net-like) staining with IgG and C3 predominately at the superficial aspect of the epidermis
OTHER HIGH YIELD POINTS
- Positive for serum **DSG1** and negative for serum DSG3
- Few cases are positive for DSG1 and DSG3
- **Associated with SLE, sarcoidosis, psoriasis, and solid tumors**
- **Can be drug induced: D-penicillamine and thiopronIne**
DIFFERENTIAL DIAGNOSIS
BULLOUS DERMATOPHYTOSIS
- Presence of fungal hyphae within the stratum corneum (PAS stain helps to visualize the fungal elements if not visible on H&E)
BULLOUS IMPETIGO
- Subcorneal bulla with few neutrophils and rare acantholytic cells
- Gram positive cocci usually seen within the bullae
STAPHYLOCOCCAL SCALDED SKIN SYNDROME
- The subcorneal split is due to exfoliative toxin A and B produced by S. aureus which result in cleavage of desmoglein-1
- Pauci-inflammatory blister (absence of neutrophils unless secondary infected) without bacterial cocci in the blister
- Lack of epidermal necrosis and dyskeratotic cells with minimal dermal infiltrate

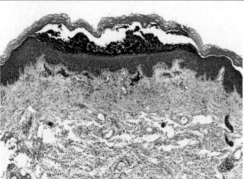

Subcorneal blister with many neutrophils

SUBCORNEAL PUSTULAR DERMATOSIS (aka Sneddon-Wilkinson disease)
CLINICAL FEATURES
- Older adults (4th to 5th decade of life)
- Recurrent crops of sterile pustules with annular or serpiginous distribution, especially in the intertriginous areas
- Usually spares the face and mucous membranes
- Flaccid pustules which can be **gravity dependent.** May be pruritic or painful
HISTOLOGIC FEATURES
- **Subcorneal** blisters with **many neutrophils (e.g., subcorneal pustule)**
- Acantholytic keratinocytes with papillary dermal edema
- Perivascular infiltrate composed of lymphocytes and neutrophils
IMMUNOFLUORESCENCE/IMMUNOHISTOCHEMISTRY
- **DIF is negative, distinguishing it from IgA pemphigus**

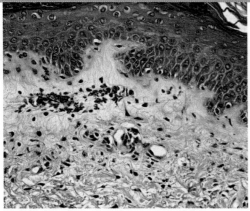

Papillary dermal edema with sparse superficial perivascular lymphocytic infiltrate and extravasted red blood cells

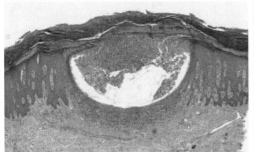

Pustular psoriasis: subcorneal and intraepidermal neutrophils, acanthosis and parakeratosis

Path Presenter

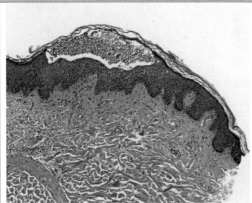

Subcorneal blister with many neutrophils

Path Presenter

OTHER HIGH YIELD POINTS
- Can be associated with **monoclonal gammopathy of IgA type** or **IgG MGUS (monoclonal gammopathy of undetermined significance)**

DIFFERENTIAL DIAGNOSIS

PUSTULAR PSORIASIS/ACUTE GENERALIZED EXANTHEMATOUS PUSTULOSIS
- Subcorneal and intraepidermal neutrophilic collections
- Acanthosis can be seen
- Parakeratosis with underlying hypogranulosis
- Dilated papillary dermal capillaries

IGA PEMPHIGUS
- DIF shows intercellular IgA deposition
- Other histologic features overlap with SPD

BULLOUS DERMATOPHYTOSIS
- Presence of fungal hyphae within the stratum corneum (PAS stain helps to visualize the fungal elements if not visible on H&E)

BULLOUS IMPETIGO
- Subcorneal bulla with few neutrophils and rare acantholytic cells
- Gram positive cocci usually seen within the bullae

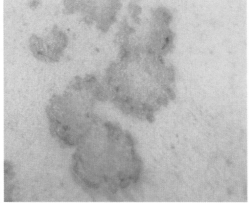

Recurrent crops of pustules with annular distribution

IGA PEMPHIGUS

CLINICAL FEATURES
- Recurrent crops of sterile pruritic pustules with **annular or serpiginous** pattern, especially in the intertriginous areas
- The pustules can be eroded, resulting in crusted plaques
- Commonly affects the trunk and proximal extremities
- No mucosal membrane involvement

HISTOLOGIC FEATURES
- **Two histologic presentations -Subcorneal pustular dermatosis or Intraepidermal neutrophilic dermatosis**
- Acantholytic keratinocytes with papillary dermal edema
- Perivascular infiltrate composed of lymphocytes and neutrophils
- Many subtypes- can histologically mimic pemphigus foliaceus, pemphigus vulgaris, subcorneal pustular dermatosis, and pemphigus vegetans

IMMUNOFLUORESCENCE/IMMUNOHISTOCHEMISTRY
- **Perilesional DIF is positive** for **intercellular deposition of IgA**

OTHER HIGH YIELD POINTS
- Can be associated with **monoclonal gammopathy of IgA type** or **IgG MGUS (monoclonal gammopathy of undetermined significance), multiple myeloma, and B-cell lymphomas**

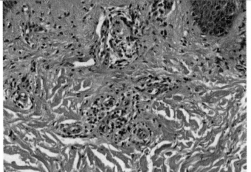

Sparse superficial perivascular lymphocytic infiltrate with rare neutrophils

DIFFERENTIAL DIAGNOSIS

PUSTULAR PSORIASIS
- Subcorneal and intraepidermal neutrophilic collections
- Acanthosis can be seen
- Parakeratosis with underlying hypogranulosis
- Dilated papillary dermal capillaries

SUBCORNEAL PUSTULAR DERMATOSIS
- Negative DIF (other histologic features overlap with IgA pemphigus)

AUTOIMMUNE BLISTERING DISORDERS (OTHERS)
- Other histologic subtypes may mimic-such as pemphigus vulgaris, pemphigus foliaceus, and pemphigus vegetans. DIF and serologies needed for confirmation

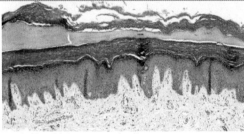

Acral skin with intra-corneal split

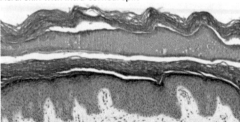

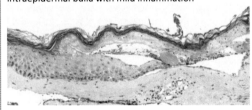

Bullous diabeticorum showing subcorneal and intraepidermal bulla with mild inflammation

Path Presenter

FRICTION BLISTER

CLINICAL FEATURES
- Tense blisters that occur at sites with combined pressure and friction
- The most common site is the heel from ill-fitting footwear

HISTOLOGIC FEATURES
- Classically, **intraepidermal split** beneath the granular cell layer, however, intra-corneal split can be also seen
- Focal to diffuse **necrosis** in the **mid-epidermis**
- Sparse superficial perivascular lymphocytic infiltrate

IMMUNOFLUORESCENCE/IMMUNOHISTOCHEMISTRY
- **DIF is negative (not required)**

OTHER HIGH YIELD POINTS
- Clinical diagnosis and biopsies are not usually needed

DIFFERENTIAL DIAGNOSIS

SUCTION BLISTER
- Subepidermal split can look similar histologically, clinical history needed

BULLOUS DIABETICORUM
- Subcorneal or intraepidermal bulla with mild inflammation
- The roof of the epidermis can have necrotic keratinocytes
- Clinical history needed

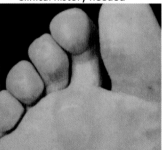

Friction blister on plantar foot

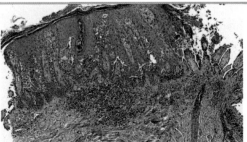

Diffuse suprabasal intraepidermal blister with acantholysis

PEMPHIGUS VULGARIS (PV)

CLINICAL FEATURES
- Autoimmune blistering disorder affecting young adults (4th-6th decade) with no gender predilection
- Flaccid blisters with predilection for the trunk, groin, axilla, scalp, and face
- **Mucosal involvement** is common (mostly oral ulcers)
- **Can be drug induced- D-penicillamine and captopril**

HISTOLOGIC FEATURES
- Diffuse **suprabasal intraepidermal blister** with **acantholysis creating a "tombstoning" effect**

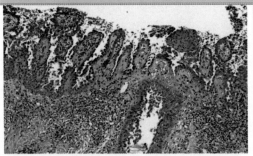
Tombstoning and follicular involvement

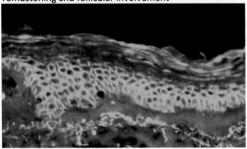
DIF is positive for intercellular (net-like) IgG and C3
Path Presenter

- **Follicular extension** of **acantholysis**
- Superficial perivascular lymphocytic infiltrate with eosinophils

IMMUNOFLUORESCENCE/IMMUNOHISTOCHEMISTRY

- **DIF** is positive for **intercellular (net-like) staining with IgG and C3**
- **Indirect immunofluorescence** on **monkey esophagus** shows **intercellular** staining with **IgG and C3**

OTHER HIGH YIELD POINTS

- **Lesional** biopsy is for routine **H&E** and **perilesional biopsy** is for **DIF**
- **Mucosal PV** is positive for **desmoglein 3** antibodies and negative for desmoglein 1
- **Mucocutaneous PV** is positive for **desmoglein 3 and desmoglein 1**
- Associated with **internal malignancies, thymoma, myasthenia gravis, Castleman's disease, and autoimmune diseases**
- **ELISA circulating antibodies to DSG3 or DSG3 and DSG1**

DIFFERENTIAL DIAGNOSIS

DARIER'S DISEASE

- Negative DIF

HAILEY-HAILEY DISEASE

- Negative DIF

PARANEOPLASTIC PEMPHIGUS

- Diffuse suprabasal intraepidermal blister with acantholysis and vacuolar or lichenoid interface changes
- DIF: **Intercellular IgG and C3** staining and **linear basement membrane** staining with **IgG and C3**

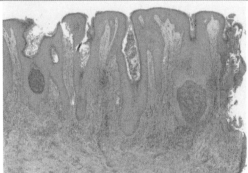
Pseudoepitheliomatous hyperlasia and acanthosis with pustules

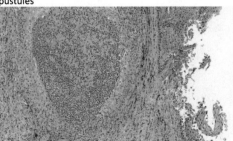
Dense intraepidermal and dermal eosinophilic infiltrate with few acantholytic cells
Path Presenter

PEMPHIGUS VEGETANS

CLINICAL FEATURES

- **Vegetative variant** of pemphigus vulgaris
- Presents with erosions and vesicles involving the oral cavity and scalp that evolve to hypertrophic verrucous plaques studded with pustules

HISTOLOGIC FEATURES

- **Prominent acanthosis** and papillomatosis with **few acantholytic cells**
- **Eosinophilic/neutrophilic pustules** present in the epidermis
- Dense infiltrate of eosinophils within the epidermis and dermis

IMMUNOFLUORESCENCE/IMMUNOHISTOCHEMISTRY

- **DIF** is positive for **intercellular (net-like) staining** with **IgG and C3**
- **Indirect immunofluorescence** on **monkey esophagus** shows **intercellular** staining with **IgG and C3**

OTHER HIGH YIELD POINTS

- Associated with inflammatory bowel disease, such as ulcerative colitis and Crohn's disease

DIFFERENTIAL DIAGNOSIS

INCONTINENTIA PIGMENTI

- Negative DIF

PARANEOPLASTIC PEMPHIGUS

- Diffuse suprabasal intraepidermal blister with acantholysis and vacuolar or lichenoid interface changes
- DIF: Intercellular IgG and C3 staining and linear basement membrane staining with IgG and C3 (pemphigus vegetans without basement membrane staining)

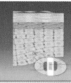
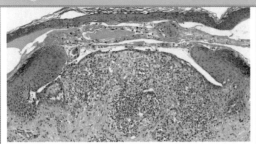

Suprabasal intraepidermal acantholysis with interface changes and lichenoid inflammation

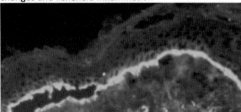

DIF is positive for intercellular (net-like) and basement membrane zone staining with IgG and C3

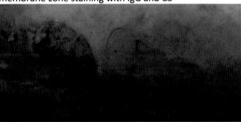

Cutaneous erosions from paraneoplastic pemphigus

Path Presenter

PARANEOPLASTIC PEMPHIGUS (PNP)
CLINICAL FEATURES
- Affects **older men** with **hematologic malignancies**
- Presents as cutaneous and **painful oral erosions** extending to the vermilion, in addition with polymorphous cutaneous lesions
- It can affect conjunctivae, esophagus, nasopharynx, vagina, or penis

HISTOLOGIC FEATURES
- Three patterns:
  1. PV-like pattern
  2. Diffuse suprabasal intraepidermal acantholysis with vacuolar or lichenoid interface changes
  3. Sometimes acantholysis is very subtle. Clue is acantholysis with lichenoid inflammation

IMMUNOFLUORESCENCE/IMMUNOHISTOCHEMISTRY
- **DIF is** positive for **intercellular (net-like) and basement membrane zone** staining with **IgG and C3**
- **Shaggy BMZ** staining with **fibrinogen**
- Indirect IF: IgG intercellular staining on **rat bladder**
- Salt split skin IF: IgG basement membrane zone staining on the epidermal aspect of split

OTHER HIGH YIELD POINTS
- Associated with **non-Hodgkin lymphoma, benign and malignant thymomas, chronic lymphocytic leukemia and Castleman's disease**
- Variable antigens are involved: **desmoplakin I** (250 kD), **BPAG1** (230 kD), **envoplakin** (210 kD) and **periplakin** (190 kD)

DIFFERENTIAL DIAGNOSIS
PEMPHIGUS VULGARIS
- No basement membrane zone staining with IgG and C3 on DIF
- No interface changes and uncommon lichenoid inflammatory infiltrate

LICHENOID DRUG ERUPTION
- Superficial and deep perivascular lymphocytic infiltrate admixed with eosinophils. Negative DIF

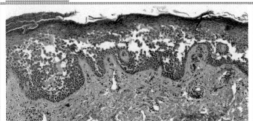

Diffuse intraepidermal acantholysis at all levels of epidermis resembling dilapidated brick wall

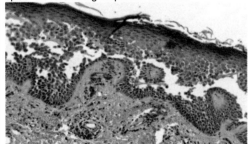

Intraepidermal acantholysis

HAILEY-HAILEY DISEASE
CLINICAL FEATURES
- Also known as benign familial pemphigus
- Onset in **young adults** in their twenties or thirties. **Predilection for intertriginous areas and axilla**
- Recurrent erythematous and vesicular red fissured plaques with subsequent crusting
- Prone to secondary infection. No mucous membrane involvement

HISTOLOGIC FEATURES
- **Diffuse intraepidermal acantholysis** at all levels of epidermis, with partial retention of cell orientation, resembling **a "dilapidated brick wall"**
- Focal dyskeratosis and perivascular lymphocytic infiltrate
- **Follicular sparing**

IMMUNOFLUORESCENCE/IMMUNOHISTOCHEMISTRY
- **DIF is negative**

OTHER HIGH YIELD POINTS
- Autosomal dominant disease with mutation in **ATP2C1** which encodes a Ca++ transport pump in the Golgi apparatus

DIFFERENTIAL DIAGNOSIS
PEMPHIGUS VULGARIS
- **Follicular involvement** by acantholysis
- **Positive DIF** (intercellular staining with IgG and C3)

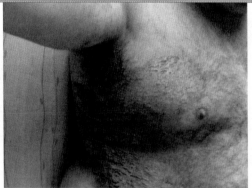

Recurrent erythematous and vesicular plaques with subsequent rupture leaving a crusted plaque

DARIER'S DISEASE

- **Presence of corps ronds and grains**
- Hyperkeratosis, acanthosis, and papillomatosis
- Predominately **suprabasal** acantholysis with dyskeratosis
- Negative DIF

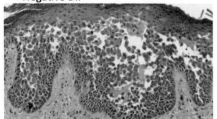

Path Presenter

Dilapidated brick wall appearance

DARIER'S DISEASE

CLINICAL FEATURES

- Also known as keratosis follicularis and dyskeratosis follicularis
- **Malodorous** greasy, red-brown papules on the trunk, face, and intertriginous areas **(seborrheic distribution)**
- Palmoplantar pits, acrokeratosis and oral cobblestone lesions
- **Nails** with longitudinal **erythro/leukonychia**, subungual hyperkeratosis, and **V-shaped nicking**

HISTOLOGIC FEATURES

- Hyperkeratosis, acanthosis, and papillomatosis
- Multiple focal **suprabasal acantholysis** with **dyskeratosis and presence of corps ronds and grains**

IMMUNOFLUORESCENCE/IMMUNOHISTOCHEMISTRY

- **DIF is negative**

OTHER HIGH YIELD POINTS

- Autosomal dominant disease with mutation in **ATP2A2** gene
- Associated with psychiatric disorders and epilepsy
- Lithium and oral steroids may exacerbate

DIFFERENTIAL DIAGNOSIS

HAILEY-HAILEY DISEASE

- Diffuse intraepidermal acantholysis at all levels of epidermis resembling a "dilapidated brick wall"
- Follicular sparing and absence of corps ronds and grains

PEMPHIGUS VULGARIS

- Diffuse suprabasal acantholysis with follicular involvement
- Positive DIF (intercellular staining with IgG and C3)

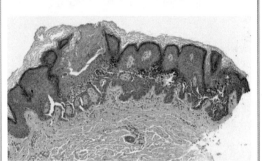

Hyperkeratosis, acanthosis and papillomatosis with suprabasal acantholysis

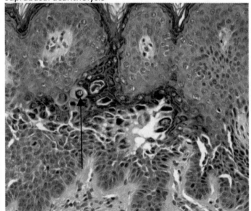

Corps ronds

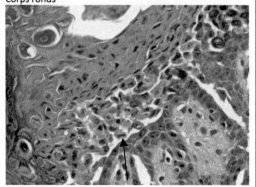

Grains

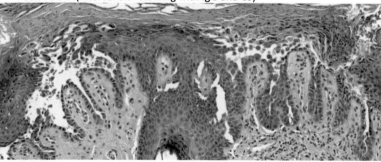

Path Presenter

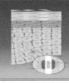
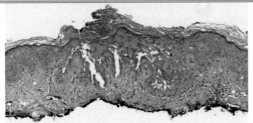

Focal acantholytic dyskeratosis with overlying parakeratosis

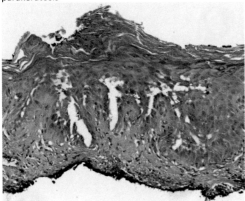

No significant dyskeratosis in this histologic variant

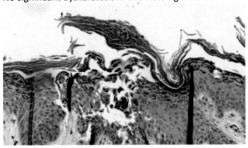

Path Presenter

GROVER'S DISEASE

CLINICAL FEATURES

- Also known as transient acantholytic dyskeratosis
- Most frequently affects middle-aged or elderly males
- Presents as **small, itchy, discrete** red-tan keratotic **papules** with a predilection for **chest and back**

HISTOLOGIC FEATURES

- **Five histologic patterns: pemphigus-like, Darier's-like, Hailey-Hailey-like, spongiotic, and superficial pemphigus-like**
- Focal acantholytic dyskeratosis with overlying parakeratosis or scale crust

IMMUNOFLUORESCENCE/IMMUNOHISTOCHEMISTRY

- **DIF is negative**

OTHER HIGH YIELD POINTS

- Requires clinical and pathologic correlation due to overlap in histologic features with Darier's disease, pemphigus vulgaris, and Hailey-Hailey disease

DIFFERENTIAL DIAGNOSIS

HAILEY-HAILEY DISEASE
- Diffuse intraepidermal acantholysis at all levels of epidermis resembling a "dilapidated brick wall"
- Follicular sparing and absence of corps ronds and grains

PEMPHIGUS VULGARIS
- Diffuse suprabasal acantholysis with follicular involvement
- Positive DIF (intercellular staining with IgG and C3)

DARIER'S DISEASE
- Hyperkeratosis, acanthosis, and papillomatosis
- Multiple focal suprabasal acantholysis with dyskeratosis and presence of corps ronds and grains

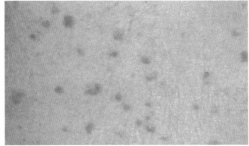

Small, discrete, red-tan keratotic papules

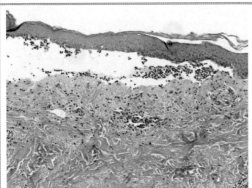

Subepidermal blisters with eosinophils

BULLOUS PEMPHIGOID (BP)

CLINICAL FEATURES

- Usually affects **older adults.** Early lesions may be papular or urticarial
- Clinically presents as **tense bullae that are exquisitely pruritic**
- **May have crusted erosions on the trunk and extremities**
- Mucosal membranes can be involved but not in most

HISTOLOGIC FEATURES

- **Subepidermal blister** with **eosinophils**
- At the edge of the blister, **eosinophilic spongiosis** is often seen as well as eosinophils lining up along the dermal-epidermal junction
- A superficial **perivascular and interstitial** inflammatory infiltrate of lymphocytes and **eosinophils** is present in the dermis
- The **urticarial** variant of BP may clinically only demonstrate eosinophilic spongiosis
- BP can also be cell poor or neutrophilic rich

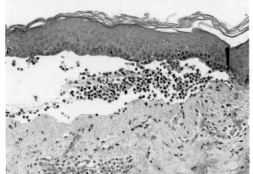

Blister cavity including many eosinophils

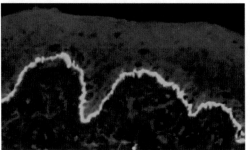

DIF is positive for linear deposition of IgG and C3 at the basement membrane zone on perilesional biopsy

Path Presenter

IMMUNOFLUORESCENCE/IMMUNOHISTOCHEMISTRY
- **DIF** is positive for **linear deposition of IgG and C3 at the basement membrane zone** on perilesional biopsy with an **N-shaped serrated pattern**
- Indirect immunofluorescence: IgG deposition at basement membrane zone
- **Salt Split Skin: IgG at basement membrane zone** on the **epidermal side** of the blister

OTHER HIGH YIELD POINTS
- Autoantibodies to **BPAG1** and **BPAG2** on **hemidesmosomes** at dermal epidermal junction
- **Intralamina lucida blister**
- **Drug-induced** pemphigoid: diuretics (**furosemide**), **captopril**, amoxicillin, etc.
- Salt-split skin can distinguish between BP and epidermolysis bullosa acquisita

DIFFERENTIAL DIAGNOSIS

LINEAR IGA BULLOUS DERMATOSIS
- Linearly aligned neutrophils along the DEJ with subepidermal blister and papillary dermal edema
- DIF is positive for linear IgA basement membrane zone staining

EPIDERMOLYSIS BULLOSA ACQUISITA
- Salt split skin shows IgG deposition at the dermal side of the blister

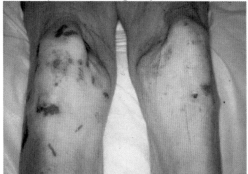

Crusted erosions on the lower legs developing after tense bullae

HERPES GESTATIONIS

CLINICAL FEATURES
- Autoimmune blistering disorder **affecting pregnant woman**
- Also known as gestational pemphigoid
- Typically affect patients in their **second or third trimester**
- Presents as pruritic erythematous or urticarial papules that evolve into vesicles and bullae around the umbilicus and then spread to the trunk and extremities
- It resolves within the first few months of the postpartum period and may recur with subsequent pregnancies

HISTOLOGIC FEATURES
- **Subepidermal blister** with **eosinophils**
- At the edge of the blister, **eosinophilic spongiosis** is often seen
- A superficial **perivascular and interstitial** inflammatory infiltrate of lymphocytes and eosinophils is present in the dermis

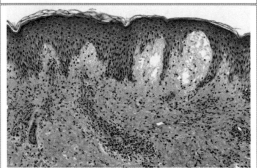

Marked subepidermal edema with superificial perivascular lymphocytic infiltrate including eosinophils

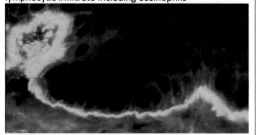

DIF is positive for linear deposition of C3 at the basement membrane zone on perilesional biopsy

IMMUNOFLUORESCENCE/IMMUNOHISTOCHEMISTRY
- **DIF** is positive for **linear deposition of C3** at the **basement membrane zone** on perilesional biopsy
- Linear basement membrane deposition of IgG in about 50% of cases

OTHER HIGH YIELD POINTS
- Autoantibodies to **BPAG1 and BPAG2** on hemidesmosomes at DEJ
- **Intralamina lucida blister. The circulating IgG antibodies are called HG factor**
- Associated with HLA-DR3, HLA-DR4 and IgG1 (fixes complement)

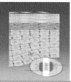

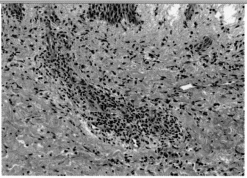

Superficial perivascular and interstitial inflammatory infiltrate with many eosinophils

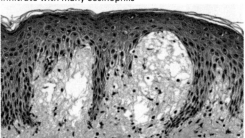

Path Presenter

- **Neonates** of affected mothers can **develop transient blistering** due to placental transfer of antibodies

DIFFERENTIAL DIAGNOSIS

PRURITIC URTICARIAL PAPULES AND PLAQUES OF PREGNANCY
- Focal parakeratosis and spongiosis
- Perivascular lymphocytic infiltrate with interstitial eosinophils
- **DIF is negative**

ARHTROPOD BITE REACTION
- Superficial and deep perivascular lymphocytic infiltrate with eosinophils
- **DIF is negative**

BULLOUS DRUG REACTION
- Superficial and deep perivascular lymphocytic infiltrate with eosinophils
- **DIF is negative**

LINEAR IGA BULLOUS DERMATOSIS
- Linearly aligned neutrophils along the DEJ with subepidermal blistering and papillary dermal edema
- DIF is positive for linear IgA basement membrane zone staining

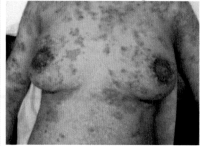

Denuded and crusted blisters on the trunk and extremities

DERMATITIS HERPETIFORMIS

CLINICAL FEATURES
- Autoimmune blistering disorder associated with **gluten-sensitive** enteropathy
- Most common in Caucasian males, usually in their second to fourth decades
- Presents as **extremely pruritic**, small blisters, urticarial papules/plaques that classically affect **elbows, buttocks**, posterior scalp, knees, and back in a symmetrical fashion
- The lesions often heal with scarring
- Mucous membrane involvement is uncommon

HISTOLOGIC FEATURES
- **Subepidermal blister** that contains predominately **neutrophils** and rare eosinophils
- **Neutrophilic microabscesses** within the **dermal papillae**
- Superficial perivascular lymphocytic infiltrate can be also seen

IMMUNOFLUORESCENCE/IMMUNOHISTOCHEMISTRY
- **Perilesional DIF** is positive for **granular IgA deposition** in the **dermal papillae**
- Linear basement membrane staining with IgA can be also seen

OTHER HIGH YIELD POINTS
- Associated with **HLA-A1, HLA-B8, HLA-DR3 and HLA-DQ2**
- Considered by many as Celiac disease of skin; however, only 10-20 percent of CD patients exhibit features of DH
- Intralamina lucida blister
- **Circulating IgA anti-endomysial antibodies to tissue transglutaminase (TTG)**

DIFFERENTIAL DIAGNOSIS

LINEAR IGA BULLOUS DERMATOSIS
- Linearly aligned neutrophils along the DEJ with subepidermal blister and papillary dermal edema

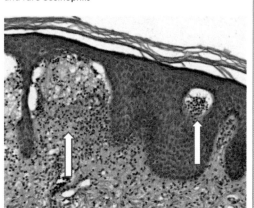

Subepidermal blister containing predominately neutrophils and rare eosinophils

Neutrophilic microabscesses within the dermal papillae

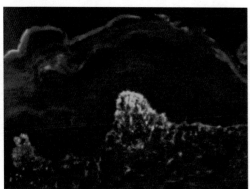

DIF is positive for granular IgA deposition in the dermal papillae

Path Presenter

- Classically lacks the neutrophilic dermal papillae microabscesses
- DIF is positive for linear IgA basement membrane zone staining

BULLOUS PEMPHIGOID

- Subepidermal blister with eosinophils
- At the edge of the blister, eosinophilic spongiosis is often seen
- DIF is positive for linear IgG and C3 deposition at the BMZ

SWEET'S SYNDROME

- Negative DIF

BULLOUS LUPUS ERYTHEMATOSUS

- **Interface changes** along with **increased dermal mucin** can be seen
- **DIF** of perilesional skin is positive for **linear and/or granular deposition of IgG and/or IgA, IgM and C3 at the basement membrane zone**

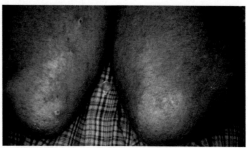

Extremely pruritic, small blisters, urticarial papules/plaques

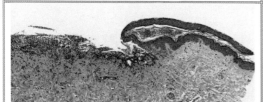

Subepidermal blister

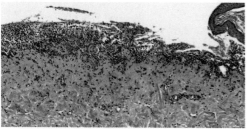

Linearly aligned neutrophils at the DEJ

LINEAR IGA BULLOUS DERMATOSIS

CLINICAL FEATURES

- Autoimmune blistering disorder commonly affecting skin and mucous membranes; can exclusively affect only mucous membranes
- Can be induced by medications, the most common being **vancomycin**
- The childhood variant is known as chronic bullous disease of childhood
- **Annular** erythematous patches with **tense blisters at the edge**, the so-called **"string of pearls"** sign
- Commonly affects the trunk and extremities
- The cutaneous lesions can mimic erythema multiforme, dermatitis herpetiformis, or bullous pemphigoid
- **Mucous membrane involvement** is **common**

HISTOLOGIC FEATURES

- **Subepidermal blister** with papillary dermal edema
- **Linearly aligned neutrophils at the DEJ**
- Superficial perivascular and interstitial neutrophilic infiltrate admixed with lymphocytes and eosinophils can also be seen

IMMUNOFLUORESCENCE/IMMUNOHISTOCHEMISTRY

- **DIF** of perilesional skin is positive for **linear IgA deposition at the basement membrane zone**
- Salt Split Skin: linear IgA deposition on both sides of the split (epidermal and dermal)

OTHER HIGH YIELD POINTS

- **Intralamina lucida blister**
- Circulating IgG autoantibodies to **BPAG1 and/or BPAG2**

DIFFERENTIAL DIAGNOSIS

BULLOUS PEMPHIGOID

- Subepidermal blister with eosinophils
- At the edge of the blister, eosinophilic spongiosis is often seen
- DIF is positive for linear IgG and C3 deposition at the basement membrane zone

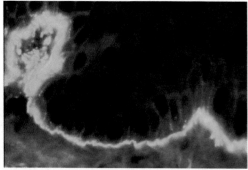

DIF of perilesional skin is positive for linear IgA deposition at the basement membrane zone

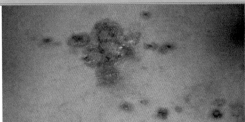

Annular plaque with blisters at the periphery, "string of pearls"

BULLOUS IMPETIGO
- Subcorneal bulla with few neutrophils and rare acantholytic cells
- Gram positive cocci usually seen withing the bullae
- DIF is negative

Path Presenter

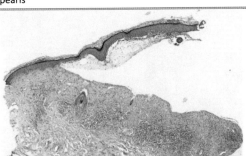

Subepidermal blister with variable inflammation and band-like inflammatory infiltrate

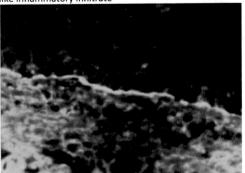

DIF of perilesional skin is positive for linear IgG and/or IgA and C3 deposition at the basement membrane zone

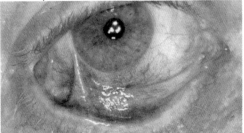

Symblepheron (conjunctival adhesion)

MUCOUS MEMBRANE PEMPHIGOID
Path Presenter

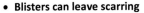

CLINICAL FEATURES
- Also known as **cicatricial pemphigoid**
- Mainly affects **elderly** people and is more common in females
- It predominately affects the **squamous mucosa** of the mouth, conjunctive, nasopharynx, genitalia, larynx, and esophagus
- **Blisters can leave scarring**
- **Can present as desquamative gingivitis**

HISTOLOGIC FEATURES
- **Subepithelial blister** with variable inflammation composed of lymphocytes, eosinophils, and/or neutrophils
- **Subepithelial fibrosis may be also seen**
- Occasionally band-like inflammatory infiltrate with plasma cells and neutrophils can be seen **(mimics lichen planus)**

IMMUNOFLUORESCENCE/IMMUNOHISTOCHEMISTRY
- **DIF of perilesional skin is positive for linear IgG and/or IgA and C3 deposition** at the **basement membrane zone**

OTHER HIGH YIELD POINTS
- Intralamina lucida blister
- Circulating IgG autoantibodies to **BPAG1 and/or BPAG2**
- **Anti-laminin 332** is strongly associated with underlying **solid organ malignancy** (the only variant that shows **dermal staining on salt-split skin**)
- **β4-subunit of α6β4 integrin** is seen exclusively in **ocular** involvement
- **Brunsting-Perry** variant: lesions limited to the cutaneous **head and neck** with **scarring alopecia** and **no mucosal involvement**

DIFFERENTIAL DIAGNOSIS
BULLOUS PEMPHIGOID
- Subepidermal blister with eosinophils
- At the edge of the blister, eosinophilic spongiosis is often seen
- DIF is positive for linear IgG and C3 deposition at the basement membrane zone

EROSIVE LICHEN PLANUS
- The histologic features may overlap with cicatricial pemphigoid
- DIF is positive for IgM and C3 in civatte bodies; however negative for linear IgG, C3, and IgA staining of the basement zone

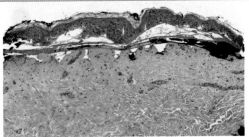

Subepidermal blister

EPIDERMOLYSIS BULLOSA ACQUISITA
CLINICAL FEATURES
- Subepidermal blistering disease that affect adults, but also has been documented in children
- Three main clinical variants: classic, inflammatory, and mucosal
- Classic variant: characterized by **trauma-induced blisters** and erosions on the **extensor surfaces** of the limbs which heals with scar and **milia formation**
- Inflammatory variant: bullous pemphigoid- like presentation
- Mucosal variant: cicatricial pemphigoid-like presentation

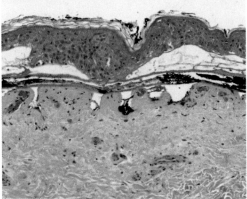

Sparse inflammation

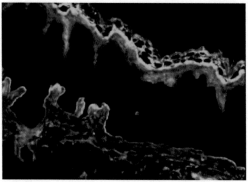

DIF of perilesional skin is positive for linear IgG and C3 deposition at the basement membrane zone in a U-shaped serrated pattern

Path Presenter

HISTOLOGIC FEATURES

- **Subepithelial cell-poor blister** with fibrin deposition on the floor of blister cavity
- **Dermal scar and milia** may be seen in **late lesions**
- Histologically can **overlap** with **bullous pemphigoid in inflammatory and mucosal variant**
- Neutrophils can be present within the inflammatory infiltrate

IMMUNOFLUORESCENCE/IMMUNOHISTOCHEMISTRY

- **DIF** of perilesional skin is positive for **linear IgG and C3 deposition at the basement membrane zone in a U-shaped serrated pattern**
- Occasional cases may have additional linear IgA deposition
- **Salt Split Skin: IgG at basement membrane** zone on the **dermal side**

OTHER HIGH YIELD POINTS

- **Sublamina densa blister**
- Circulating IgG autoantibodies to **collagen type VII**

DIFFERENTIAL DIAGNOSIS

BULLOUS PEMPHIGOID

- **Subepidermal blister** with **eosinophils**
- **DIF: U-serrated pattern** of linear IgG and C3 deposition at the BMZ
- **Salt Split Skin:** IgG at basement membrane zone on the **epidermal side** of the blister

CICATRICIAL PEMPHIGOID

- **Subepithelial blister** with variable inflammation composed of lymphocytes, eosinophils, and/or neutrophils
- **DIF** of perilesional skin is positive for **linear IgG and/or IgA and C3 deposition** at the **basement membrane zone**

LINEAR IGA BULLOUS DERMATOSIS

- Subepidermal blister with papillary dermal edema
- Linearly aligned neutrophils at the DEJ
- **DIF positive for linear IgA deposition** at the **basement membrane zone**

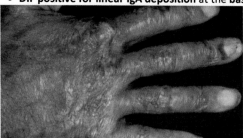

Trauma-induced blisters and erosions which heals with scar and milia formation

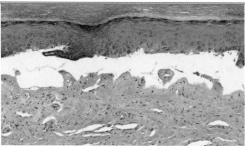

Festooning of the dermal papillae and solar elastosis

Path Presenter

PORPHYRIA CUTANEA TARDA (PCT)

CLINICAL FEATURES

- Reduced activity of **uroporphyrinogen decarboxylase enzyme (UROD)**
- **Sporadic/acquired variant** has dysfunctional enzyme in liver only
- **Autosomal dominant variant** has dysfunctional enzyme in all tissue
- Skin fragility with blistering, erosions, and crust
- Associated with **photosensitivity, hypertrichosis, scarring alopecia** and **sclerodermoid** changes
- Predominant on dorsal hands; however, can affect any sun-exposed or mechanically stressed site
- The skin lesions heal with **scarring** and **milia formation**

HISTOLOGIC FEATURES

- **Subepithelial blister** with **festooning of the dermal papillae**
- Sparse perivascular and interstitial lymphoid infiltrate

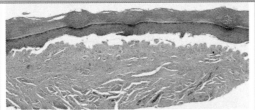
Pauci-inflammatory subepidermal blister

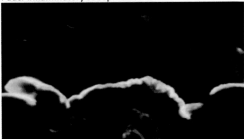
DIF positive for linear C3 at the basement membrane zone and occasionally IgG, IgM, and IgA

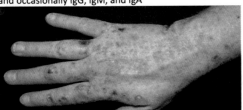
Tense blisters, erosions, and crusts that heal with scarring and milia formation

- Prominent solar elastosis and the presence of caterpillar bodies (pink basement membrane material in the epidermis)
- Thickened vessel walls within the papillary dermis, can be highlighted by PAS stain

IMMUNOFLUORESCENCE/IMMUNOHISTOCHEMISTRY
- DIF positive for linear C3 around dermal vessels and occasionally at the basement membrane zone. Occasionally may also stain with IgG, IgM, and IgA

OTHER HIGH YIELD POINTS
- Intralamina lucida blister
- Elevated total porphyrin levels in urine (24-hour urine testing needed)
- Patient's urine will get darker after exposure of natural light and will fluoresce under Wood's lamp light
- Isocoproporphyrin in feces
- Raised serum ferritin in most patients
- Associated with hemochromatosis, hepatitis C infection, and hepatocellular carcinoma

DIFFERENTIAL DIAGNOSIS
PSEUDOPORPHYRIA
- Histologic features can overlap with PCT
- Normal UROD enzyme activity

EPIDERMOLYSIS BULLOSA ACQUISITA
- Histologic features can overlap with PCT
- DIF positive for linear deposition of IgG and C3 at the basement membrane zone
- Salt split skin shows IgG deposition at the dermal side of the blister

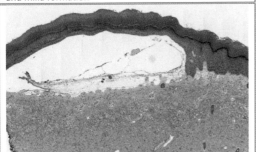
Subepidermal blister

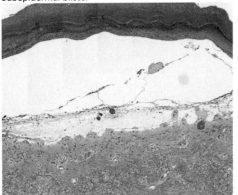
No significant inflammatory infiltrate and prominent solar elastosis

PSEUDOPORPHYRIA
CLINICAL FEATURES
- Normal activity of uroporphyrinogen decarboxylase (UROD)
- Similar presentation to PCT with photo distributed blisters with scar and milia formation. The hypertrichosis and sclerodermatous changes of PCT are NOT seen
- Commonly seen in patients undergoing hemodialysis and chronic renal insufficiency
- Commonly associated drugs: NSAIDs (naproxen), thiazides, furosemide, nalidixic acid and tetracycline

HISTOLOGIC FEATURES
- Subepidermal blister with minimal inflammation
- Prominent solar elastosis and thickened vessel walls in papillary dermis, highlighted by PAS stain

IMMUNOFLUORESCENCE/IMMUNOHISTOCHEMISTRY
- DIF is positive for C3 and/or IgG staining around the dermal vessels and/or the basement membrane zone staining

DIFFERENTIAL DIAGNOSIS
PORPHYRIA CUTANEA TARDA
- Histologic features can overlap with pseudoporphyria
- Prominent solar elastosis and thickened vessel walls in the papillary dermis
- Reduced UROD enzyme activity

EPIDERMOLYSIS BULLOSA ACQUISITA
- Histologic features can overlap with pseudoporphyria
- DIF of perilesional skin is positive for linear deposition of IgG and C3 at the basement membrane zone

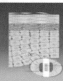

Path Presenter

- **Salt split skin** shows **IgG deposition at the dermal side** of the blister

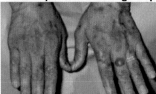

Tense blisters, erosions, and crusts that heal with scarring and milia formation

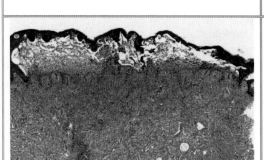

Subepidermal blister with neutrophils within the papillary dermis in a diffuse pattern

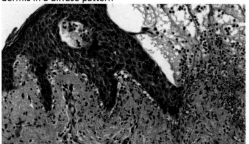

Interface changes and prominent neutrophils within the papillar dermis

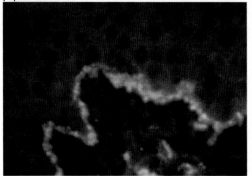

DIF with positive linear and/or granular deposition of IgG and/or IgA, IgM and C3 at the basement membrane zone

BULLOUS SYSTEMIC LUPUS ERYTHEMATOSUS
CLINICAL FEATURES
- Most commonly affects young black females
- Tense herpetiform bullae that affect predominately sun-exposed skin
- Trunk and flexural sites are commonly affected
- Oral lesions can occur

HISTOLOGIC FEATURES
- **Subepidermal blister** with **neutrophils (often numerous)** within the papillary dermis in a diffuse pattern
- **Interface changes** can be seen
- Superficial perivascular and periadnexal inflammatory infiltrate with occasional neutrophils and **increased dermal mucin**
- Rarely leukocytoclastic vasculitis

IMMUNOFLUORESCENCE/IMMUNOHISTOCHEMISTRY
- **DIF** of perilesional skin is positive **linear and/or granular deposition of IgG and/or IgA, IgM, and C3 at the basement membrane zone**
- **Salt Split Skin: IgG** deposition at the **basement membrane zone** at the **dermal side** of the split

OTHER HIGH YIELD POINTS
- **Sublamina densa blister**
- Circulating IgG autoantibodies against **type VII collagen**

DIFFERENTIAL DIAGNOSIS

EPIDERMOLYSIS BULLOSA ACQUISITA
- **Subepidermal blister** with fibrin deposition on the floor of blister cavity
- Neutrophils can be present within the inflammatory infiltrate
- **No increase in dermal mucin**

LINEAR IGA BULLOUS DERMATOSIS
- Subepidermal blister with papillary dermal edema
- Linearly aligned neutrophils at the DEJ
- **DIF** of perilesional skin is positive for **linear IgA deposition** at the **basement membrane zone**

Path Presenter

COMA BLISTERS
CLINICAL FEATURES
- Large tense blisters at the **pressure sites** of **comatose patients**
- Most common affected sites are sacrum, hand, wrists, knee, legs, and heels
- Can be associated with **barbiturate overdose** and other sedative drugs
- Pressure, friction, and local hypoxia have been implicated

HISTOLOGIC FEATURES
- **Subepidermal blister** often with full thickness necrosis of the epidermis/blister roof

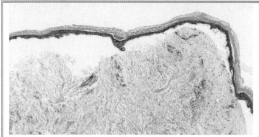

Pauci-inflammatory subepidermal blister

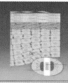
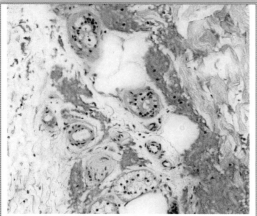

Eccrine glands with ischemic changes

Path Presenter

- **Necrosis of the eccrine glands** and occasionally the **pilosebaceous units**
- Sparse perivascular and interstitial lymphocytic and neutrophilic inflammatory infiltrate

IMMUNOFLUORESCENCE/IMMUNOHISTOCHEMISTRY

- **DIF is negative**

OTHER HIGH YIELD POINTS

- Intralamina lucida blister

DIFFERENTIAL DIAGNOSIS

FRICTION BLISTER

- **Intraepidermal split** beneath the granular cell layer
- Focal to diffuse necrosis in the mid aspect of the epidermis
- No necrosis of the eccrine glands

BULLOUS DIABETICORUM

- **Subcorneal or intraepidermal bulla** with mild inflammation
- The roof of the epidermis can have necrotic keratinocytes
- No necrosis of the eccrine glands

PORPHYRIA CUTANEA TARDA AND PSEUDOPORPHYRIA

- Subepidermal blister with minimal inflammation
- Prominent solar elastosis and thickened vessel walls in the papillary dermis
- No necrosis of the eccrine glands

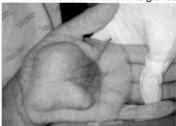

Large tense bulla in a comatosed patient

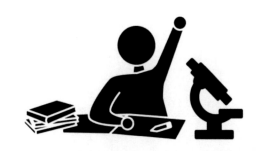

CHAPTER 18: GRANULOMATOUS REACTION PATTERN

CHRISTINE AHN, MD
MICHAEL GREAS, MD

GRANULOMATOUS REACTION PATTERN

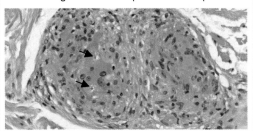
Well-formed granulomas in superficial and deep dermis

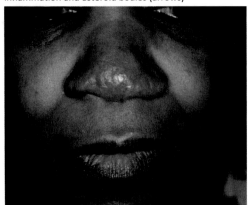
Epithelioid histiocytes forming granulomas with scant inflammation and asteroid bodies (arrows)

Red-brown thickening and papules on the nose, prominent along the alar rim

Path Presenter

SARCOIDOSIS

CLINICAL FEATURES

- Multisystem granulomatous disease, can involve **lungs** (up to 90%), lymph nodes, eyes, liver/spleen, heart, CNS, bones, joints, kidneys
- Seen in adults, increased incidence in African Americans
- Red-brown to violaceous papules and plaques, most often on face (favors nose and lips), neck, upper extremities, within scars and tattoos
- Under diascopy, lesions have "apple jelly" appearance
- Associated with erythema nodosum

HISTOLOGIC FEATURES

- Superficial and deep dermal well-formed granulomas, epithelioid histiocytes with minimal associated inflammation ("**naked granulomas**")
- **Asteroid bodies** (engulfed collagen) within multinucleated histiocytes and **Schaumann bodies** (calcified laminated collections of degenerating lysosomes)

OTHER HIGH YIELD POINTS

- **Löfgren syndrome**: acute form with erythema nodosum and hilar adenopathy
- **Darier-Roussy**: subcutaneous sarcoid
- **Blau syndrome**: *NOD2/CARD15*, sarcoid-like granulomatous disease of skin, uveal tract, and joints

DIFFERENTIAL DIAGNOSIS

- Infection – special stains for acid-fast and fungal organisms, PCR to exclude mycobacterial
- Tuberculoid leprosy – granulomas follow course of nerves, horizontal or elongated "sausage-shaped" contour
- Foreign body reaction (zirconium, beryllium, silica, tattoo ink, soft tissue fillers) – polarize to exclude birefringent foreign material
- Granulomatous rosacea – more tuberculoid than "naked" sarcoidal granulomas, vascular dilation, folliculocentric inflammation
- Melkerson-Rosenthal syndrome – dermal edema, mixed perivascular inflammatory infiltrate with lymphocytes, plasma cells, histiocytes, eosinophils, granulomas more centered around vessels
- Granulomatous mycosis fungoides – infiltrate of atypical lymphocytes
- Necrobiosis lipoidica – diffuse palisading or interstitial granulomatous inflammation, necrobiosis, extracellular lipid, vascular changes
- Cutaneous Crohn disease – granulomas with more inflammation, admixed neutrophils, clinical association with inflammatory bowel disease
- Granuloma annulare – palisading or interstitial granulomatous inflammation, necrobiosis, and mucin present

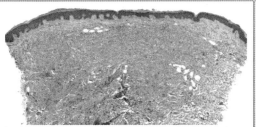
Interstitial pattern with "busy dermis" appearance of blue histiocytes between collagen bundles

GRANULOMA ANNULARE

CLINICAL FEATURES

- Arciform or annular erythematous to violaceous plaques, favor dorsal hands and feet
- Other variants include subcutaneous, macular, and perforating
- Usually localized, self-limited; can be photo-distributed or disseminated
- Affects young adults, increased incidence in women

HISTOLOGIC FEATURES

- Histiocytic dermal infiltrate in two main patterns: (1) **interstitial**- histiocytes between collagen fibers with minimal degeneration; (2) **palisaded**- central collagen degeneration surrounded by palisading granulomas and lymphocytes
- Eosinophils can be present but not necessary
- Mucin deposition between collagen fibers or center of palisaded granulomas

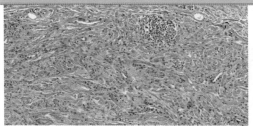

Interstitial histiocytes, some multinucleated, and mucin deposition

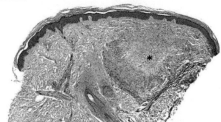

Palisaded pattern with area of collagen degeneration (*)

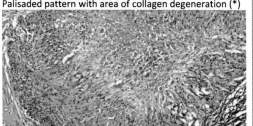

Collagen degeneration and mucin with surrounding palisade of histiocytes and lymphocytes

- Fibrin, neutrophils, karyorrhexis may be present

SPECIAL STAINS

- Alcian blue or colloidal iron can highlight mucin

DIFFERENTIAL DIAGNOSIS

- Granulomatous mycosis fungoides – presence of atypical lymphocytic infiltrate
- Epithelioid sarcoma – central necrosis surrounded by polygonal cells with eosinophilic cytoplasm
- Necrobiosis lipoidica – horizontally oriented eosinophilic necrobiosis with intervening granulomatous inflammation, fibrosis and plasma cells present
- Actinic granuloma (annular elastolytic giant cell granuloma) – less organized granulomas, more multinucleated cells, elastophagocytosis, minimal mucin
- Sarcoidosis – eosinophils and mucin absent

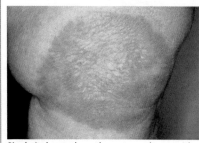
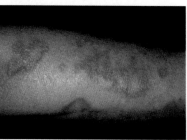

Single indurated, erythematous plaque with raised border

Multiple red-brown indurated papules and plaques with elevated border

Path Presenter

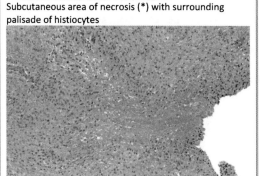

Subcutaneous area of necrosis (*) with surrounding palisade of histiocytes

SUBCUTANEOUS GRANULOMA ANNULARE

CLINICAL FEATURES

- Large, painless, skin-colored nodules located on the hands, palms, legs, feet, buttocks, and scalp
- Usually seen in children < 10 years old

HISTOLOGIC FEATURES

- Deep dermal and/or subcutaneous nodules with larger areas of necrobiosis than superficial type surrounded by palisade of lymphocytes and histiocytes
- Eosinophils frequently seen; mucin less prominent than superficial type of granuloma annulare

DIFFERENTIAL DIAGNOSIS

- Rheumatoid/pseudorheumatoid nodule – fibrinous eosinophilic necrobiosis, more giant cells

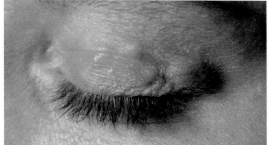

Central necrosis with palisading histiocytes and lymphocytes

Subcutaneous, skin-colored nodules on the upper eyelid

Path Presenter

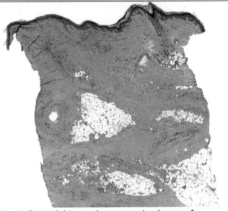

"Square" punch biopsy demonstrating layers of inflammation between areas of necrobiosis, affecting full thickness of dermis extending into subcutaneous fat

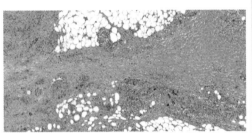

Dermal fibrosis, necrobiosis, and inflammation with histiocytes (numerous multinucleated)

NECROBIOSIS LIPOIDICA

CLINICAL FEATURES

- Red papules or plaques enlarge radially with atrophic yellow-brown center
- Most common on anterior legs, can occur on forearms, hands
- Affects young adults, women more than men

HISTOLOGIC FEATURES

- Tiers of chronic inflammation and sclerosis create a layered appearance
- Superficial and deep perivascular and interstitial mixed inflammatory infiltrate involving full thickness dermis and subcutis
- Inflammatory areas show histiocytes (including multinucleated) admixed with plasma cells and lymphoid aggregates
- Areas of necrobiosis and dermal sclerosis
- Endothelial swelling and lymphocytic vasculitis seen in deeper vessels

IMMUNOFLUORESCENCE

- IgM and C3 can be seen in blood vessel walls, fibrin in necrobiotic areas

DIFFERENTIAL DIAGNOSIS

- Granuloma annulare – lacks broad zones of eosinophilic necrobiosis
- Erythema nodosum – lacks dermal changes of NL

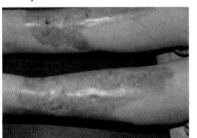

Bilateral shiny plaques on the anterior legs with yellow-brown, atrophic center

Path Presenter

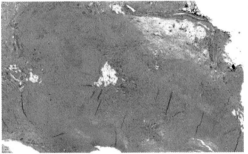

Deep subcutaneous zones of eosinophilic necrobiosis

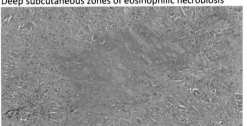

Necrobiotic zone surrounded by elongated histiocytes and other inflammatory cells

RHEUMATOID NODULE

CLINICAL FEATURES

- Firm, semi-mobile subcutaneous nodules most often in periarticular distribution
- Seen in 20% of patients with rheumatoid arthritis
- **Accelerated rheumatoid nodulosis** – eruption of multiple small nodules in hands, feet, ears after initiation of methotrexate or TNF-α inhibitors

HISTOLOGIC FEATURES

- Central zone of eosinophilic necrobiosis with fibrin situated in the deep dermis or subcutis surrounded by palisade of elongated histiocytes, lymphocytes, neutrophils, mast cells, foreign body giant cells, and occasional plasma cells
- Early lesions may show interstitial neutrophilic infiltrate and leukocytoclastic vasculitis
- Established lesions show fibrosis, clefts, degeneration of necrobiotic foci

DIFFERENTIAL DIAGNOSIS

- Subcutaneous GA – necrobiosis more pale, mucinous, basophilic
- Palisaded and neutrophilic granulomatous dermatitis (PNGD) – overlap with early rheumatoid nodules, lack necrobiosis

Path Presenter

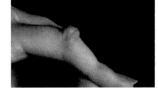

Firm subcutaneous nodule overlying joint

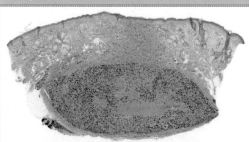

Well-formed granuloma in the mid dermis

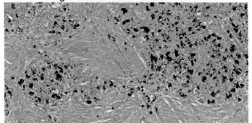

Histiocytes with foreign body giant cells forming around graphite pigment deposition

FOREIGN BODY REACTION

CLINICAL FEATURES

- Foreign material producing sarcoidal granulomas include silica, silicone, sodium bisulfate (in ophthalmic drops), tattoo pigment, zirconium, beryllium, zinc, sea-urchin spines, interferon injection sites
- Skin-colored or red-brown papule or nodule arising within area of trauma or exposure
- Nonsarcoidal granulomas - more common presentation

HISTOLOGIC FEATURES

- Sarcoidal granulomas within the dermis and sparse perigranulomatous infiltrate
- Nonsarcoidal granulomas - variable mixture of macrophages, lymphocytes, Langerhans giant cells and neutrophils

DIFFERENTIAL DIAGNOSIS

- Sarcoidosis – clinical history important, true differentiation can be difficult as granulomas can develop in scars and contain birefringent crystals in sarcoid

Path Presenter

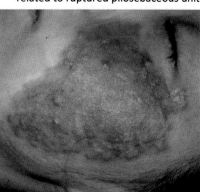

Superficial telangiectasias, dermal edema, and inflammation centered around components of hair follicle

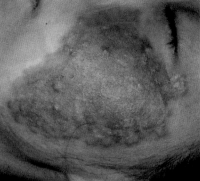

Granulomatous inflammation with accompanying lymphocytes around sebaceous glands and hair follicles

ROSACEA

CLINICAL FEATURES

- Persistent erythema and telangiectasia of central face
- Granulomatous form characterized by more monomorphic skin-colored to red-brown dome-shaped papules

HISTOLOGIC FEATURES

- Noncaseating epithelioid granulomas within the dermis, may be centered around ruptured hair follicles or located diffusely throughout dermis
- Superficial dermal telangiectasias and dermal edema are an accompanying finding - sometimes may be the only finding
- Plasma cells are often seen

OTHER HIGH YIELD POINTS

- Granulomas may represent response to *Demodex* organisms or lipids

DIFFERENTIAL DIAGNOSIS

- Lupus vulgaris – tuberculoid granulomas with epithelioid histiocytes and rim of lymphocytes and plasma cells, special stains can help distinguish
- Lupus miliaris disseminatus faciei (LMDF) – characteristic caseation necrosis related to ruptured pilosebaceous unit

Erythematous plaque with red-brown papules within the plaque and raised border

Path Presenter

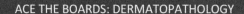

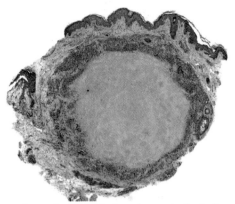

Large focus of eosinophilic dermal necrosis situated in the superficial dermis with surrounding infiltrate of histiocytes and lymphocytes

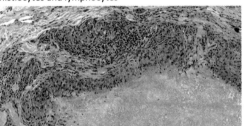

Palisade of epithelioid histiocytes, multinucleate giant cells, and lymphocytes surrounding central necrosis

LUPUS MILIARIS DISSEMINATUS FACIEI

CLINICAL FEATURES
- Yellow-brown papules on the central face, less often with extrafacial involvement (neck, extremities, axilla)
- Seen in adolescents and young adults

HISTOLOGIC FEATURES
- Superficial dermal necrosis (caseation) surrounded by epithelioid histiocytes, multinucleate giant cells, lymphocytes
- Often associated with pilosebaceous units
- Late lesions may show associated dermal fibrosis

OTHER HIGH YIELD POINTS
- *Facial idiopathic granulomas with regressive evolution* (FIGURE) is a proposed alternative term for this entity

DIFFERENTIAL DIAGNOSIS
- Rosacea – overlap with LMDF that show perifollicular granulomas without caseation
- Granuloma annulare – relationship to hair follicles not observed
- Tuberculosis – special stains highlight presence of acid-fast organisms
- Sarcoidosis – do not demonstrate necrobiosis

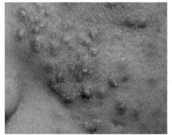

Path Presenter   Yellowish red papules and nodules located on the central face

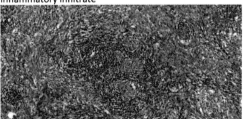

Ulcerated nodule with numerous granulomas throughout the dermis and dense collections of superficial and deep inflammatory infiltrate

Tuberculoid granulomas with surrounding cuff of lymphocytes

CUTANEOUS CROHN DISEASE

CLINICAL FEATURES
- Cutaneous Crohn disease can be the presenting finding in 20% of patients
- Genital involvement presents with linear ulceration within body folds, can develop into sinus tracts, fissures, ulcers, and vegetating plaques
- Oral findings include cobble-stoning of buccal mucosa, aphthae-like ulcers, linear ulcerations, angular cheilitis, indurated fissuring of lower lip, gingival hyperplasia, pyostomatitis vegetans
- Non-genital involvement presents as dusky erythematous plaques on legs, trunk, and upper extremities, can also develop into ulcers, draining sinuses and fistulas, and resultant scarring

HISTOLOGIC FEATURES
- Findings can be variable
- Noncaseating, tuberculoid granulomas with cuff of lymphocytes
- Dense collections of superficial and deep perivascular mixed inflammatory infiltrate with lymphocytes, histiocytes, and eosinophils
- Can sometimes present with neutrophils in dermis

OTHER HIGH YIELD POINTS
- No consistent correlation between mucocutaneous disease activity and gastrointestinal disease activity

DIFFERENTIAL DIAGNOSIS
- Sarcoidosis-sarcoidal granulomas
- Foreign body granuloma-suppurative and granulomatous inflammation
- Infectious granuloma-suppurative and granulomatous inflammation

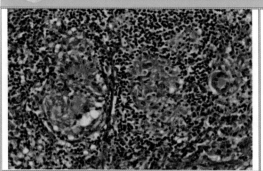

- Pyoderma gangrenosum – can have overlapping features and clinical context but granulomatous inflammation rarely observed

 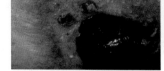 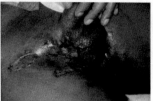

Path Presenter   Eroded nodule with surrounding small nodules and hyperpigmentation   Ulcers and fissures in the genital region

MELKERSSON-ROSENTHAL SYNDROME
CLINICAL FEATURES
- Triad: chronic orofacial swelling (lips), recurrent facial nerve palsy, fissured tongue (lingua plica)
- Complete triad only observed in 25%
- Granulomatous cheilitis, orofacial granulomatosis – terms used to describe monosymptomatic form of localized episodic swelling of lips

HISTOLOGIC FEATURES
- Marked dermal edema, perivascular infiltrate of lymphocytes, plasma cells, histiocytes, eosinophils
- "Naked" epithelioid granulomas, tuberculoid granulomas, or isolated multinucleate giant cells
- Dilated lymphatics, inflammation related to dermal vessels

DIFFERENTIAL DIAGNOSIS
- Sarcoidosis – vessels uninvolved, primarily "naked" epithelioid granulomas
- Crohn's disease – no reliable features can distinguish, clinical context paramount
- Intravascular histiocytosis – intravascular/intralymphatic, no granulomas as seen in Melkersson-Rosenthal syndrome

Dermal edema and perivascular and periadnexal inflammatory infiltrate

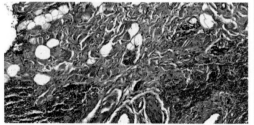

Scattered collections of histiocytes and granulomas and perivascular lymphocytic inflammation

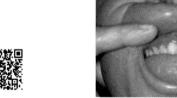

Path Presenter   Swelling of the lip and fissured tongue

INTERSTITIAL GRANULOMATOUS DERMATITIS/PALISADED AND NEUTROPHILIC GRANULOMATOUS DERMATITIS
CLINICAL FEATURES
- Granulomatous dermatitis seen in the context of autoimmune diseases, seen in two major patterns
- Interstitial granulomatous dermatitis (IGD): skin-colored or erythematous annular or linear cords ("rope sign"), most often on trunk, proximal extremities
- Palisaded neutrophilic and granulomatous dermatitis (PNGD): skin-colored to erythematous umbilicated papules, affect extensor extremities

HISTOLOGIC FEATURES
- Two major patterns described
  - Interstitial and perivascular dermal infiltrate of neutrophils, histiocytes, lymphocytes, and karyorrhexis
  - Palisaded histiocytes and lymphocytes surrounding neutrophils
- Leukocytoclastic vasculitis can be seen

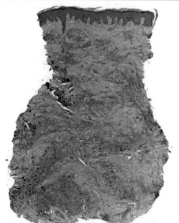

"Bottom heavy" interstitial infiltrate of histiocytes

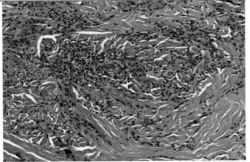
Interstitial infiltrate of histiocytes, mucin absent

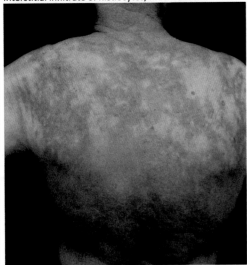
Erythematous and annular plaques on the trunk in patient with IGD

- Rosettes of histiocytes surrounding empty spaces with degenerated collagen bundles
- "Bottom-heavy," dense, dermal interstitial infiltrate, mucin usually absent

IMMUNOFLUORESCENCE

- C3, IgM, fibrinogen deposition in dermal blood vessels in some cases

OTHER HIGH YIELD POINTS

- Associated with systemic illnesses: rheumatoid arthritis, lupus erythematosus, autoimmune hepatitis, sarcoidosis, among others

DIFFERENTIAL DIAGNOSIS

- Granuloma annulare – close resemblance to interstitial form, more focal infiltrates, neutrophils and leukocytoclasia not typically seen, "top-heavy" infiltrate, mucin deposition
- Interstitial granulomatous drug reaction – more likely to have eosinophils and interface changes, neutrophils absent, minimal collagen degeneration, no vasculitis
- Necrobiosis lipoidica – inflammation in layers, neutrophils less prominent
- Rheumatoid nodules – central eosinophilia and subcutaneous location

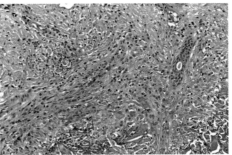
Palisaded histiocytes, neutrophils, karryorhexis in the dermis in a case of PNGD

Path Presenter

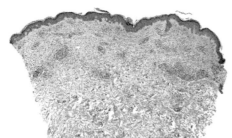
Interstitial and perivascular infiltrate of histiocytes and lymphocytes

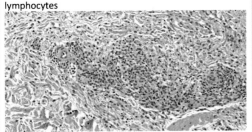
Numerous scattered eosinophhils admixed with interstitial infiltrate

INTERSTITIAL GRANULOMATOUS DRUG REACTION

CLINICAL FEATURES

- Erythematous to violaceous plaques, often annular
- Most often affect inner arms, medial thighs, intertriginous sites, and trunk

HISTOLOGIC FEATURES

- Interstitial infiltrate of lymphocytes and histiocytes, occasional multinucleate giant cells and eosinophils
- Mild interface changes (vacuolar change, apoptotic keratinocytes)
- Variable mucin deposition, epidermotropism, and extravasation of erythrocytes, no vasculitis

OTHER HIGH YIELD POINTS

- Implicated drugs: **calcium channel blockers**, **statins**, **TNF-α inhibitors**, ACE inhibitors, β blockers, furosemide, antihistamines

DIFFERENTIAL DIAGNOSIS

- Granuloma annulare – presence of necrobiosis, predominance of histiocytes or lymphocytes, absence of significant eosinophils, and interface changes

Path Presenter

CHAPTER 18: GRANULOMATOUS REACTION PATTERN

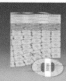

Clear spaces Inflammation

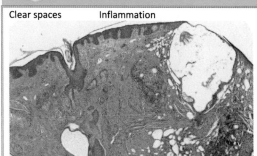

Granulomatous inflammation Giant cells

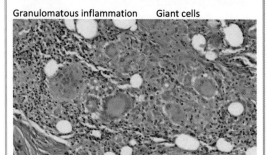

CHALAZION
CLINICAL FEATURES
- Solitary, painless lesion of eyelid due to blocked sebaceous gland

HISTOLOGIC FEATURES
- Granulomatous inflammation with mixed tuberculoid and foreign body features surrounding clear space where lipids from sebaceous gland released
- Chronic inflammation surrounding granulomas composed of lymphocytes, plasma cells, and occasionally collections of neutrophils (suppuration)

OTHER HIGH YIELD POINTS
- Recurrent lesions associated with seborrheic dermatitis and rosacea

DIFFERENTIAL DIAGNOSIS
- Infection – special stains and clinical history can distinguish

Path Presenter

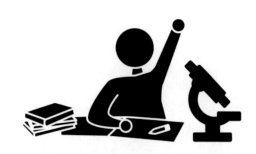

ACE MY PATH
Come Ace With Us!

CHAPTER 19: VASCULITIS AND
VASCULOPATHIC REACTION
PATTERN

POOJA SRIVASTAVA, MD
FRANCHESCA CHOI, MD
ASHLEY ELSENSOHN, MD

PERIVASCULAR INFLAMMATION

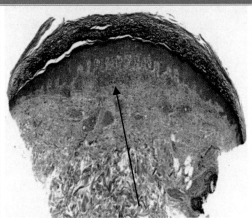
Superficial perivascular infiltrate of lymphocytes

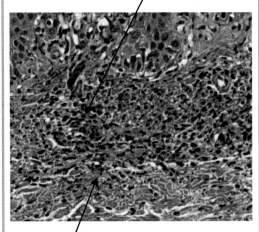
Extravasated erythrocytes

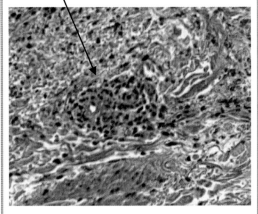

PIGMENTED PURPURIC DERMATOSES (PPD) / CAPILLARITIS

CLINICAL FEATURES
- Telangiectatic punctate macules to patches with classic red brown **cayenne-pepper** appearance
- With **pigmentation** as a result of **hemosiderin** deposition
- Usually limited to lower extremities, but may involve upper extremities and trunk
- See Other High Yield Points for clinical sub-types

HISTOLOGIC FEATURES
- Superficial **perivascular infiltrate of lymphocytes** (sometimes minimal) in the **papillary dermis**
- **Extravasated erythrocytes**
- **Hemosiderin**-laden macrophages
- Epidermis usually normal, may show spongiosis with lymphocytic exocytosis

OTHER HIGH YIELD POINTS
- Four main clinical variants. On pathology these are indistinguishable:
    1. Purpura annularis telangiectodes of Majocchi: Annular purpuric macules
    2. Progressive pigmentary dermatosis of Schamberg
    3. Pigmented purpuric dermatitis of Gougerot and Blum: More prominent lichenoid inflammation compared to perivascular inflammation
    4. Eczematoid-like purpura of Doucas and Kapetanakis: More spongiosis with scale
- Schamberg disease: pigmentation predominates
- **Lichen aureus** is a localized variant (patches composed of closely set, flat rust, copper or orange papules); male predilection; peak in fourth decade
- Venous insufficiency may be a factor as stasis changes have been noted
- Also reported as initial manifestation of T-cell lymphoproliferative disease

DIFFERENTIAL DIAGNOSIS
LICHENOID DERMATITIS (LICHEN PLANUS, LICHEN STRIATUS)
- Lichenoid dermatitis has an interface pattern with the dermoepidermal junction. Civatte bodies or basal layer vasculopathy present

STASIS DERMATITIS
- Stasis dermatitis has 'cannonball' proliferation of capillaries with minimal red blood cell extravasation or hemosiderin
- More pronounced epidermal changes and fibrosis of the dermis

CUTANEOUS T CELL LYMPHOMA (CTCL)
- CTCL with migration of atypical, angulated lymphocytes into the epidermis (epidermotropism)
- Demonstrates clonality with typical ratio CD4:CD8 cell > 4:1; TCR gene rearrangement positive (although can be false positives)

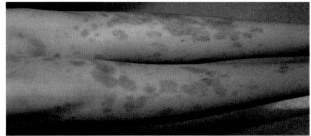
Telangiectatic macules and patches with cayenne-pepper like pigmentation

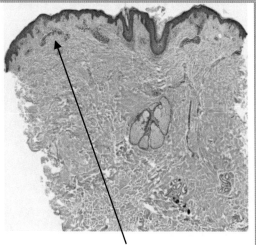

Superficial perivascular "coat-sleeve" lymphocytic infiltrate

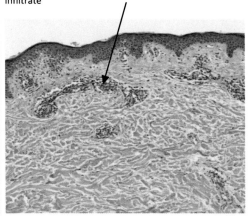

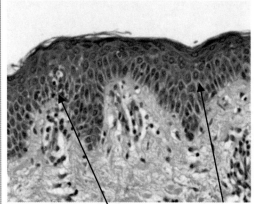

Focal extravasation of erythrocytes and spongiosis

Path Presenter

ERYTHEMA ANNULARE CENTRIFUGUM (EAC)

CLINICAL FEATURES

- Superficial (scale) and deep (no scale) clinical variants
- Expanding erythematous ring that can be oval or polycyclic
- **Superficial variant:** with characteristic **trailing scale** (scale on the innermost portion of the rim rather than outermost like in tinea)
- **Deep variant:** palpable erythema with central clearing; **no surface changes**
- Predilection for trunk and proximal extremities of adults

HISTOLOGIC FEATURES

- Erythematous ring corresponds to a focus of superficial perivascular tightly cuffed **("coat-sleeve") lymphocytic infiltrate**
- Superficial variant: focal epidermal spongiosis and parakeratosis; infiltrate, spongiotic, and parakeratotic foci line up at about a **45-degree angle**
- Deep variant: also has deep coat-sleeve perivascular lymphocytic infiltrate with occasional focal vacuolar alteration of the basal layer keratinocytes

OTHER HIGH YIELD POINTS

- Most cases resolve spontaneously within several weeks to months
- May be related to occult infections, dermatophytosis, candidiasis, medications, hormonal changes, foods (blue cheese, tomatoes), and, rarely, an underlying malignancy. The aforementioned should be ruled out

DIFFERENTIAL DIAGNOSIS

SECONDARY SYPHILIS

- Syphilis with **plasma cells** and histiocytes, **swollen endothelial cells**
- Immunohistochemistry (Spirochete) or Special stain (Steiner) positive for **spirochetes**

TUMID LUPUS ERYTHEMATOSUS

- Tumid lupus can appear similar to deep EAC (superficial and deep perivascular lymphocytic inflammation). Lupus will have an increased deposit of **mucin** (Colloidal Iron stain) in an interstitial pattern between collagen bundles

Superficial EAC with classic annular plaque with "trailing scale "

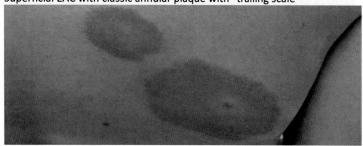

Deep EAC with annular plaques showing central clearing No surface changes

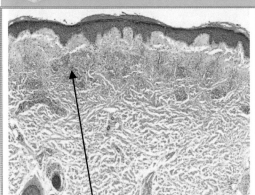

Moderate, superficial and deep perivascular and periadnexal lymphocytic infiltrate

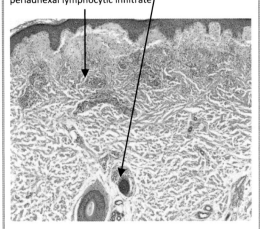

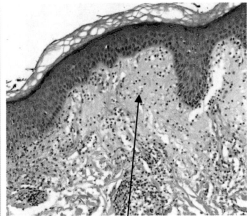

Marked papillary dermis edema

Path Presenter

POLYMORPHOUS LIGHT ERUPTION (PMLE)

CLINICAL FEATURES

- Transient, intermittent, symmetrical eruption of nonscarring, erythematous, itchy papules, plaques, or vesicles
- Usually appears hours to 1-2 days after sun exposure. Typically seasonal
- Lasts for hours, days, or rarely weeks before resolving. Often recurs
- Presents with several morphologies (papular, eczematous, blistering, urticarial, annular) but always the same morphology in the same patient

HISTOLOGIC FEATURES

- Very early lesions: mild spongiosis with focal lymphocyte exocytosis; mild or occasionally moderate, **superficial and deep perivascular lymphocytic** inflammatory cell infiltrate (CD3/CD4 positive)
- Predominantly lymphocytes but may be admixed histiocytes, neutrophils and eosinophils
- As lesions progress: **marked edema of the papillary dermis** and more prominent dermal inflammation and spongiosis; **focal interface change**; mild hydropic basal cell degeneration
- There are often lymphocytes in the epidermis (exocytosis)
- Focal dyskeratosis may be noted

OTHER HIGH YIELD POINTS

- More common in women with typical onset ages 20-40 years
- Presents more often in climates that have less sunlight exposure

DIFFERENTIAL DIAGNOSIS

CUTANEOUS LUPUS

- More prominent interface change
- **Dermal mucin** will be present in **lupus**, not increased in PMLE
- Papillary dermal edema usually not present in lupus
- Increased **CD123+ plasmacytoid** dendritic cells (PDCs) in **lupus** infiltrate

ACTINIC PRURIGO

- Variable epidermal hyperplasia, **more prominent** spongiosis, and **lymphocyte exocytosis**
- Usually **absent dermal edema**; excoriation changes

CHILBLAINS

- Similar histology but clinically distinct location on **fingers**

ROSACEA

- Rosacea with typically less robust lymphocytic dermal infiltrate
- Absent epidermal changes, no dermal edema, superficial inflammation

CUTANEOUS T-CELL LYMPHOMA (CTCL)

- CTCL typically without marked dermal edema. Shows migration of atypical, angulated lymphocytes into the epidermis (epidermotropism)
- Usually **absent dermal edema**

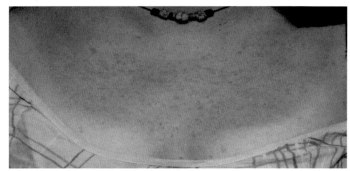

Erythematous papular eruption on the upper chest

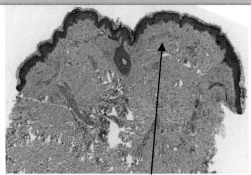

Superficial perivascular lymphocytic inflammation

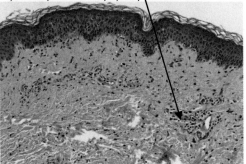

Path Presenter

VIRAL EXANTHEM

CLINICAL FEATURES
- Non-specific erythematous macular or morbilliform eruption

HISTOLOGIC FEATURES
- Mild superficial perivascular lymphocytic inflammation with focal exocytosis
- May see basilar keratinocyte vacuolar destruction
- May see rare epidermal dyskeratotic cells

DIFFERENTIAL DIAGNOSIS

DERMATOMYOSITIS
- Dermatomyositis may have **flattened rete** ridges, a thickened basement membrane zone, and increased dermal **mucin** deposition (Colloidal Iron)

GRAFT VERSUS HOST DISEASE
- More marked dyskeratotic keratinocytes with **satellite cell necrosis** (necrotic cells with surrounding lymphocytes) in epidermis AND follicular epithelium

DRUG ERUPTION
- Superficial and deep perivascular lymphocytic infiltrate with **eosinophils**

Non-specific macular-papular erythematous drug rash

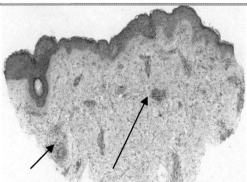

Periadnexal, perivascular lymphocytic infiltrate

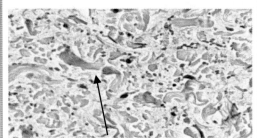

Increased dermal mucin

RETICULAR ERYTHEMATOSUS MUCINOSIS (REM)

CLINICAL FEATURES
- **Erythematous, reticulated (net-like)** macules to papules to patches with irregular but well-defined margins, usually in **center of chest and upper back**
- Usually asymptomatic but may be pruritic. Young to middle-aged women

HISTOLOGIC FEATURES
- Mild/moderate **perivascular and periadnexal lymphocytic infiltrate** (helper T cell)
- Increased **dermal mucin.** Mucin may be absent in macular lesions
- Epidermal changes absent

IMMUNOFLUORESCENCE
- Fine granular deposits of IgM, IgA, and C3 along basal layer in some cases

OTHER HIGH YIELD POINTS
- May be presenting sign of lupus, overlap with tumid lupus

DIFFERENTIAL DIAGNOSIS

JESSNER LYMPHOCYTIC INFILTRATE
- Typically, a **denser lymphocytic** infiltrate with **less mucin**

TUMID LUPUS ERYTHEMATOSUS
- **May not be possible to distinguish**, but may show vacuolar changes in basal layer of epidermis and follicular units of lupus

Path Presenter

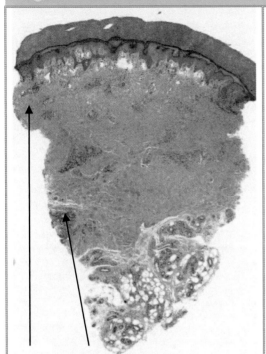

Superficial and deep perivascular inflammation on acral location (note thick stratum corneum)

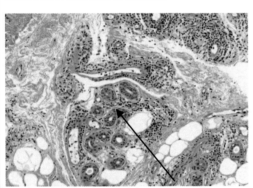

Lymphocytic infiltrate around deep eccrine coils

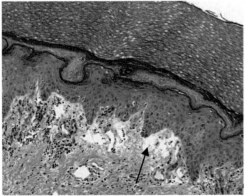

Marked papillary dermal edema

PERNIOSIS (CHILBLAINS)

CLINICAL FEATURES

- Erythematous and violaceous papules, plaques, and/or nodules, affecting **distal sites of the body,** including the fingers, toes, heels, ears, and nose
- May progress to bullae and erosions
- Pruritic, burning, and/or painful

HISTOLOGIC FEATURES

- Moderate to dense, **superficial and deep perivascular lymphocytic** infiltrate in dermis and subcutaneous fat; accentuation around the **deep eccrine coils**
- Prominent **papillary dermal edema**
- **Lymphocytic vasculitis** (endothelial cell swelling, edema and infiltration of the vessel walls by lymphocytes) **without fibrinoid necrosis**
- Rarely thrombi may be noted in vessels

OTHER HIGH YIELD POINTS

- May be presenting sign of lupus, has significant overlap with tumid lupus

DIFFERENTIAL DIAGNOSIS

ERYTHEMA MULTIFORME

- No deep infiltrate or papillary dermal edema

CHILBLAIN LUPUS ERYTHEMATOSUS

- May not be possible to distinguish histologically, but lupus may also show effacing interface dermatitis and increased dermal mucin

CUTANEOUS LYMPHOMA

- Lymphocytic atypia; no superficial dermal edema

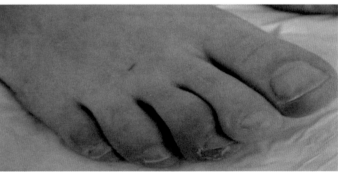

Painful, violaceous patches on the toes

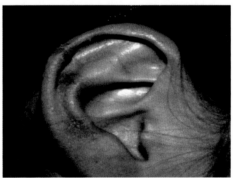

Painful, erythematous patch of the right ear

Path Presenter

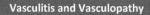
Vasculitis and Vasculopathy

POLYARTERITIS NODOSA (PAN)

CLINICAL FEATURES

- Two clinical presentations: Limited to skin (Cutaneous PAN) or associated with systemic symptoms (Systemic PAN)
- Tender subcutaneous nodules that may ulcerate, can show a background of livedo reticularis
- May show bullae or atrophie blanche-like lesions
- Most often on the lower legs in men; women less commonly affected
- End-stage lesions include gangrene of toes and fingers

HISTOLOGIC FEATURES

- **Small to medium vessels vasculitis** with **fibrinoid degeneration of small to medium** sized arteries. Vessels at **different stages** of involvement is characteristic
- Necrotizing leukocytoclastic vasculitis involving a **medium artery** in **deep dermis or subcutaneous tissue**, often with surrounding **fat lobular necrosis**
- **Early** lesions: partial to complete destruction of external and internal elastic laminae with **neutrophilic infiltrate**, leukocytoclasis with some eosinophils and deposition of **fibrinoid material**
- **Late** lesions: intimal proliferation and **thrombosis** lead to lumen occlusion and surrounding fibrosis with ischemia and possible **ulceration**, mixed infiltrate

IMMUNOFLUORESCENCE/IMMUNOHISTOCHEMISTRY

- **C3 and IgM** may be found in **vessel walls** for direct immunofluorescence

OTHER HIGH YIELD POINTS

- **Systemic PAN-renal involvement** (present in 75%) is most common cause of death
- Fever, malaise, weight loss, weakness, myalgias, arthralgias, and anorexia are common symptoms
- Joint, nervous system, kidney, gastrointestinal, cardiac involvement possible
- **Arteriography** of visceral arteries often show **multiple aneurysms** that are highly suggestive of PAN

DIFFERENTIAL DIAGNOSIS

MICROSCOPIC POLYANGIITIS (MPA)

- Not distinguishable histologically, but clinically MPA causes glomerulonephritis
- ANCA+ and there is a lack of arteriography findings

KAWASAKI DISEASE

- PAN like changes in coronary vessels

OTHER VASCULITIS

- Histologically may be indistinguishable with vasculitis caused by infection, connective tissue disease, temporal arteritis, ANCA-associated vasculitis

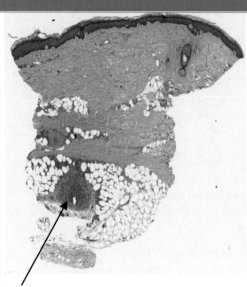

Vasculitis of medium-sized vessel

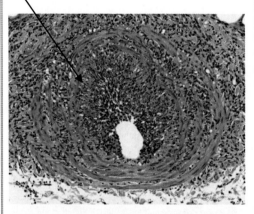

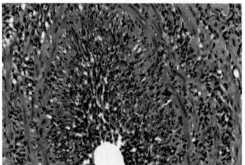

Destruction of external & internal elastic laminae
Neutrophilic infiltrate and fibrinoid deposition

Path Presenter

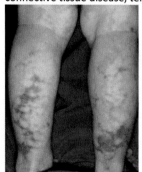

PAN with retiform "netlike" morphology

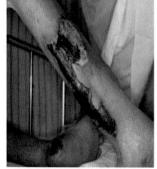

Late PAN showing eschars

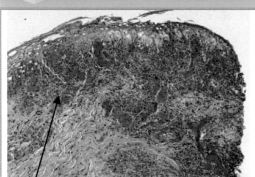

RBC extravasation into perivascular tissue

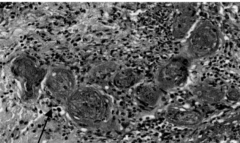

Intravascular fibrin thrombi

Path Presenter

DISSEMINATED INTRAVASCULAR COAGULATION (DIC) / THROMBOTIC THROMBOCYTOPENIC PURPURA (TTP) / AND OTHER COAGULOPATHIES

CLINICAL FEATURES
- Mild forms: petechiae; severe forms: purpura, hemorrhagic bullae, acral cyanosis, localized necrosis

HISTOLOGIC FEATURES
- Little or no inflammation
- Mild forms: extravasation of RBCs into perivascular connective tissue
- Moderate forms: intravascular fibrin thrombi in dermal vessels
- Severe forms: thrombotic vascular occlusion leads to hemorrhagic infarcts, epidermal and dermal necrosis, blister formation

IMMUNOFLUORESCENCE/IMMUNOHISTOCHEMISTRY
- **Fibrin** in **vessel walls** for early lesions of direct immunofluorescence
- **Late** stages with various immunoglobulins and complement around vessels

DIFFERENTIAL DIAGNOSIS
DEEP FUNGAL INFECTION
- Will show fungal hyphae many times in vessel walls
ECTHYMA GANGRENOSUM
- Necrosis and bluish tinge created by bacterial colonies around vessel walls

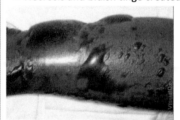

Purpuric, hemorrhagic bullae (late)   Retiform "netlike" erythema (early)

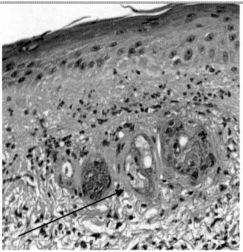

Fibrinoid material in vessel wall; hemorrhage

Path Presenter

ATROPHIE BLANCHE / LIVEDOID OR SEGMENTAL HYALINIZING VASCULITIS

CLINICAL FEATURES
- Purpuric macules and papules usually on **ankles and dorsal feet in middle-aged to older females**, may develop into small painful ulcers with tendency to recur
- Healing of the ulcers results in irregularly outlined **white atrophic scars** with peripheral hyperpigmentation and telangiectasia

HISTOLOGIC FEATURES
- **Early** lesions: **fibrinoid** material in vessel wall or lumen, **hemorrhage**
- **Late** atrophic lesions: thinned epidermis, sclerotic dermis, little to no cellular infiltrate; dermal **vessel wall intima** may show **thickening and hyalinization, thrombi within vessels, extravasated red blood cells**
- **PAS+** thickening of vessel walls

OTHER HIGH YIELD POINTS
- May be associated with hypercoagulable states such as lupus antiphospholipid, protein C deficiency, factor V Leiden mutations, homocysteinemia and essential cryoglobulinemia

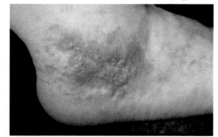

Atrophic, stellate scars with surrounding telangiectasia

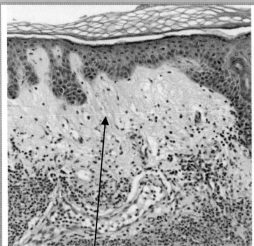

Marked papillary edema

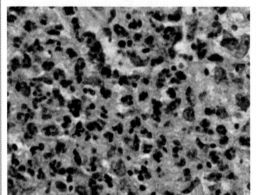

Neutrophilic infiltrate with karyorrhexis

Sheets of neutrophils in the dermis

Path Presenter

SWEET SYNDROME / ACUTE FEBRILE NEUTROPHILIC DERMATOSIS

CLINICAL FEATURES

- Red, tender erythematous plaques
- Fever, peripheral leukocytosis
- Usually preceded by upper respiratory infection
- About **10%** of patients have an associated **myeloproliferative disorder**
- Often on **face or extremities**, only rarely involves trunk

HISTOLOGIC FEATURES

- Nodular and diffuse perivascular infiltrates of **neutrophils** with karyorrhexis
- Marked papillary **dermal edema**
- **Admixed lymphocytes, histiocytes and eosinophils may be noted**

OTHER HIGH YIELD POINTS

- Vascular alterations may be secondary to the massive extravasation of activated neutrophils
- Incidental leukocytoclasia, no vasculitis
- Can have "histiocytoid" Sweet Syndrome where neutrophils look like histiocytes; stain with Myeloperoxidase (MPO) to prove neutrophils

DIFFERENTIAL DIAGNOSIS

PYODERMA GANGRENOSUM

- No karyorrhexis in pyoderma gangrenosum, ulceration often present
- No marked papillary dermal edema

BOWEL-ASSOCIATED DERMATOSIS-ARTHRITIS SYNDROME (BADAS)

- Clinicopathological correlation

INFECTION

- Obtain Gram Stain and PAS to rule out infection

NEUTROPHILIC DERMATOSIS OF DORSAL HANDS

- Histology similar but limited to dorsal hands

RHEUMATOID NEUTROPHILIC DERMATOSIS

- Similar histology, may show admixed plasma cells; associated with Rheumatoid Arthritis

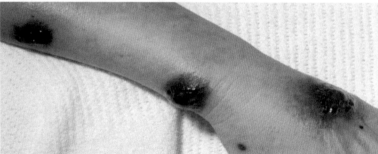

Violaceous, edematous nodules

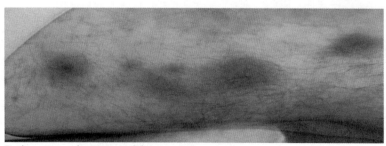

Erythematous, edematous nodules

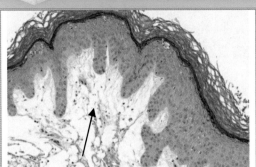

Marked papillary edema

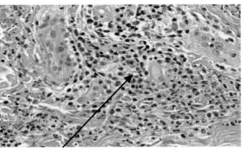

Dense neutrophilic infiltrate

Path Presenter

BOWEL-ASSOCIATED DERMATOSIS-ARTHRITIS SYNDROME (BADAS)

CLINICAL FEATURES

- Associated with **bowel disease** and blind loop after peptic ulcer surgery
- Papules developing into **pustules** on purpuric base; lesions last 1-2 weeks and have tendency to recur in months; **upper part of body** especially **arms**
- May be accompanied by **fever, myalgias and arthralgias**

HISTOLOGIC FEATURES

- Nodular and diffuse perivascular infiltrates of **neutrophils** with **karyorrhexis**
- Marked papillary **dermal edema**
- Little or no vasculitis seen

OTHER HIGH YIELD POINTS

- Thought to be related to peptidoglycan antigens of **group A strep**

DIFFERENTIAL DIAGNOSIS

SWEET SYNDROME

Clinicopathological correlation

PYODERMA GANGRENOSUM

- No karyorrhexis in pyoderma gangrenosum, ulceration often present
- No marked papillary dermal edema

INFECTION

- Obtain Gram Stain and PAS to rule out infection

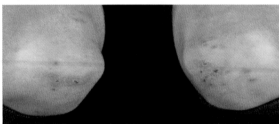

Papulopustules on the elbows

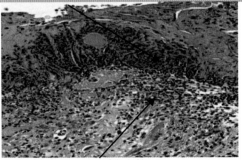

Ulcer with dense neutrophilic infiltrate

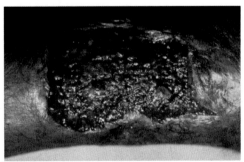

Ulcer with undermined borders

PYODERMA GANGRENOSUM

CLINICAL FEATURES

- Typically begins as tender papulopustules that enlarge and ulcerate
- **Ulcers** typically have raised, **undermined border** with **dusky purple** color
- Often displays **pathergy**, tissue breakdown in response to minor trauma

HISTOLOGIC FEATURES

- Nonspecific histologic findings, clinical pathologic diagnosis of exclusion

- Epidermis usually focally necrotic, sometimes with subepidermal blister
- **Early** lesions: **suppurative folliculitis** or **neutrophilic dermatitis**
- **Late** lesions: **ulceration** with mixed infiltrate
- Deep and extensive inflammation with predominance of neutrophils

OTHER HIGH YIELD POINTS

- May be associated with inflammatory bowel disease, lymphoproliferative disease, and connective tissue disease
- Surgical debridement or trauma worsens wound

DIFFERENTIAL DIAGNOSIS

SWEET SYNDROME

- Sweets often with marked papillary dermal edema

INFECTION

- Obtain Gram Stain and PAS to rule out infection

Path Presenter

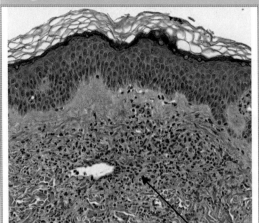
Perivascular mixed inflammatory infiltrate

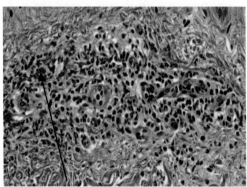
Red blood cell extravasation surrounding post capillary venules with mixed inflammation

Neutrophilic karyorrhexis

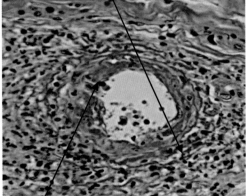
Fibrinoid necrosis of blood vessel walls

Path Presenter

LEUKOCYTOCLASTIC VASCULITIS (LCV)

CLINICAL FEATURES
- Typically presents as palpable purpura on the lower extremities; can be painful

HISTOLOGIC FEATURES
- Small vessel vasculitis, which primarily involves **post-capillary venules**
- **Fibrinoid necrosis** of blood **vessel walls**
- Endothelial cell swelling
- Perivascular mixed inflammatory infiltrate but with **neutrophil predominance**
- **Karyorrhexis (leukocytoclasis)** of neutrophils
- Red blood cell extravasation
- Epidermis normal but can sometimes show bulla formation and necrosis

OTHER HIGH YIELD POINTS
- Numerous underlying etiologies (medication, infection, autoimmune, etc.)
- **"Little 5 LCV"**; post capillary venules only – Drug, Henoch Schoenlein Purpura (HSP), Mixed Cryoglobulinemia (not Type 1), Serum Sickness, Urticarial Vasculitis. Also connective tissue disease (minus Rheumatoid Arthritis)
- **"Big 5 LCV"**; post capillary venules + deeper – Rheumatoid Arthritis, Granulomatosis with Polyangiitis, Microscopic Polyangiitis, Eosinophilic Granulomatosis with polyangiitis, Septic Vasculitis

IMMUNOFLUORESCENCE/IMMUNOHISTOCHEMISTRY
- Immunofluorescence may be useful to confirm vascular damage
- Deposition of **fibrinogen, C3, IgG and IgM** can be seen within **vessel walls**
- **HSP** with deposition of **IgA** in vessel walls

DIFFERENTIAL DIAGNOSIS
SWEET SYNDROME
- Sweets often with marked papillary **dermal edema** and **diffuse neutrophils** in the dermis

BOWEL-ASSOCIATED DERMATOSIS-ARTHRITIS SYNDROME
- **Little to no vasculitis** in BADAS; may have papillary **dermal edema** and **diffuse neutrophils** in the dermis

LIVEDOID VASCULOPATHY
- **No perivascular neutrophils or karyorrhexis.** Will have fibrin deposition around vessels and wedge shaped devitalized collagen

GRANULOMA FACIALE
- **Facial** skin, **mixed inflammation** with neutrophils, eosinophils, lymphocytes and histiocytes. **Grenz zone** of sparing may be present

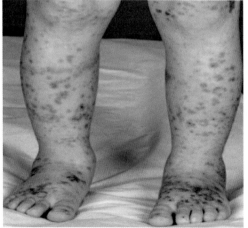
Palpable purpura of lower legs and feet

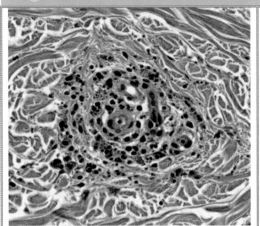

Leukocytoclastic vasculitis

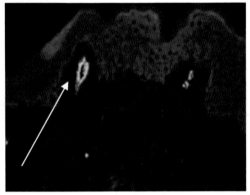

IgA deposits around vessel wall on DIF

Path Presenter

HENOCH SCHOENLEIN PURPURA (HSP)

CLINICAL FEATURES

- Most common in children, HSP is also known as IgA vasculitis
- Inflammation of small blood vessels in skin, joints, intestines, and kidneys
- In addition to typical lower extremity palpable purpura, often extends to buttocks and abdomen
- Characterized by abdominal pain, arthralgia, hematuria, and palpable purpura. May develop after a variety of infections or can be a drug reaction

HISTOLOGIC FEATURES

- **Leukocytoclastic vasculitis** (see above)

IMMUNOFLUORESCENCE/IMMUNOHISTOCHEMISTRY

- **IgA** deposits in **vessel walls** on direct immunofluorescence (DIF) diagnostic
- **Fibrinogen and C3** may also be present on DIF

OTHER HIGH YIELD POINTS

- Abdominal imaging if gastrointestinal symptoms present (e.g., radiography, ultrasonography)
- Doppler flow studies or radionuclide scans in case of scrotal symptoms to rule out testicular torsion

DIFFERENTIAL DIAGNOSIS

OTHER LEUKOCYTOCLASTIC VASCULITIS

- Presence of IgA deposits in vessels walls distinguishes HSP

ACUTE HEMORRHAGIC EDEMA OF INFANCY

- Children less than 3 years of age, presents with fever and edema of face and extremities, bright red purpuric ears
- No IgA present

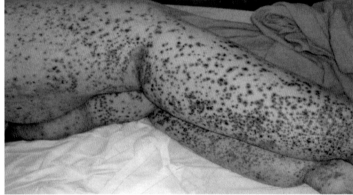

Palpable purpura cover the lower extremities

SEPTIC VASCULITIS

CLINICAL FEATURES

- Septic vasculitis is associated with **septicemia** caused by different microorganisms (**meningococcus, gonococcus, pseudomonas**, etc.)
- Cutaneous lesions are variable and include **peripheral gangrene** and **purpuric generalized rash** with papules, nodules, pustules, and/or bullae
- Features of **disseminated intravascular coagulation** are present with purpura especially of the **extremities** and **dependent areas**

HISTOLOGIC FEATURES

- Mild **leukocytoclastic vasculitis** with **deep dermal** and **subcutaneous** involvement
- Often associated with **vasculopathy** in the form of **thrombi in vessels**
- Epidermal spongiosis with neutrophilic abscesses common
- **Necrosis** of dermal adnexa may be seen
- **Microorganisms** may be seen in **acute stage**

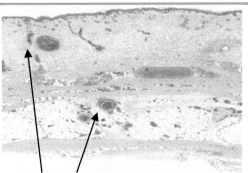

Superficial and deep perivascular inflammation of small and medium-sized vessels

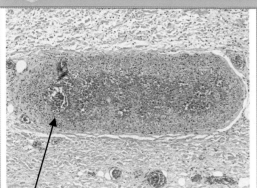

Medium vessel vasculitis in deep dermis

Path Presenter

DIFFERENTIAL DIAGNOSIS

OTHER LEUKOCYTOCLASTIC VASCULITIS
- Microorganisms may be seen in acute stages
- Deep inflammation with adnexal necrosis
- May be histologically indistinguishable from other "Big 5" LCV and clinical correlation necessary

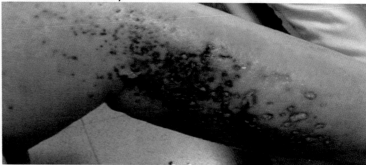

Palpable purpura with areas of eschar and impending cutaneous necrosis

EOSINOPHILIC GRANULOMATOSIS WITH POLYANGIITIS (EGP)

CLINICAL FEATURES
- Associated with **necrotizing vasculitis** and **asthma**
- Clinical presentation includes asthma, fever, multisystem necrotizing vasculitis, extravascular granuloma, and **hypereosinophilia**
- 40-70% patients develop cutaneous lesions. This may include petechiae, purpura, nodules, livedo reticularis, and ulceration
- Positive for **anti MPO (55-60%) (p-ANCA)**

HISTOLOGIC FEATURES
- **Leukocytoclastic vasculitis** with **numerous eosinophils**
- **Granulomatous** inflammation
- Inflammation often **palisades around degenerating collagen fibers**

OTHER HIGH YIELD POINTS
- Previously known as **Churg-Strauss Syndrome**
- Imaging of upper and lower respiratory tract (e.g. high-resolution CT scan), may be needed for workup and/or diagnosis

DIFFERENTIAL DIAGNOSIS

POLYARTERITIS NODOSA
- Necrotizing vasculitis with large vessel vasculitis and fibrinoid necrosis of small to mid-sized arteries
- Mixed inflammatory infiltrate that may have **secondary panniculitis**
- **Vessels at different stages** of involvement is characteristic
- Typically, **fewer eosinophils** than EGP, less granulomatous inflammation

OTHER LEUKOCYTOCLASTIC VASCULITIS
- May be histologically indistinguishable from other "Big 5" LCV and clinical correlation necessary. Typically other LCVs with fewer eosinophils

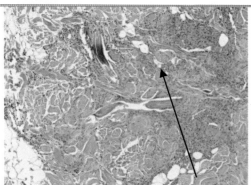

Deep granulomatous inflammation with palisading around collagen fibers

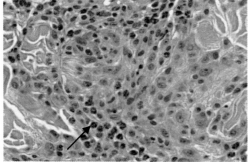

Numerous eosinophils amidst granulomatous inflammation

Path Presenter

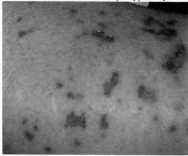 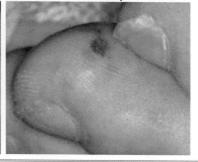

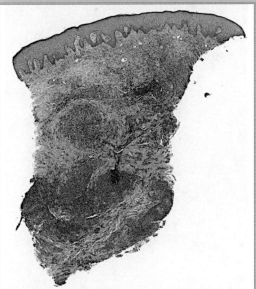

Superficial and deep inflammation

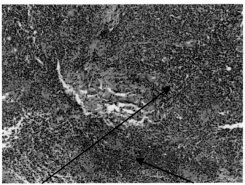

Dense granulomatous inflammation with red blood cell extravasation

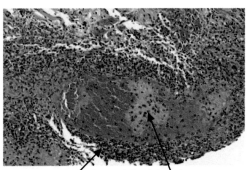

Medium vessel vasculitis with focal thrombus

Path Presenter

GRANULOMATOSIS WITH POLYANGIITIS (GPA)

CLINICAL FEATURES

- **Classic Triad**
  1. **Glomerulonephritis**
  2. Focal **vasculitis of the lung**
  3. Necrotizing **granulomatou**s lesions of the **upper and/or less often lower respiratory tract**
- The cutaneous findings include **purpura**, bruising, nodules, **oral ulcers**, **saddle-nose deformity**, gingival hyperplasia, and livedo reticularis
- Associated with **c-ANCA** in most cases

HISTOLOGIC FEATURES

- Epidermis frequently shows focal ulceration and/or necrosis
- Histologic findings are often non-specific, showing leukocytoclastic vasculitis
- Some cases show classic **necrotizing, granulomatous vasculitis** of small and medium-sized dermal vessels
- Extensive **necrosis of the dermis**
- **Older lesions** showing **palisading granulomas**
- **Thrombi** in vessels

OTHER HIGH YIELD POINTS

- Previously known as **Wegener's Granulomatosis**
- Imaging of upper and lower respiratory tract (e.g. high-resolution CT scan), may be needed for workup and/or diagnosis

DIFFERENTIAL DIAGNOSIS

POLYARTERITIS NODOSA

- Necrotizing vasculitis with large vessel vasculitis and fibrinoid necrosis of small to mid-sized arteries
- Mixed inflammatory infiltrate that may have **secondary panniculitis**
- **Vessels at different stages** of involvement is characteristic
- Typically, **fewer granulomas** than GPA

MICROSCOPIC POLYANGIITTIS:

- Presence of p-ANCA and associated kidney disease

OTHER LEUKOCYTOCLASTIC VASCULITIS

- May be histologically indistinguishable from other "Big 5" LCV and clinical correlation necessary Typically **other LCVs less granulomatous**

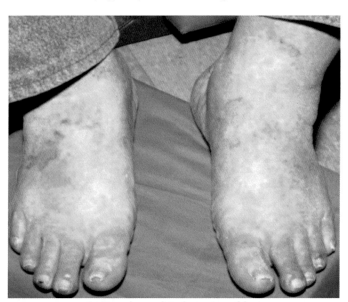

Scattered, angulated purpura of feet

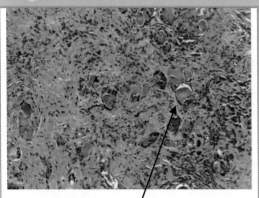

Type I Cryoglobulinemia: glassy material in small dermal blood vessels with little inflammation

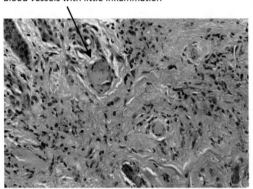

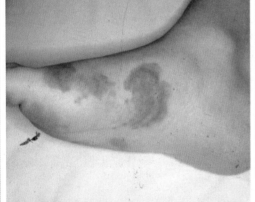

CRYOGLOBULINEMIA

CLINICAL FEATURES

- Type 1 Cryoglobulinemia
  - Patients generally **asymptomatic**
  - Cutaneous findings include purpura of the extremities with ulceration, livedo, Raynaud's phenomenon, and infarction of the digits, ears, and nose
  - **History of malignancy** such as Waldenström macroglobulinemia or multiple myeloma, or monoclonal gammopathy of uncertain significance (MGUS)
- Mixed Cryoglobulinemia (Type II and III)
  - Patients usually **symptomatic** with myalgias, arthralgias, **peripheral neuropathy** and **membranoproliferative glomerulonephritis**
  - Cutaneous findings include macules, papules, purpura with hemorrhagic crusts or ulcers, Raynaud phenomenon and livedo reticularis
  - Associated with Hepatitis, EBV

HISTOLOGIC FEATURES

- Type 1 Cryoglobulinemia
  - **Glassy material** ("jello jigglers") in **small dermal vessels** with little or **no inflammation**. Material is **PAS+**
- Mixed Cryoglobulinemia
  - **Thrombi in small dermal vessels** with associated **small vessel leukocytoclastic vasculitis.**

DIFFERENTIAL DIAGNOSIS (TYPE 1 CRYOGLOBULINEMIA)

DISSEMINATED INTRAVASCULAR COAGULAPATHY

- **Thrombin** in dermal vessels (rather than PAS+ glassy material, in Cryoglobulinemia Type 1.) Epidermal and dermal atrophy common in coumadin necrosis

MIXED CRYOGLOBULINEMIA

- **Thrombin** in dermal vessels with associated **LCV**

DIFFERENTIAL DIAGNOSIS (MIXED CRYOGLOBULINEMIA)

OTHER LEUKOCYTOCLASTIC VASCULITIS

- May be histologically indistinguishable from other "Little 5" LCV and clinical correlation is necessary

Path Presenter

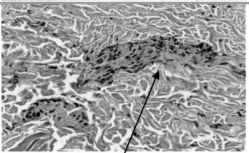

Low grade leukocytoclastic vasculitis

URTICARIAL VASCULITIS

CLINICAL FEATURES

- Clinically **resembles urticaria** but histologically shows LCV
- Systemic symptoms may include angioedema, **arthralgias**, pulmonary disease, abdominal pain
- Differs clinically from urticaria in that individual lesions may be **tender or burning**, have a **bruise-like color** and **last longer than 24 hours**

HISTOLOGIC FEATURES

- Early to **low grade leukocytoclastic vasculitis**, usually not fully developed. Admixed eosinophils
- In **later lesions, lymphocytic vasculitis** may be seen
- Karyorrhexis or fibrinoid necrosis, with or without RBC extravasation

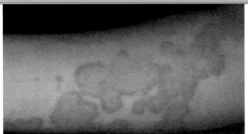

Urticarial-like plaques

Path Presenter

OTHER HIGH YIELD POINTS
- Subgroup has **hypocomplementemia** which correlates with systemic involvement and have **more severe disease**
- **Schnitzler's** syndrome: **urticarial vasculitis** + monoclonal **IgM gammopathy**

DIFFERENTIAL DIAGNOSIS
OTHER LEUKOCYTOCLASTIC VASCULITIS
- May be histologically indistinguishable from other "Little 5" LCV. Typically LCV in urticarial vasculitis not fully developed

URTICARIA
- **No karyorrhexis** in urticaria and mild **dermal edema**

ARTHROPOD ASSAULT
- **Eosinophils** are a prominent finding in arthropod assault, and can be seen **away from the vessels** and in the **deeper dermis**
- **Epidermis** is variably **spongiotic** in arthropod assault

---

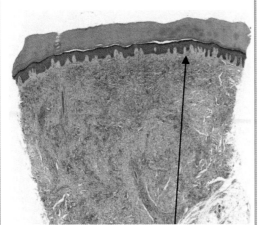

Nodular, dense inflammation with Grenz zone on acral skin

Mixed infiltrate with predominance of neutrophils

Path Presenter

ERYTHEMA ELEVATUM DIUTINUM
CLINICAL FEATURES
- Persistent, symmetric red or purple to yellow papules and plaques over the extensor surface of joints, especially the elbows, knees, hands, and feet
- May have arthralgia
- Asymptomatic to painful

HISTOLOGIC FEATURES
- Nodular, dense mixed infiltrate with **predominant neutrophils** and admixed lymphocytes and plasma cells
- **Early-stage lesions** show **leukocytoclastic vasculitis-like** appearance with predominance of **neutrophils**
- **Older** lesions show capillary proliferation with **neutrophilic** infiltrate, extracellular **cholesterol cleft deposits** and **onion-skinning fibrosis** surrounding vessels
- May have a Grenz Zone

OTHER HIGH YIELD POINTS
- Frequently associated with paraproteinemia; **IgA monoclonal gammopathy**

DIFFERENTIAL DIAGNOSIS
GRANULOMA FACIALE
- Facial skin, mixed infiltrate with **eosinophils**, neutrophils, lymphocytes, and plasma cells often in a **perivascular pattern**

SWEET SYNDROME
- Sweets often with marked papillary **dermal edema** and **diffuse neutrophils** in the dermis. Focal leukocytoclastic vasculitis but **no fibrinoid necrosis**

LEUKOCYTOCLASTIC VASCULITIS
- **Perivascular pattern** of inflammation in LCV

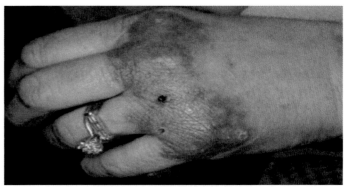

Red-brown plaque on dorsal hand

Grenz zone

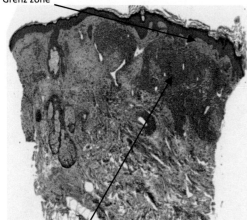

Dense, nodular perivascular inflammation

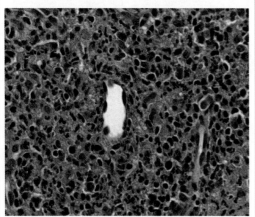

Mixed inflammation with eosinophils, neutrophils, lymphocytes, and plasma cells

Path Presenter

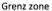

GRANULOMA FACIALE
CLINICAL FEATURES
- Most often occurs in middle-aged adult males
- Single or multiple red to brown firm papules and/or plaques
- Most commonly on the face (nose, malar prominence, forehead, and ear)

HISTOLOGIC FEATURES
- Nodular, dense mixed infiltrate with **eosinophils, neutrophils, lymphocytes, and plasma cells** often in a **perivascular pattern**
- **Grenz zone** often present
- **Leukocytoclastic vasculitis** in **early** lesions
- Concentric **fibrosis** surrounding dermal capillaries is **later** lesions

IMMUNOFLUORESCENCE/IMMUNOHISTOCHEMISTRY
- IgG, IgA, IgM and C3 within blood vessel walls on direct immunofluorescence

DIFFERENTIAL DIAGNOSIS
ERYTHEMA ELEVATUM DIUTINUM
- **Non-facial skin, neutrophil predominant,** later stages with lipid deposits/**cholesterol clefts**

SWEET SYNDROME
- Sweets often with marked papillary **dermal edema** and **diffuse neutrophils** in the dermis. Fewer to no eosinophils compared to granuloma faciale

ARTHROPOD ASSAULT
- **Eosinophils** are a prominent finding in arthropod assault, and can be seen **away from the vessels** and in the **deeper dermis**
- **Epidermis** is variably **spongiotic** in arthropod assault and it has a **wedge-shaped appearance** architecturally

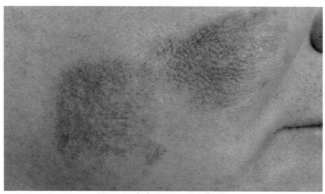

Firm, red plaque on the cheek

DEGOS DISEASE (MALIGNANT ATROPHIC PAPULOSIS)
CLINICAL FEATURES
- Small red macules that heal as white atrophic papules, commonly on trunk
- Historically related to a cutaneointestinal syndrome associated with abdominal pain that often led to intestinal perforations and death

HISTOLOGIC FEATURES
- Wedge-shaped area of altered dermis covered by atrophic epidermis with slight hyperkeratosis
- Vascular alterations: endothelial swelling, lymphocytic vasculitis, or intravascular fibrin thrombi
- Loss of adnexa with dermal sclerosis in older lesions
- Increased mucin in dermis
- Base of wedge in deep dermis may show thrombosed arterioles with minimal lymphocytic inflammation (may need multiple sections to visualize)

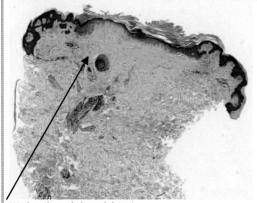

Wedge-shaped altered dermis

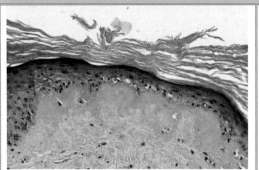

Hyperkeratosis overlying an atrophic epidermis

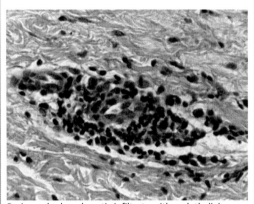

Perivascular lymphocytic infiltrate with endothelial swelling

HIGH YIELD POINTS
- 50% mortality usually related to brain or bowel infarcts
- Considered to be variant of connective tissue disease

DIFFERENTIAL DIAGNOSIS

SCAR
- Usually lacks atrophic epidermis and increased mucin

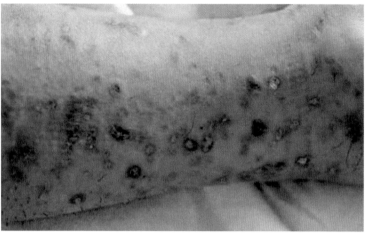

Red macules healing as atrophic white papules

Path Presenter

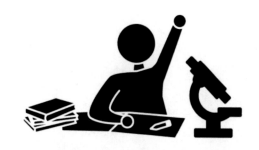

ACE MY PATH
Come Ace With Us!

CHAPTER 20: PANNICULITIS

ASHLEY ELSENSOHN, MD

PANNICULITIS

Septal Panniculitis

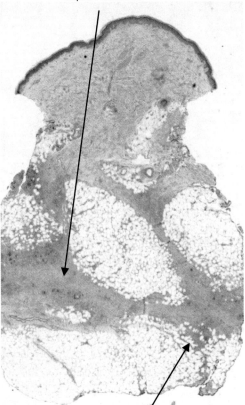

Minimal "spill-over "lace like lobular inflammation

Path Presenter

ERYTHEMA NODOSUM

CLINICAL FEATURES

- Scattered, red to purple tender nodules that do not ulcerate
- Most commonly involving the pretibial area of young adult women
- Clinical Differential Diagnosis: Polyarteritis Nodosa, Lymphoma Cutis, Morphea, Arthropod Assault, Bechet's Syndrome

HISTOLOGIC FEATURES

- **Septal panniculitis** with thickened fibrotic septa and lace-like infiltration into lobules. Fat lobules intact (same shape and size) – no necrosis
- Acute – Neutrophils and suppuration in septum
- Chronic – Eosinophils, lymphocytes, and granulomas
- **Miescher's radial granulomas** – septal granulomas that form in response to septal thickening and vessel degeneration

OTHER HIGH YIELD POINTS

- Majority of cases are idiopathic
- Typically **resolve in 3-6 weeks**
- Associated with **streptococcus infection** in kids, inflammatory bowel disease, **sarcoidosis** (Lofgren's), medications (iodides, bromides, sulfonamides), oral contraceptive pills (**OCPs**), and lymphoma

DIFFERENTIAL DIAGNOSIS

- SARCOIDAL PANNICULITIS – Non-caseating epithelioid granulomas in dermis and/or subcutaneous tissue with minimal lymphocytic infiltrate
- INFECTIVE PANNICULITIS – Lobular and septal panniculitis with neutrophilic and granulomatous inflammation. Abscess formation, hemorrhage, vasculitis and necrosis may also be present
- ERYTHEMA INDURATUM – Septal panniculitis +/- lobular panniculitis. Suppurative and granulomatous inflammation with vasculitis in the septa

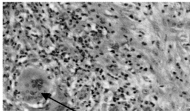 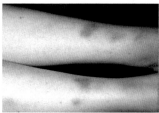

Multinucleated "Miescher's granuloma"   Tender subcutaneous nodules on shins

Mixed septal and lobular panniculitis

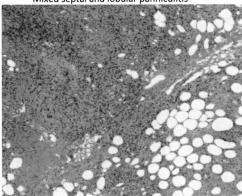

NODULAR VASCULITIS/ERYTHEMA INDURATUM

CLINICAL FEATURES

- Usually bilateral and involves the **calves of middle-aged women**
- Lesions ulcerate and drain liquefied fat/oil
- Clinical Differential Diagnosis: Infective panniculitis, erythema nodosum, polyarteritis nodosa

HISTOLOGIC FEATURES

- **Mixed septal and lobular panniculitis**
- Suppurative and granulomatous inflammation
- **Caseating granulomas** may be seen in lobules or septum
- **Vasculitis** in septa with inflammation around vessels and fibrinoid necrosis

OTHER HIGH YIELD POINTS

- Nodular vasculitis – tuberculosis is <u>**not**</u> present (type III)
- Erythema induratum – tuberculosis is present (type IV)
- Body's response to tuberculosis, high degree of immunity
- Erythema induratum improves with treatment of tuberculosis

Mixed septal and lobular panniculitis

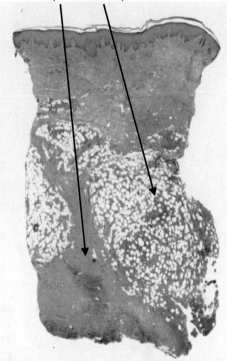

DIFFERENTIAL DIAGNOSIS

- **ALPHA1 ANTITRYPSIN DEFICIENCY** – Septal necrosis with associated lobular panniculitis. Vasculitis is not a typical feature. Neutrophilic infiltrate with admixed lymphocytes and macrophages
- **ERYTHEMA NODOSUM** – Septal panniculitis with lace-like infiltration into lobules. Acute phase can be neutrophil predominant. Vasculitis not typical
- **INFECTIVE PANNICULITIS** – Lobular and septal panniculitis with neutrophilic and granulomatous inflammation. Abscess formation, hemorrhage, vasculitis, and necrosis may also be present. Special stains and/or tissue cultures needed to confirm

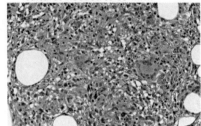
Suppurative and granulomatous infiltrate

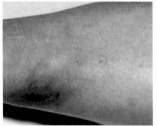
Tender subcutaneous nodule on the calf with evidence of early ulceration

Path Presenter

Lobular panniculitis

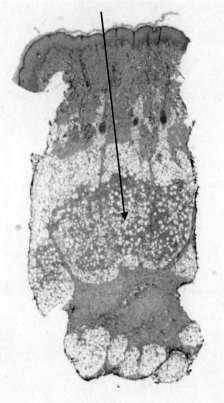

SUBCUTANEOUS FAT NECROSIS OF THE NEWBORN
CLINICAL FEATURES

- **Full term infants** with firm to rubbery, erythematous nodules, usually on the upper back, buttocks, cheeks, or proximal extremities
- Occurs within the first few weeks of life and resolves spontaneously within 3 months. No scarring
- Clinical Differential Diagnosis: Post-Steroid Panniculitis, Sclerema Neonatorum, Cellulitis, Farber's Lipogranulomatosis

HISTOLOGIC FEATURES

- **Lobular Panniculitis**
- **Dense** infiltrate of neutrophils, lymphocytes, plasma cells, and numerous multinucleated giant cells
- Fat necrosis with **needle shaped radial clefts** in lipocytes
- **Calcification** and fibrosis common

OTHER HIGH YIELD POINTS

- Crystals due to higher **oleic acid** – crystallized rosettes are not calcium like in pancreatic panniculitis (triglycerides)
- Granulomatous infiltrate most prominent at the periphery of the lobules
- Associated with hypercalcemia in a significant number of patients

DIFFERENTIAL DIAGNOSIS

- SCLEREMA NEONATORUM – Minimal inflammation and fat necrosis. Needle-shaped crystals arranged radially in adipocytes can be seen in both Sclerema neonatorum and subcutaneous fat necrosis of the newborn
- POST-STEROID PANNICULITIS – Lobular panniculitis with patchy infiltrate of macrophages, giant cells, lymphocytes, eosinophils, and neutrophils. Characteristic needle shaped crystals in radial fashion within lipocytes
- CUTANEOUS OXALOSIS – Presence of translucent polyhedral, rhomboid, and fan-like calcium oxalate crystals

Dense inflammatory infiltrate with neutrophils, giant cells, lymphocytes, and plasma cells

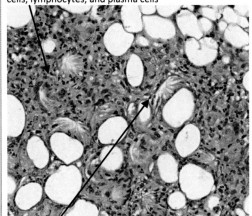

Needle shaped clefts in adipocytes

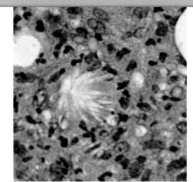

Needle shaped radial clefts in lipocytes

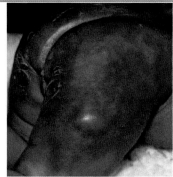

Full term infant with firm subcutaneous plaque on buttocks and upper legs

Path Presenter

Lobular panniculitis with minimal inflammation

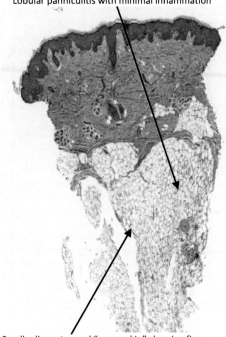

Small adipocytes and "young skin" showing fine, non-sun damaged reticular collagen bundles

Path Presenter

SCLEREMA NEONATORUM
CLINICAL FEATURES
- **Ill premature neonates** in the first few days of life. The skin begins to harden on the buttocks and lower extremities before rapidly spreading to the rest of the body
- Clinical Differential Diagnosis: Cold Panniculitis, Panniculitis of the Newborn, Post-Steroid Panniculitis, Subcutaneous Fat Necrosis of Newborn

HISTOLOGIC FEATURES
- **Lobular panniculitis**, **minimal inflammation,** and fibrotic septa
- **Needle shaped clefts** radially arranged within enlarged lipocytes
- Fibrosis and calcification "Young skin" with small adipocytes

OTHER HIGH YIELD POINTS
- Clinically **prognosis is very poor**

DIFFERENTIAL DIAGNOSIS
- POST-STEROID PANNICULITIS – Lobular panniculitis with patchy infiltrate of macrophages, giant cells, lymphocytes, eosinophils, and neutrophils. Needle-shaped crystals in radial fashion within lipocytes— this is also present in Sclerema neonatorum and subcutaneous fat necrosis of the newborn
- SUBCUTANEOUS FAT NECROSIS OF THE NEWBORN – Lobular panniculitis with dense infiltrate of neutrophils, lymphocytes, plasma cells, and numerous multinucleated giant cells. More inflammatory than Sclerema neonatorum although needle shaped clefts in lipocytes also present

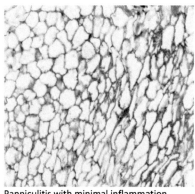

Panniculitis with minimal inflammation

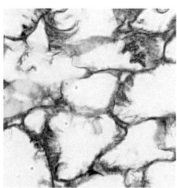

Needle shaped clefts within lipocytes

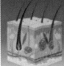

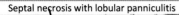
Septal necrosis with lobular panniculitis

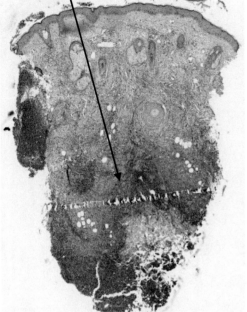

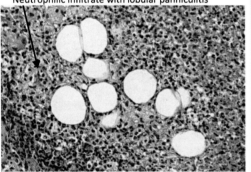
Neutrophilic infiltrate with lobular panniculitis

Path Presenter

ALPHA-1 ANTITRYPSIN DEFICIENCY
CLINICAL FEATURES
- Typically appears between **ages 20 to 40** but can occur in childhood after minor trauma
- Presents as painful nodules on the extremities or trunk that **drain an oily, brown liquid**
- Clinical Differential Diagnosis: Erythema Induratum, Infectious Panniculitis, Pancreatic Panniculitis, Pyoderma Gangrenosum, Sweet's Syndrome

HISTOLOGIC FEATURES
- **Septal necrosis** with associated **lobular panniculitis**
- Fat necrosis within lobules and liquefactive necrosis of fibrous septa
- **Neutrophilic** infiltrate with admixed lymphocytes and macrophages
- Characteristically affected areas in the fat with adjacent normal areas

OTHER HIGH YIELD POINTS
- Classic histologic description is necrosis and **liquefaction of the septa**, with fat lobules floating in a sea of red (necrotic septal material)
- Deficiency also results in **emphysema** and **liver disease**

DIFFERENTIAL DIAGNOSIS
- INFECTIVE PANNICULITIS – Lobular and septal panniculitis with neutrophilic and granulomatous inflammation. Abscess formation, hemorrhage, vasculitis, and necrosis may also be present. Special stains and/or tissue cultures needed to confirm diagnosis
- FACTICIAL PANNICULITIS – Lobular Panniculitis. May be foreign material in dermis and/or subcutis with associated fat necrosis. Suppurative and granulomatous response
- PANCREATIC PANNICULITIS – Lobular Panniculitis. Early disease can have neutrophilic infiltrate. Characteristic ghost cell and calcium saponification

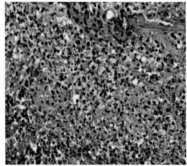
Dense neutrophilic inflammation

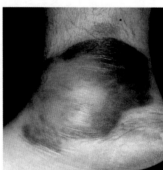
Subcutaneous induration with necrosis

CYTOPHAGIC HISTIOCYTIC PANNICULITIS (CHP)
CLINICAL FEATURES
- **Multisystem disease** that presents with widespread erythematous, painful subcutaneous nodules, which may become **ecchymotic or ulcerated**
- Other clinical features include **fever**, hepatosplenomegaly, pancytopenia, **hypertriglyceridemia**, and liver dysfunction
- Clinical Differential Diagnosis: Malignant histiocytosis, subcutaneous T-cell lymphoma, calciphylaxis, Infection

HISTOLOGIC FEATURES
- **Lobular panniculitis** Predominance of lymphocytes with admixed macrophages, neutrophils, and plasma cells
- **Cytophagocytosis**- macrophages engulfing erythrocytes, lymphocytes and karyorrhectic debris (**bean bag cells**)
- Rim of atypical lymphocytes around adipocytes

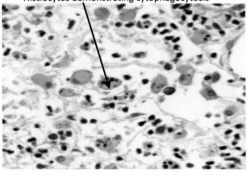
Histiocytes demonstrating cytophagocytosis

Lobular panniculitis

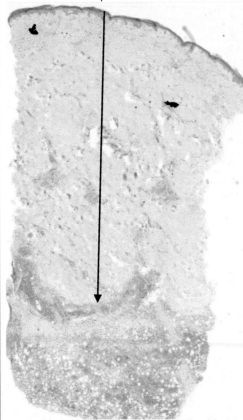

OTHER HIGH YIELD POINTS
- Some cases post-viral, others are caused by malignant clone of lymphocytes that secrete cytokines that cause the histiocytes to phagocytize
- "Bean bag cells" can also be seen in lupus profundus
- Prednisone and Cyclosporine responsive if CHP and not lymphoma

DIFFERENTIAL DIAGNOSIS
- SUBCUTANEOUS PANNICULITIS-LIKE T CELL LYMPHOMA – Atypical, clonal lymphocytes that rim adipocytes. Cytophagocytosis not present
- LUPUS PROFUNDUS – Lobular, lymphocytic panniculitis. May have interface changes present at the dermoepidermal junction and the presence of lymphoid follicles helps diagnose lupus profundus. "bean bag cell" may also be seen in lupus profundus, although fewer than in CHP
- ROSAI-DORMAN – Emperipolesis which can look similar to CHP, but Rosai-Dorfman is not limited to the fat and is S100+ (CHP S100-)

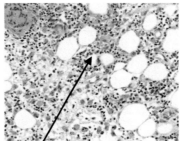

Atypical lymphocytes around adipocytes Admixed histocytes and plasma cells   Cytophagocytosis "bean bag cells"

Path Presenter

PANCREATIC PANNICULITIS

CLINICAL FEATURES
- Tender or painless erythematous subcutaneous nodules most commonly on the **lower leg** in patients with either **pancreatitis** or **pancreatic cancer**
- May ulcerate and drain a brown, oily material
- Clinical Differential Diagnosis: Alpha-1 Antitrypsin Deficiency Panniculitis, Erythema Induratum, Erythema Nodosum, Infectious Panniculitis, Factitial Panniculitis, Subcutaneous Panniculitis Like T Cell Lymphoma

HISTOLOGIC FEATURES
- **Lobular panniculitis** with mixed infiltrate of foamy histiocytes, lymphocytes and neutrophils
- Fat necrosis with **ghost-like fat cells** (amorphous pink cells; honeycomb-like; no contrast and loss of nuclear detail)
- **Calcium saponification** – basophilic granular deposits in adipocytes

OTHER HIGH YIELD POINTS
- In nearly half of cases, panniculitis is the first sign of the pancreatic pathology
- Patients often also report arthritis
- Increased risk in Down's syndrome

DIFFERENTIAL DIAGNOSIS
- INFECTIVE PANNICULITIS – Lobular and septal panniculitis with neutrophilic and granulomatous inflammation. Abscess formation, hemorrhage, vasculitis and necrosis may also be present
- ALPHA1 ANTITRYPSIN DEFICIENCY – Septal necrosis with associated lobular panniculitis. Neutrophilic infiltrate with admixed lymphocytes and macrophages. Ghost-like fat cells and calcium saponification not present

Lobular panniculitis

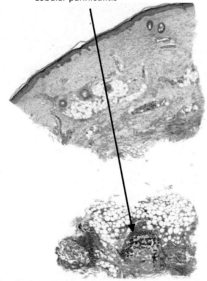

Path Presenter

Lobular panniculitis with calcium saponification

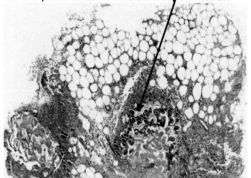

- CALCIPHYLAXIS – Lobular Panniculitis. Can have stippled calcifications on elastic fibers, eccrine glands, around adipocytes, and in small blood vessels. Variable fibrin thrombi

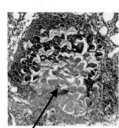
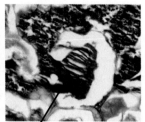
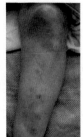

Ghost cells   Calcium saponification

Lobular panniculitis

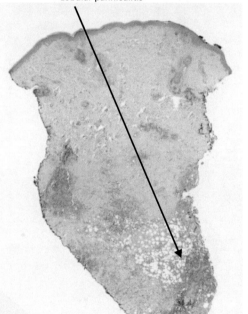

LUPUS PANNICULITIS

CLINICAL FEATURES

- Firm, usually **non-tender** subcutaneous nodules on the proximal extremities
- Healing results in depression and hyperpigmentation
- Similar to other forms of lupus, **women** between the **ages of 20 and 45** are most affected
- Clinical Differential Diagnosis: Atrophoderma of Pasini and Pierini, Erythema Induratum, Erythema Nodosum, Morphea Profunda, Subcutaneous Panniculitis Like T Cell Lymphoma

HISTOLOGIC FEATURES

- **Lobular panniculitis** with **lymphocytic nodules** and admixed plasma cells
- **Hyalinization** of fat lobules
- Dermis may have morphea-like sclerosis. Calcification may be seen
- May or may not have **associated changes of lupus** in dermis and at the **DEJ**

OTHER HIGH YIELD POINTS

- Lupus Panniculitis also called **lupus profundus**
- Positive DIF with granular deposits at the dermal-epidermal junction if there is interface change. **Lymphoma can look similar.** Worry about atypical lymphocytes around adipocytes
- CD123 positive plasmacytoid dendritic cells favor connective tissue disease

DIFFERENTIAL DIAGNOSIS

- SUBCUTANEOUS PANNICULITIS-LIKE T CELL LYMPHOMA – Atypical, clonal lymphocytes that rim adipocytes. No interface changes present
- ERYTHEMA INDURATUM – Septal panniculitis +/- lobular panniculitis. Neutrophilic and granulomatous inflammation with vasculitis in the septa

Hyalinization of fat

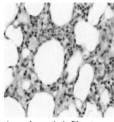
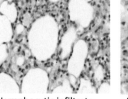
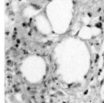
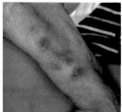

Lymphocytic infiltrate   Hyaline necrosis   Non-tender nodules proximal arm

Path Presenter

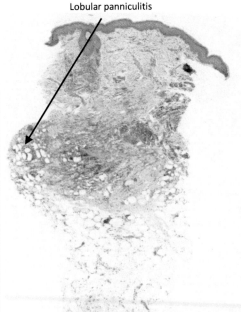
Lobular panniculitis

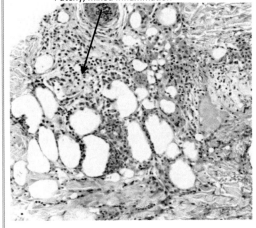
Patchy, mixed inflammation

POST-STEROID PANNICULITIS

CLINICAL FEATURES

- Firm subcutaneous nodules on the cheeks, trunk, and proximal extremities within a month of **tapering systemic corticosteroids**
- Clinical Differential Diagnosis: Cold Panniculitis, Panniculitis of the Newborn, Sclerema Neonatorum

HISTOLOGIC FEATURES

- **Lobular panniculitis** with patchy infiltrate of macrophages, giant cells, lymphocytes, eosinophils, and neutrophils
- Characteristic **needle shaped crystals** in radial fashion within lipocytes and macrophages

OTHER HIGH YIELD POINTS

- Most commonly develops in children on high doses of systemic corticosteroids that are rapidly withdrawn

DIFFERENTIAL DIAGNOSIS

- INFECTIVE PANNICULITIS – Lobular and septal panniculitis with neutrophilic and granulomatous inflammation. Abscess formation, hemorrhage, vasculitis and necrosis may also be present
- FACTITIAL PANNICULITIS – Lobular Panniculitis. May be foreign material in dermis and/or subcutis with associated fat necrosis. Suppurative and granulomatous response

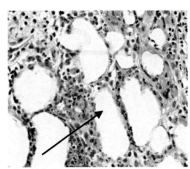
Mixed lobular inflammation

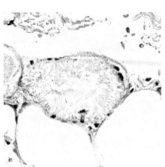
Needle shaped radially arranged crystals

Path Presenter

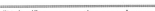
"Naked" non-caseating granulomas

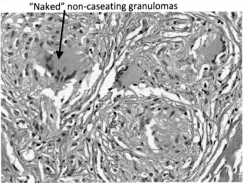

SUBCUTANEOUS SARCOIDOSIS

CLINICAL FEATURES

- Most commonly presents as a **systemic disorder** with uveitis, bilateral hilar lymphadenopathy, and pulmonary infiltration
- Cutaneous lesions are generally plaques with a red-brown-violaceous color that looks like "**apple jelly**" when blanched
- Clinical Differential Diagnosis: Gouty Tophi, Epidermoid Cyst, Interstitial Granulomatous Dermatitis, Morphea, Lipoma, Rheumatoid Nodule, Subcutaneous Panniculitis T Cell Lymphoma

HISTOLOGIC FEATURES

- **Non-caseating** epithelioid **granulomas** in dermis and/or subcutaneous tissue with **minimal lymphocytic infiltrate ("naked" granulomas)**
- **Schaumann bodies** (may be present) – calcium and protein inclusions in the cytoplasm of giant cells

Dermal and subcutaneous granulomas

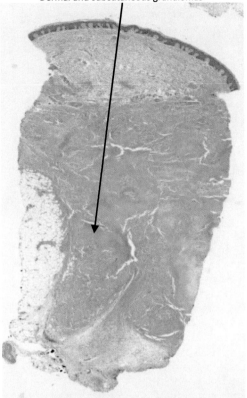

- **Asteroid bodies** (may be present) – eosinophilic, stellate or spider-like inclusions in the cytoplasm of giant cells

OTHER HIGH YIELD POINTS

- Sarcoidosis is a **diagnosis of exclusion.** Must rule out infection (negative fungal, mycobacterial staining) and foreign body granuloma

DIFFERENTIAL DIAGNOSIS

- INFECTIVE PANNICULITIS – Lobular and septal panniculitis with neutrophilic and granulomatous inflammation. Abscess formation, hemorrhage, vasculitis, and necrosis may also be present. Special stains and/or tissue cultures needed to confirm
- FACTITIAL PANNICULITIS – Lobular Panniculitis. May be foreign material in dermis and subcutis with associated fat necrosis. Suppurative and granulomatous

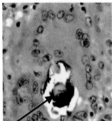
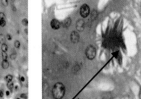
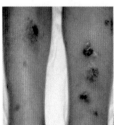

Schaumann body   Asteroid body   Red-brown nodules and plaques

Path Presenter

LIPODERMATOSCLEROSIS

CLINICAL FEATURES

- Early – erythematous tender subcutaneous nodules or plaques on legs that resemble erythema nodosum
- Late – woody induration of legs resulting in an **inverted champagne bottle appearance** to the medial lower legs
- Clinical Differential Diagnosis: Cellulitis, Stasis Dermatitis, Eosinophilic Cellulitis, Erythema Nodosum, Nephrogenic Systemic Sclerosis, Pretibial Myxedema

HISTOLOGIC FEATURES

- **Lobular panniculitis** with dermal changes of **stasis dermatitis**
- Sclerotic septa with mild to moderate chronic inflammation and siderophages
- **Fat necrosis** with **lipomembranous changes**

OTHER HIGH YIELD POINTS

- Clinically, induration can be seen without obvious inflammatory panniculitis
- Location on **medial malleolus** helps distinguish from erythema nodosum (shins) and from most other panniculitides (posterior mid calves)
- Gradual progression from ankles proximally also helps distinguish from other lobular panniculitis

DIFFERENTIAL DIAGNOSIS

- LUPUS PROFUNDUS – Lobular, lymphocytic panniculitis. May have interface changes present at the dermoepidermal junction and the presence of lymphoid follicles helps diagnose lupus profundus
- MORPHEA PROFUNDUS – Thickened and hyalinized collagen bundles in the deep dermis and subcutis with a moderate lymphocytic infiltrate. Loss of CD34 with immunohistochemical staining

Lobular panniculitis

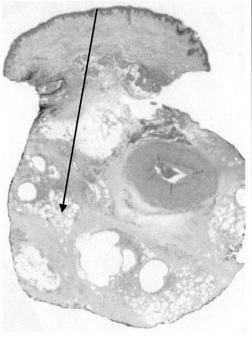

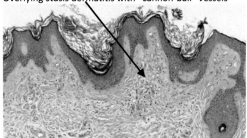
Overlying stasis dermatitis with "cannon-ball" vessels

Path Presenter

- ERYTHEMA NODOSUM – Septal panniculitis with lace-like infiltration into lobules. Acute phase can be neutrophil predominant. Vasculitis not a typical feature

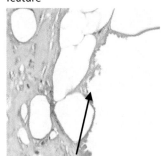
Lipomembranous changes

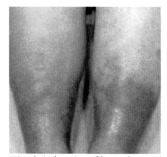
Woody induration of lower legs with "inverted champagne bottle" appearance

TRAUMATIC/FACTICIAL PANNICULITIS

CLINICAL FEATURES

- Occurs most commonly on the **shins, thighs, breasts, arms, and buttock** of **women.** Initially there is often bruising followed by induration at injury site
- Clinical Differential Diagnosis: Erythema nodosum, lupus profundus, infective panniculitis, Atrophoderma of Pasini and Pierini

HISTOLOGIC FEATURES

- **Lobular** panniculitis
- Early – fat microcysts surrounded by histiocytes, collections of foam cells, and inflammatory cells
- Late – fibrosis, **lipomembranous changes**, or dystrophic **calcium** deposits
- May be **foreign material** in dermis and/or subcutis with associated fat necrosis if factitial. Suppurative and granulomatous response

OTHER HIGH YIELD POINTS

- A **suture reaction** can cause some traumatic/foreign body reaction in the fat
- Can show **lipophages** – foamy histiocytes in adipose tissue that are full of fat – in any traumatic panniculitis

DIFFERENTIAL DIAGNOSIS

- SCLEROSING LIPOGRANULOMA – granulomatous subcutaneous reaction with extensive fibrosis and hyalinization. "Swiss-cheese" like appearance from injection of oily substance
- SILICONE – "Swiss-cheese" like appearance. Foreign body granulomatous inflammation with giant cells that have refractile and non-birefringent particles

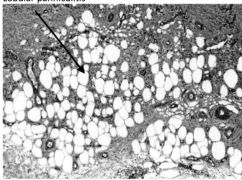
Lobular panniculitis

Path Presenter

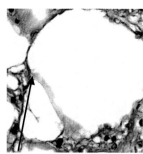
Lipomembranous changes

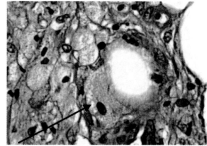
Lipophages (lipid laden foamy histiocytes)

Lobular and septal panniculitis

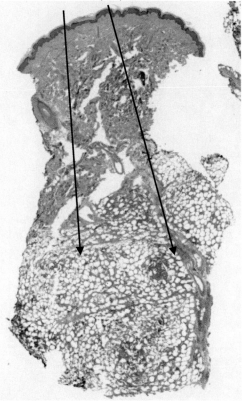

INFECTIVE PANNICULITIS

CLINICAL FEATURES

- Presents similar to other panniculitides as often painful, red deep subcutaneous nodules on the legs, arms, and trunk
- Clinical Differential Diagnosis: Cellulitis, Alpha-1 Antitrypsin Deficiency Panniculitis, Erythema Induratum, Erythema Nodosum, Traumatic Panniculitis, Pancreatic Panniculitis

HISTOLOGIC FEATURES

- **Lobular and septal** panniculitis
- **Neutrophilic** and **granulomatous** inflammation
- **Abscess** formation, hemorrhage, **vasculitis** and necrosis

OTHER HIGH YIELD POINTS

- **Neutrophilic** panniculitis includes infectious causes, early pancreatic panniculitis, alpha 1 antitrypsin, erythema induratum, traumatic/factitial, bowel bypass, and Behcet's Syndrome

DIFFERENTIAL DIAGNOSIS

- ALPHA1 ANTITRYPSIN DEFICIENCY – Septal necrosis with associated lobular panniculitis. Vasculitis not a typical feature. Neutrophilic infiltrate with admixed lymphocytes and macrophages
- ERYTHEMA INDURATUM – Septal panniculitis +/- lobular panniculitis. Suppurative and granulomatous inflammation with presence of vasculitis in the septa
- PANCREATIC PANNICULITIS – Lobular Panniculitis. Early disease can have neutrophilic infiltrate. Characteristic ghost cell and calcium saponification

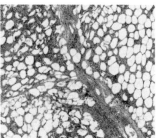 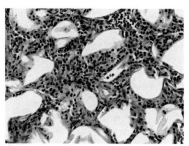

Lobular and septal panniculitis   Mixed inflammation with neutrophils and histiocytes

Lobular Panniculitis with numerous eosinophils

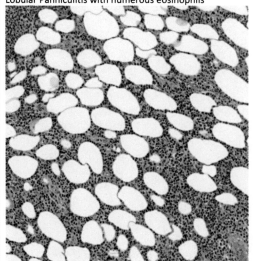

EOSINOPHILIC PANNICULITIS

CLINICAL FEATURES

- Presents similar to other panniculitides as often painful, red deep subcutaneous nodules
- Clinical Differential Diagnosis: Cellulitis, infective panniculitis, erythema induratum, traumatic panniculitis, morphea profundus

HISTOLOGIC FEATURES

- **Lobular panniculitis** with **eosinophils** predominating the infiltrate
- **Flame figures** often present – degranulated **major basic protein** from eosinophils on collagen bundles

OTHER HIGH YIELD POINTS

- Eosinophilic panniculitis is a histologic pattern that is seen in a diverse range of disease entities— parasites, hypereosinophilic syndrome, arthropod assaults, eosinophilic granulomatosis with polyangiitis, Wells Syndrome, etc.

DIFFERENTIAL DIAGNOSIS

- EOSINOPHILIC GRANULOMATOSIS WITH POLYANGITIS – Small to medium vessel necrotizing vasculitis with eosinophils. Flame figures may be present
- ARTHROPOD BITE – Wedge shaped superficial and deep mixed inflammatory infiltrate often with overlying spongiosis. Typically, eosinophils perivascular and interstitial. Flame figures, dermal edema and vasculitis may be present

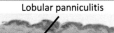

Lobular panniculitis

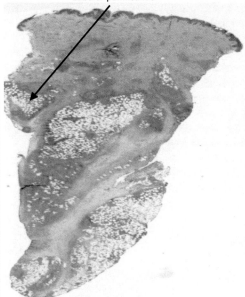

- WELLS SYNDROME – Diffuse, superficial and deep dermal infiltrate of perivascular and interstitial eosinophils. Flame figures may be present. No vasculitis present

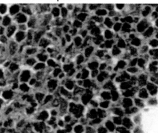

Numerous eosinophils

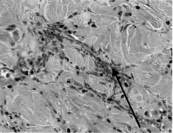

"Flame figure" from degranulate eosinophilic major basic protein on collagen bundles

Path Presenter

Lobular panniculitis

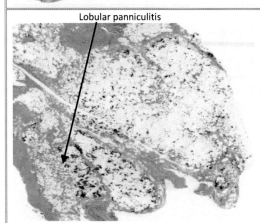

Scattered calcification and subcutaneous fat

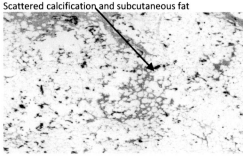

Path Presenter

CALCIPHYLAXIS

CLINICAL FEATURES

- Occurs in patients with **renal failure** and **secondary hyperparathyroidism**
- Tender, **livedoid** erythematous plaques or nodules most commonly on the buttocks, abdomen, and breasts
- Clinical Differential Diagnosis: Antiphospholipid Antibody Syndrome, Warfarin Necrosis, Heparin Necrosis, Disseminated Intravascular Coagulation

HISTOLOGIC FEATURES

- **Lobular panniculitis** with fat necrosis and dermal necrosis
- Mural **calcification** and intimal proliferation within small vessels of deep dermis and subcutaneous fat with **variable fibrin thrombi**
- Can have **stippled calcifications** on **elastic fibers**, **eccrine glands**, around adipocytes, and in small blood vessels

OTHER HIGH YIELD POINTS

- Calcification can be subtle and the use of a **von Kossa stain** might be helpful

DIFFERENTIAL DIAGNOSIS

- CALCINOSIS CUTIS – Calcium present. Unlike calciphylaxis, there is NO mural calcification in the small vessels in the subcutaneous fat
- CUTANEOUS OXALOSIS – Presence of translucent polyhedral, rhomboid, and fan-like calcium oxalate crystals
- PANCREATIC PANNICULITIS – Lobular Panniculitis. Early disease can have neutrophilic infiltrate. Characteristic ghost cell and calcium saponification

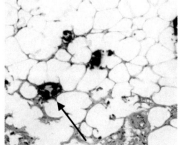

Calcification of small vessels in fat

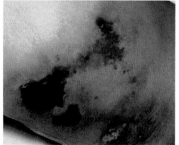

Livedoid, necrotic plaque

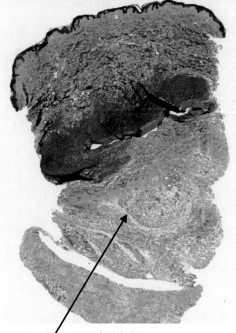

Atrophic subcutaneous fat lobules

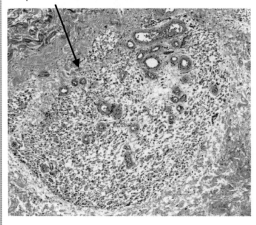

LIPOATROPHY-LIPODYSTROPHY

CLINICAL FEATURES

- Subcutaneous fat is markedly reduced
- Lipodystrophies can be generalized, partial, or localized, and may be congenital or acquired. **Hypertriglyceridemia** and **diabetes mellitus** with insulin resistance occur in many cases
- **Acquired** lipodystrophy is associated with Highly Active Antiretroviral Therapy (**HAART**) for **HIV**
- Clinical Differential Diagnosis: Atrophoderma of Pasini and Pierini, Cachexia, Cushing Syndrome, Lupus, Parry-Romberg Syndrome

HISTOLOGIC FEATURES

- Atrophic subcutaneous nodules with **small lipocytes**, intervening hyalinized connective tissue with increased capillaries
- Sometimes associated with mild inflammation

OTHER HIGH YIELD POINTS

- Looks like "baby fat" histologically because small adipocytes and lobules but in an adult

DIFFERENTIAL DIAGNOSIS

- LIPODERMATOSCLEROSIS – Lobular panniculitis with dermal changes of stasis dermatitis. Sclerotic septa with mild to moderate chronic inflammation and siderophages. Fat necrosis with lipomembranous changes
- FOCAL DERMAL HYPOPLASIA – adipose tissue high in the dermis. Can be subepidermal, mid-dermal, perivascular, or involved the entire dermis

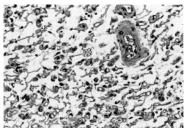

Small lipocytes with increased capillaries

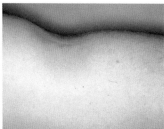

Markedly reduced subcutaneous fat

Path Presenter

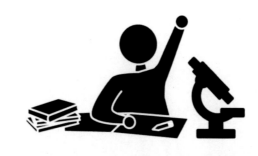

ACE MY PATH
Come Ace With Us!

CHAPTER 21: INFECTIONS AND
INFESTATIONS

SNEHAL SONAWANE, MD
POOJA SRIVASTAVA, MD

BACTERIAL INFECTIONS

Epidermal ulceration

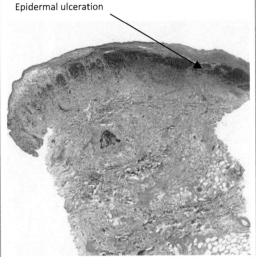

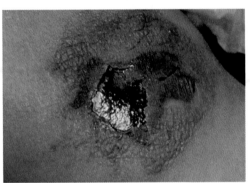

Thick adherent crusts over punched out ulcers

ECTHYMA
CLINICAL FEATURES
- This is a deeper version of impetigo that mostly occurs on the lower extremities
- There are thick adherent crusts over punched out ulcers with indurated borders, usually associated with Streptococcus pyogenes

HISTOLOGICAL FEATURES
- Epidermal ulceration with scale crust
- Heavy neutrophilic infiltrate in dermis
- Gram positive cocci within inflammatory crust may be seen

OTHER HIGH YIELD POINTS
- Clinical differential diagnosis includes Ecthyma Gangrenosum, Pyoderma Gangrenosum, Anthrax

DIFFERENTIAL DIAGNOSIS
- Cellulitis: Dermal edema with diffuse interstitial neutrophilic infiltrate. Epidermis may show ulceration. Bacteria may be seen in some cases within the dermal infiltrate
- Bullous Impetigo: Subcorneal bulla with few neutrophils and rare acantholytic cells. Gram positive cocci may be seen within the bulla
- Herpes: Dermal edema with ballooning degeneration of keratinocytes with acantholysis followed by intradermal vesicle formation; Multinucleation of keratinocytes (fusing of adjacent cells), molding and margination of nuclear chromatin; Intranuclear and cytoplasmic basophilic and/or pale ground-glass inclusions; Background of neutrophilic inflammation; Dermal vessels can demonstrate features of leukocytoclastic vasculitis; HSV infection of the hair follicle epithelium can result in herpes folliculitis

Path Presenter

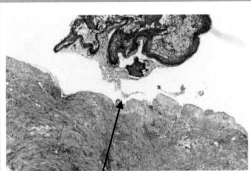

Epidermal ulceration

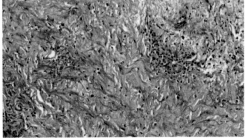

Interstitial neutrophilic infiltrate

CELLULITIS
CLINICAL FEATURES
- Ill-defined expanding erythema with warmth, edema and tenderness characterize cellulitis
- The lower extremities are most commonly affected in adults, usually at a site of trauma
- Commonly due to Group A streptococci, Staphylococcus aureus and other bacteria, cultures may be positive in 10 percent of cases

HISTOLOGICAL FEATURES
- Dermal edema with diffuse interstitial neutrophilic infiltrate
- Epidermis may show ulceration
- Bacteria may be seen in some cases within the dermal infiltrate

OTHER HIGH YIELD POINTS
- Clinical differential diagnosis includes Lipodermatosclerosis, Erysipelas, Allergic Contact Dermatitis, Arthropod Bite Reaction, Calciphylaxis
- This is primarily a clinical diagnosis
- Skin biopsy can be performed if there is any question about the diagnosis

DIFFERENTIAL DIAGNOSIS
- Erysipelas: Cellulitis of face, usually has a sharply demarcated elevated border. Dermal edema with perivascular and interstitial neutrophilic infiltrate, Dermal foci of suppurative necrosis may be present

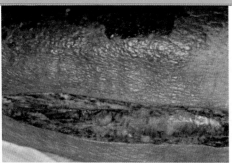
Necrotizing Fasciitis

- Necrotizing Fasciitis: Dense infiltration of soft tissue and fascia with neutrophils and lymphocytes amidst necrosis and hemorrhage
- Atypical Mycobacterial Infection: Histologic findings are variable, ranging from acute suppurative poorly formed granulomas to chronic well-formed tuberculoid granulomas, typically located within the dermis, epidermal changes range from acanthosis, pseudoepitheliomatous hyperplasia to ulceration. AFB/Fite stain will reveal rare organisms in immunocompetent hosts

Path Presenter

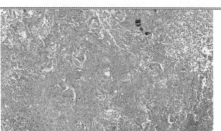
Necrosis & hemorrhage

Neutrophils, lymphocytes amidst necrosis & hemorrhage

Path Presenter

NECROTIZING FASCIITIS
CLINICAL FEATURES
- This rapidly progressing deep infection has been referred to as "flesh eating bacteria
- The lower extremities are the most common site
- The initial cellulitis-like presentation can progress quickly to a dusky violaceous color with cutaneous anesthesia but deep pain out of proportion to the clinical findings
- Systemic toxicity is notable

HISTOLOGICAL FEATURES
- Dense infiltration of soft tissue and fascia with neutrophils and lymphocytes amidst necrosis and hemorrhage
- Secondary vasculitis and vasculopathy (thrombosis)

OTHER HIGH YIELD POINTS
- This is a potentially life threatening surgical and medical emergency
- Often related to immunosuppression, diabetes, drug abuse, injury, peripheral vascular disease

DIFFERENTIAL DIAGNOSIS
- Pyoderma Gangrenosum: Epidermal ulceration and focal dermal necrosis, pseudoepitheliomatous hyperplasia. Characterized by diffuse neutrophilic infiltrate with abscess formation and occasionally admixed giant cells
- Cellulitis: Dermal edema with diffuse interstitial neutrophilic infiltrate. Epidermis may show ulceration. Bacteria may be seen in some cases within the dermal infiltrate

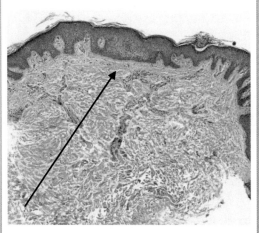

ERYTHRASMA
CLINICAL FEATURES
- This corynebacterial infection (Corynebacterium minutissimum) presents as a well-defined red-brown finely scaly patch in an intertriginous area

HISTOLOGICAL FEATURES
- Filamentous Gram-positive rods in stratum corneum, also seen on H&E
- Minimal inflammation

OTHER HIGH YIELD POINTS
- "Wood's lamp examination demonstrating coral red fluorescence is diagnostic
- Washing of area before Wood's lamp examination may lead to false negativity
- Skin scraping for KOH preparation to exclude superficial fungal infection
- Skin biopsy can be performed if there is any question about the diagnosis

DIFFERENTIAL DIAGNOSIS
- Dermatophytosis: The organisms are hyphae and spores, better visualized with PAS or GMS stain
- Candidiasis: Epidermal hyperplasia, with parakeratosis and neutrophils in the cornified layer. Hyphae often in vertical orientation, with spores

Minimal inflammation
Filamentous Gram-positive rods in stratum corneum

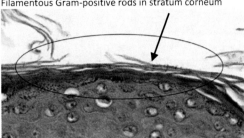

- Allergic Contact Dermatitis

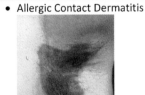

red-brown finely scaly patch   Wood's lamp exam   Path Presenter

Gram-positive coccobacilli in stratum corneum

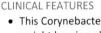

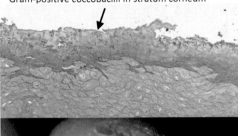

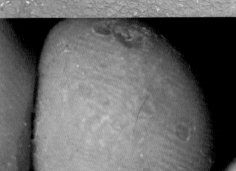

Path Presenter

PITTED KERATOLYSIS
CLINICAL FEATURES
- This Corynebacterium infection (Micrococcus Sedentarius) occurs on the weight bearing plantar surface as shallow pits and erosions, associated with hyperhidrosis and odor
HISTOLOGICAL FEATURES
- Small pits in partially macerated stratum corneum with Gram positive coccobacilli or filaments
OTHER HIGH YIELD POINTS
- This is primarily a clinical diagnosis
- Skin biopsy can be performed if there is any question about the diagnosis
DIFFERENTIAL DIAGNOSIS
- Dermatophytosis: The hallmark feature of dermatophytosis is the presence of hyphae in the stratum corneum. Hyphae may be apparent on H&E and are usually highlighted with PAS or GMS staining. Varying degrees of inflammation and spongiosis may be seen in the underlying epidermis and dermis. Neutrophils may be present and it is not uncommon to see neutrophils admixed in the parakeratotic horn
- Candidiasis: Epidermal hyperplasia, with parakeratosis and neutrophils in the cornified layer. Hyphae often in vertical orientation, with spores
- Darier's Disease: Abnormal keratinocyte-keratinocyte adhesion and aberrant epidermal keratinization are the primary histologic features. Hyperkeratosis, acanthosis, and papillomatosis present. Suprabasal acantholysis with dyskeratosis forming corps ronds and grains

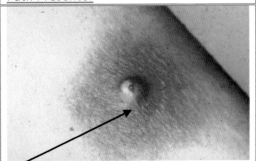

Erythematous purulent nodule

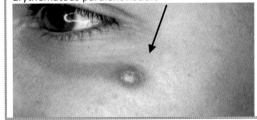

FURUNCLE/CARBUNCLE
CLINICAL FEATURES
- This is an acute tender erythematous purulent nodule
- Predilection for the posterior neck, axilla, thigh, perineum and buttocks as well as any hair bearing site
HISTOLOGICAL FEATURES
- Acute infection predominantly involving follicle below infundibulum
- Perifollicular inflammation, focal necrosis, dermal abscess inflammation and occasional subcorneal pustule
CARBUNCLE
CLINICAL FEATURES
- This is a collection of furuncles with multiple draining tracts that extend into the deep subcutaneous tissue
HISTOLOGICAL FEATURES
- Multiple inflamed follicles with suppurative inflammation below infundibulum
- Some follicles may be ruptured with surrounding foreign body reaction
OTHER HIGH YIELD POINTS
- Correlate clinical findings with culture studies and Gram stain
- Skin biopsy in resistant cases or if there is any question about the diagnosis

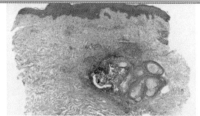
Inflammation in and around follicle

DIFFERENTIAL DIAGNOSIS

- Suppurative Folliculitis: Acute and chronic inflammatory infiltrate in association with a hair follicle
- Fungal Folliculitis: Intra and perifollicular neutrophilic infiltrate with or without eosinophils. Hyphae within follicle and overlying stratum corneum

Path Presenter

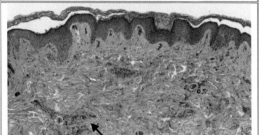
Vasculitis and vasculopathy with associated necrosis

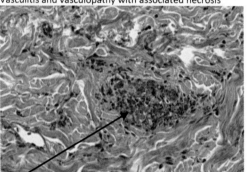
Vasculitis and vasculopathy with associated necrosis

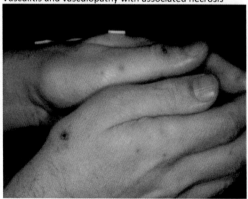

MENINGOCOCCEMIA
CLINICAL FEATURES

- This occurs most in children and young adults with fever, chills, hypotension, and meningitis
- Acral petechial lesions and ecchymoses are common and gray infarctive lesions with an erythematous halo are characteristic

HISTOLOGICAL FEATURES

- Acute cases-vasculitis and vasculopathy with associated necrosis, hemorrhage, and thrombosis
- Gram negative diplococci (Neisseria meningitidis) may be seen in and around vessels
- Chronic cases- Perivascular lymphocytic infiltrate with neutrophils
- Gram negative diplococci in vessels

OTHER HIGH YIELD POINTS

- Blood culture, Skin biopsy, Gram stain and tissue culture. Cultures of cerebrospinal fluid should be sent if meningitis is a clinical concern
- Throat culture. Cultures of other aspirates of clinically indicated
- PCR tests available
- Latex agglutination test
- Other laboratory workup may include CBC with differential, complete metabolic panel including renal and hepatic function tests, coagulation studies (PT, PTT, platelet count, fibrinogen, fibrin degradation products, D dimer), urinalysis
- Chest Xray, echocardiogram and other investigations, MRI to determine extent of disease and organ involvement; sometimes even shock in adrenocortical insufficiency (Waterhouse-Friderichsen syndrome)

DIFFERENTIAL DIAGNOSIS

- Gonococcemia: Histology similar to meningococcemia
- Viral Exanthem: usually no vasculitis. Dyskeratosis in epidermis
- Rocky Mountain Spotted Fever: Predominantly a lymphocytic vasculitis

Path Presenter

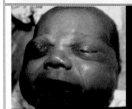
Vesiculopustule

GONOCOCCEMIA
CLINICAL FEATURES

- This is a multisystem illness due to dissemination from the primary sexually transmitted mucosal infection
- Features include fever, arthralgia, and arthritis
- The skin lesions are acral small erythematous macules that become vesiculopustules on a purpuric base

HISTOLOGICAL FEATURES

- Focal epidermal necrosis, intraepidermal and subepidermal neutrophilic micro abscesses

Leukocytoclastic vasculitis

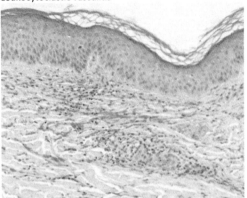

- Leukocytoclastic vasculitis with hemorrhage and thrombosis
- Gram negative diplococci may be noted

OTHER HIGH YIELD POINTS

- Blood culture, Skin biopsy, Gram stain and tissue culture. Cultures of cerebrospinal fluid should be sent if meningitis is a clinical concern

DIFFERENTIAL DIAGNOSIS

- Leukocytoclastic Vasculitis: Usually no organisms noted
- Meningococcemia: Histology similar
- Rocky Mountain Spotted Fever: Predominantly lymphocytic vasculitis

Path Presenter

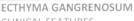

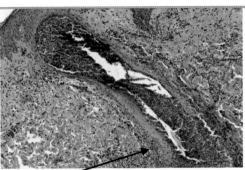

Broken follicular epithelium with acute inflammation

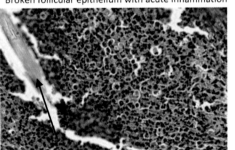

Naked hair shaft and acute inflammation

Path Presenter

PSEUDOMONAL FOLLICULITIS

CLINICAL FEATURES

- This is also known as hot tub folliculitis due to exposure to organisms in the heated water
- The eruption presents a few days after exposure as pruritic erythematous follicular papules and pustules on the trunk

HISTOLOGICAL FEATURES

- Also known as Hot tub folliculitis
- Broken follicular epithelium surrounded by acute inflammation and secondary vasculitis

OTHER HIGH YIELD POINTS

- Culture and Gram stain of pustules. Skin biopsy can be performed if there is any question about the diagnosis
- This is usually a self-limited condition, and treatment is generally not necessary in immunocompetent patients
- In immunocompromised patients, more severe cases

DIFFERENTIAL DIAGNOSIS

- Bacterial Folliculitis: Spongiosis of the follicular epithelium with neutrophil accumulation and pustule formation. Bacterial colonies within follicular orifice. May have follicular rupture with dermal abscess formation or granulomatous inflammation
- Suppurative Folliculitis: Acute and chronic inflammatory infiltrate in association with a hair follicle
- Majocchi's Granuloma: Hyphae and spores within hair follicle and surrounding dermis, with rupture of follicular epithelium. Dense suppurative and granulomatous mixed inflammatory infiltrate within the surrounding dermis

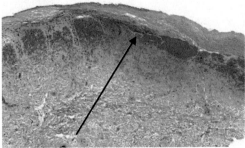

Necrosis and ulceration of epidermis

ECTHYMA GANGRENOSUM

CLINICAL FEATURES

- This bacterial infection is most often due to Pseudomonas aeruginosa septicemia
- Red to purple macules ulcerate and develop black eschar
- The anogenital region and extremities are sites of predilection

HISTOLOGICAL FEATURES

- Necrosis and ulceration of epidermis
- Focal necrosis of dermis with sparse inflammation, sometimes with vasculitis and vasculopathy

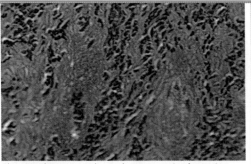

Blue-grey haze around vessels representing bacteria
Path Presenter

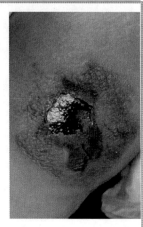

- Blue-grey haze in dermis consisting of sheets of Gram-negative bacilli

OTHER HIGH YIELD POINTS
- Skin biopsy with Gram stain
- Tissue and blood cultures

DIFFERENTIAL DIAGNOSIS
- Cellulitis: Dermal edema with diffuse interstitial neutrophilic infiltrate. Epidermis may show ulceration. Bacteria may be seen in some cases within the dermal infiltrate
- Pyoderma Gangrenosum: Findings are variable depending on the site biopsied and the stage of the lesion. Dense neutrophilic infiltrate. No bacteria noted
- Mucor: Broad based fungi noted

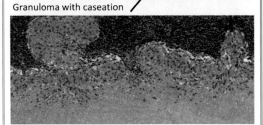

Granuloma with caseation

Path Presenter

TUBERCULOSIS (TUBERCULOSIS VERRUCOSA CUTIS)
- AFB bacilli usually present

CLINICAL FEATURES
- This occurs after direct inoculation into the skin in a person with some immunity or active infection elsewhere
- An indurated nodule develops a keratotic warty surface that expands but focally involutes
- The knees, elbows, hands, feet and buttocks are common sites of involvement

HISTOLOGICAL FEATURES
- Hyperkeratosis, papillomatosis, acanthosis with intraepidermal neutrophilic abscesses
- Suppurative and granulomatous inflammation in dermis
- Granulomas may or may not show caseation

OTHER HIGH YIELD POINTS
- Skin biopsy for acid fast bacilli stain and mycobacterial culture
- PCR for detection of mycobacterial DNA can be performed in tissue
- Chest Xray Sputum acid fast bacilli smear and culture
- Skin purified protein derivative (PPD test) and interferon-γ release assay
- HIV testing for all patients diagnosed with tuberculosis

DIFFERENTIAL DIAGNOSIS
- Verruca Vulgaris: Papillated epidermal hyperplasia with hypergranulosis. No neutrophilic abscesses
- Deep Fungal Infection: Granulomatous and suppurative inflammation, often with overlying pseudoepitheliomatous hyperplasia. Fungal elements highlighted by PAS and GMS stains within the infiltrate

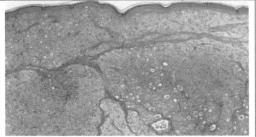

Diffuse dermal infiltrate of foamy macrophages

LEPROSY
Lepromatous Leprosy
CLINICAL FEATURES
- This is seen typically in patients who have a poor cell mediated immunity to Mycobacterium leprae
- Lesions are symmetric, firm and nodular with a predilection for the cooler face and dorsal hands
- Loss of eyebrow hair is common
- The lesions become anesthetic due to neural involvement

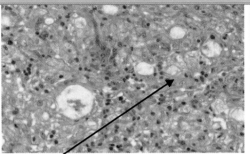
Diffuse dermal infiltrate of foamy macrophages

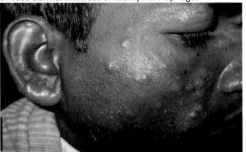
Lesions are symmetric, firm and nodular

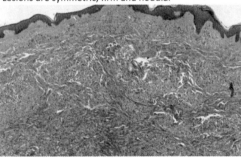
Histoid Leprosy: Nodular proliferation of spindled cells with some polygonal cells

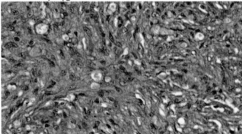
Histoid Leprosy: Nodular proliferation of spindled cells with some polygonal cells

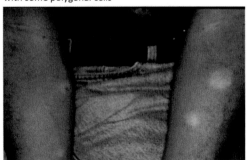

HISTOLOGICAL FEATURES
- Grenz zone separating a diffuse dermal infiltrate of foamy macrophages from epidermis
- Numerous AFB and Fite positive organisms in clusters (globi)

OTHER HIGH YIELD POINTS
- Clinical features may highly suggest the diagnosis
- Skin biopsy for histologic examination and special stains to detect organisms. Skin smear, Tissue culture to rule out other mycobacterial infections
- PCR to detect M leprae DNA from tissue. Nerve biopsy may be useful in ruling out neuropathic forms of leprosy. Serum antiPGL-1 antibodies (not available in the US) are only sensitive for the diagnosis of leprosy in the setting of multibacillary disease, and not helpful in the diagnosis of tuberculoid leprosy VDRL and FTAABS (false positivity)
- HLAB*13:01 recently reported to be associated with development of hypersensitivity syndrome to dapsone among leprosy patients

DIFFERENTIAL DIAGNOSIS
- Sarcoidosis: Diagnosis of exclusion. Infection stains negative
- Granular Cell Tumor: Cells positive for S100 and CD68
- Atypical Mycobacterial Infection: Histologic findings are variable, ranging from acute suppurative poorly formed granulomas to chronic well-formed tuberculoid granulomas, typically located within the dermis. Epidermal changes range from acanthosis, pseudoepitheliomatous hyperplasia to ulceration. AFB stain will reveal rare organisms in immunocompetent hosts

Histoid Leprosy

CLINICAL FEATURES
- This variant occurs in patients with lepromatous leprosy with development of numerous cutaneous and subcutaneous nodules and plaques, especially on bony areas like the elbows and knees

HISTOLOGICAL FEATURES
- Nodular proliferation of spindle cells with some polygonal cells
- Many organisms within these cells seen with Fite stain
- Admixed foamy macrophages may be present

OTHER HIGH YIELD POINTS
- Clinical features may highly suggest the diagnosis
- Skin biopsy for histologic examination and special stains to detect organisms
- Skin smear
- Tissue culture to rule out other mycobacterial infections
- PCR to detect M leprae DNA from tissue
- Nerve biopsy may be useful in ruling out neuropathic forms of leprosy
- Serum antiPGL-1 antibodies (not available in the US) are only sensitive for the diagnosis of leprosy in the setting of multibacillary disease, and not helpful in the diagnosis of tuberculoid leprosy
- VDRL and FTAABS (false positivity)
- HLAB*13:01 recently reported to be associated with development of hypersensitivity syndrome to dapsone among leprosy patients

DIFFERENTIAL DIAGNOSIS
- Dermatofibroma: No associated inflammation or organisms
- Sarcoidosis: Naked granulomas, stains negative

Path Presenter   Path Presenter

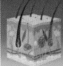
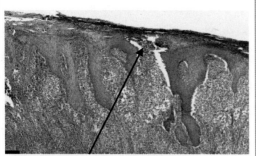
Central ulceration with pseudoepitheliomatous hyperplasia

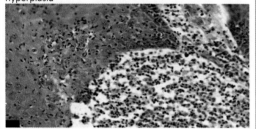
Suppurative inflammation with micro abscesses

Path Presenter

GRANULOMA INGUINALE

CLINICAL FEATURES

- This sexually transmitted disease, due to Klebsiella granulomatis, results in beefy red friable painless ulcers of the perineum

HISTOLOGICAL FEATURES

- Central ulceration with surrounding pseudoepitheliomatous hyperplasia
- Suppurative and granulomatous inflammation with admixed histiocytes, plasma cells and scattered neutrophilic micro abscesses
- Large macrophages can show the gram-negative organisms (Donovan bodies) Warthin starry and Giemsa stains can highlight the organisms. Bipolar staining will highlight organisms showing a safety pin appearance (1-2 microns)

OTHER HIGH YIELD POINTS

- Identification of intracytoplasmic inclusion bodies (Donovan bodies) on tissue smears with the assistance of special stains (Giemsa, Wright, or Leishman)
- Screening for other sexually transmitted diseases should be considered

DIFFERENTIAL DIAGNOSIS

Syphilis: Variable findings depending on the morphology of the biopsied lesion. May see: Combined psoriasiform epidermal hyperplasia with hyperkeratosis and parakeratosis. Superficial and deep perivascular and periadnexal lymphocytic infiltrate with admixed plasma cells, sometimes in a lichenoid Interface/vacuolar change. Long thin rete ridges. Variable spongiosis. Neutrophils in the granular layer and/or stratum corneum. Immunohistochemical stain will show spirochetes in 70-90% of cases

Malakoplakia: Macrophages show granules that stain with Von Kossa, Iron stains

Chancroid: Shows zones of inflammation under ulceration-necrotic debris and neutrophils on surface, granulation tissue in middle and deeper plasma cells and lymphocytes

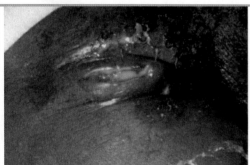

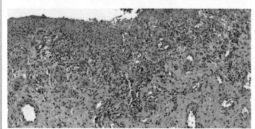
Ulceration with underlying neutrophils and plasma cells

Path Presenter

CHANCROID

CLINICAL FEATURES

- This sexually transmitted disease, due to Gram negative coccobacilli-Haemophilus ducreyi, results in a painful punched-out tender ulcer with purulent base, nonindurated (soft chancre)
- Suppurative unilateral lymphadenopathy

HISTOLOGICAL FEATURES

- Ulcer with fibrin and neutrophils in base. Underlying granulation tissue with the deepest layers showing dense infiltrate of plasma cells and neutrophils
- Coccobacilli may be seen within the topmost neutrophilic zone

OTHER HIGH YIELD POINTS

- Identification of organism on special culture media
- Exclusion of other infectious causes for genital ulcer (e.g., syphilis, herpesvirus, etc.)
- Screening for other sexually transmitted infections should be considered

DIFFERENTIAL DIAGNOSIS

- Syphilitic Chancre: Significant admixed plasma cells and spirochete positive bacilli
- Herpes: Dermal edema with ballooning degeneration of keratinocytes with acantholysis followed by intradermal vesicle formation, Multinucleation of keratinocytes (fusing of adjacent cells), molding and margination of nuclear chromatin. Intranuclear and cytoplasmic basophilic and/or pale ground-glass inclusions. Background of neutrophilic inflammation
- Lymphogranuloma Venereum: Genital ulcers related to Chlamydia trachomatis L1, L2, and L3 serovars. Granulomatous inflammation associated with perifollicular infiltrates composed of lymphocytes, histiocytes and plasma cells. Associated neural hyperplasia and fibrosis

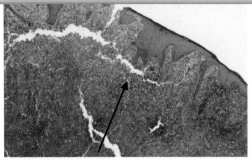

Inflammation with hemorrhage

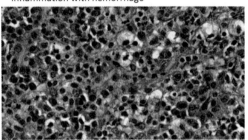

Macrophages with admixed plasma cells

RHINOSCLEROMA

CLINICAL FEATURES

- This bacterial infection (Klebsiella rhinoscleromatis) most commonly affects the nasal cavity in tropical areas
- What starts as rhinitis becomes swollen blue-red mucosa with intranasal rubbery nodules and polyps and eventuates in deformity and destruction of the nasal cartilage

HISTOLOGICAL FEATURES

- Dense infiltrate of macrophages, neutrophils, lymphocytes with admixed plasma cells and Russell bodies
- Some of the larger macrophages (Mikulicz cells) contain a large number of Gram-negative bacilli. Bacilli visible on H&E, PAS and Giemsa stains
- Pseudoepitheliomatous hyperplasia and fibrosis in older lesions

OTHER HIGH YIELD POINTS   Path Presenter

- Skin biopsy
- Tissue culture
- Head and neck CT and MRI imaging

DIFFERENTIAL DIAGNOSIS

- Histoplasma Capsulatum: Granulomatous dermatitis with admixed macrophages, lymphocytes, neutrophils, and plasma cells. Intracellular organisms with round, basophilic nuclei and rod-like kinetoplast scattered haphazardly and filling the macrophages

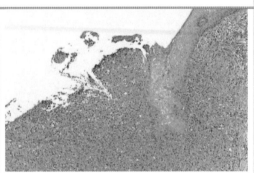

Sheets of histiocytes, admixed with neutrophils, plasma cells, lymphocytes, and granulation tissue

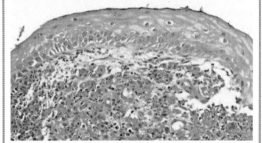

Characteristic basophilic bodies containing calcium

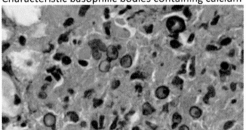

MALAKOPLAKIA

CLINICAL FEATURES

- Mostly seen in immunocompromised patients. Poor ability of macrophages to digest E coli
- The condition most commonly affects the urinary tract but can also involve the GI tract, lymph nodes, brain, bone, adrenals, and skin
- Presentation of the disease can vary and may include papules, plaques, polyps, ulcers, and sinuses. Skin lesions associated with this condition are non-progressive but persist as firm nodules
- Some skin lesions may exhibit a central dimple or draining sinus

HISTOLOGICAL FEATURES

- Sheets of histiocytes (Granular von Hansemann histiocytes) other inflammatory cells are present, including neutrophils, plasma cells, lymphocytes, and granulation tissue
- Within the histiocytes, characteristic basophilic round laminated structures (Michaelis Gutmann bodies) noted. Stain with Von Kossa, Iron and PAS

OTHER HIGH YIELD POINTS

- When dealing with E coli infections, a combination of antibiotic therapy and surgery is often the most effective approach

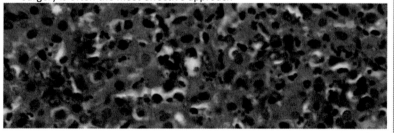

Path Presenter

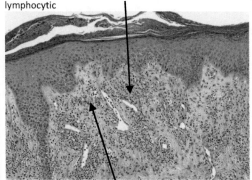

Mild leukocytoclastic vasculitis, predominantly lymphocytic

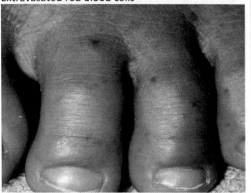

Extravasated red blood cells

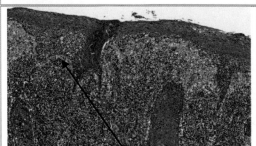

Path Presenter

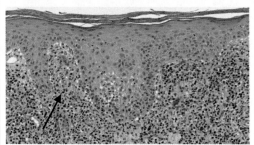

Psoriasiform hyperplasia with thin rete ridges

Lichenoid and perivascular inflammation with plasma cells

ROCKY MOUNTAIN SPOTTED FEVER

CLINICAL FEATURES

- This tick born infection (caused by gram negative coccobacillus, Rickettsia rickettsii) presents with fever, myalgias, headache and petechial rash starting on the ankles/wrists and palms/soles with centripetal spread
- Infectious vasculitis results in potentially fatal systemic involvement

HISTOLOGICAL FEATURES

- Mild leukocytoclastic vasculitis, predominantly lymphocytic with occasional fibrin microthrombi in vessels
- Extravasated red blood cells common
- Epidermis may show ulceration, lymphocytic exocytosis, scattered apoptosis and vacuolar alteration at the DEJ
- Organisms may be seen in vessels on Giemsa stain

OTHER HIGH YIELD POINTS

- Clinical appearance with history of a tick bite may suggest the diagnosis and treatment should be initiated immediately when there is high clinical suspicion
- Serologic studies may be unreliable in early stages of infection
- Skin biopsy can be performed for routine histology
- Immunofluorescent or immunoperoxidase staining of R. rickettsii performed on frozen tissue can be used for rapid histologic diagnosis, however this is not a very sensitive method.
- Laboratory workup includes CBC with differential, basic metabolic panel including renal function tests, liver function tests, coagulation panel
- Serologic diagnosis (via indirect immunofluorescent antibody, latex agglutination, or enzyme immunoassay) is usually retrospective, because antibodies become positive in the 2nd or 3rd week of disease, and delaying treatment until serologic confirmation may result in death
- PCR studies may be helpful

DIFFERENTIAL DIAGNOSIS

- Viral Exanthem: usually no vasculitis or vasculopathy
- Meningococcemia: gram negative coccobacilli noted

SECONDARY SYPHILIS

CLINICAL FEATURES

- Generalized papulosquamous rash that involves palms and soles, and/or the mouth and anogenital regions
- Eruption commonly manifests as symmetric, non-pruritic, variably scaly, pink to copper-colored discrete macules and papules
- Palm and sole lesions may be tender on palpation ("Ollendorff's sign")
- Patchy "moth-eaten" alopecia may be noted
- Condyloma lata may be seen in the anogenital folds or in the mouth. Highly infectious
- Mucosal lesions are often eroded erythematous macules and patches
- Patients may have systemic symptoms, including malaise, fever, chills, headache, anorexia, myalgias, photophobia, conjunctival injection, arthralgias, splenomegaly, sore throat, among other findings
- Lymphadenopathy almost always present (particularly at epitrochlear nodes)
- Secondary syphilis occurs approximately 1-3 months after a primary syphilis chancre, upon hematogenous and lymphatic dissemination of the spirochete
- Secondary syphilis lesions heal within 2-10 weeks, with or without treatment If left untreated, approximately ¼ of patients will relapse within 2 years

HISTOLOGICAL FEATURES

- Can present with variable findings depending on the morphology of the biopsied lesion
- Combined psoriasiform epidermal hyperplasia with hyperkeratosis and

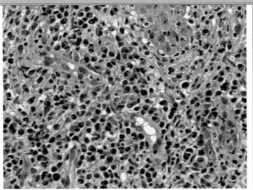

Numerous plasma cells with lymphocytes

Noduloulcerative lesions

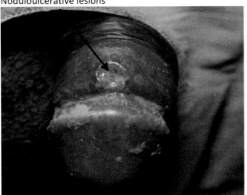

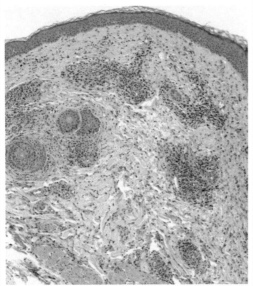

Superficial and deep perivascular and periadnexal infiltrate

Path Presenter

- parakeratosis
- Superficial and deep perivascular and periadnexal lymphocytic infiltrate with admixed plasma cells, sometimes in a lichenoid fashion
- Interface/vacuolar change
- Long thin rete ridges
- Variable spongiosis
- Neutrophils in the granular layer and/or stratum corneum
- Endothelial cell swelling
- Immunohistochemical stain will show spirochetes in 70-90% of cases

OTHER HIGH YIELD POINTS

- Serologic testing
- Traditionally, nontreponemal serology screening (e.g., VDRL, RPR) is performed first, with all positive cases confirmed with a specific treponemal test (e.g., FTAABS, MHATP, TPPA, TPEIA). All patients should be tested for HIV (repeat testing in 3 months if first test is negative) and be evaluated for other sexually transmitted diseases
- Some laboratories reverse the order of testing, with starting with treponemal enzyme and chemiluminescence immunoassays (EIA/CIA) and followed by testing all reactive sera with quantitative nontreponemal test
- False negative results may occur with nontreponemal serology testing, particularly in the setting of HIV, and retesting is indicated
- False negativity can also occur due to prozone phenomenon, and if syphilis is strongly suspected, the serum should be diluted and test should be rerun
- False positive results can occur with nontreponemal test due to various reasons: collagen vascular disease, endocarditis, liver disease, intravenous drug use, multiple blood transfusions, pregnancy, lymphomas, non-syphilis treponemal infection, rickettsial infections, tuberculosis, etc.
- False positive results with treponemal tests are less common, but can occur in various settings: lupus erythematosus (including drug induced), pregnancy, genital herpes infections, rheumatoid arthritis, scleroderma, smallpox vaccination, hypergammaglobulinemia, non-syphilis treponemal infection
- Nontreponemal test titers generally reflect disease activity and therefore may be used to monitor efficacy of treatment
- Treponemal tests remain positive for life and cannot distinguish past successfully treated infection versus current active infection
- PCR can also be performed from affected tissue
- Direct identification of spirochetes can be attempted by darkfield microscopy or direct fluorescent antibody testing, however, may be difficult at this stage
- Darkfield microscopy should not be performed on oral mucosa lesions because it cannot distinguish commensal spirochetes of the oral mucosa from T pallidum
- Skin biopsy can also be helpful and can rule out other alternative possibilities. Immunohistochemical stain for T pallidum and silver stains to detect spirochetes are available
- Full history and physical examination. Patients may require examination and additional procedures by subspecialists (e.g., ophthalmologic examination, neurologic examination, cardiologic and vascular evaluation)
- Patients with late syphilis should be given a CSF examination before initiating treatment. Imaging tests may be indicated to evaluate involvement of other organs (e.g., bones, CNS, heart, great vessels)

DIFFERENTIAL DIAGNOSIS

- Drug Eruption: Eosinophils are more predominant and epidermal changes less evident
- Lyme Disease: Epidermal Changes less prominent, clinicopathological correlation helpful. Serology for Lyme

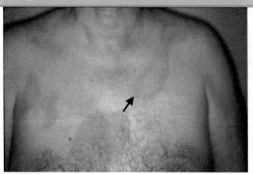

Erythematous papule with extending annular erythema that clears centrally

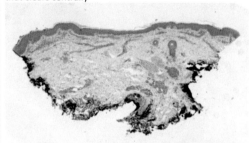

Superficial and deep perivascular lymphocytic infiltrate

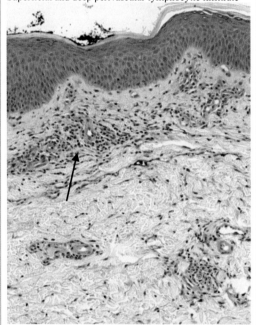

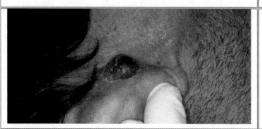

Perivascular lymphocytic infiltrate with plasma cells

ERYTHEMA MIGRANS (Lyme Disease)
CLINICAL FEATURES

- Erythema Migrans is the characteristic eruption of Lyme disease
- It starts at the tick bite site as an erythematous papule with extending annular erythema that clears centrally
- Multiple lesions can appear with dissemination but are smaller and less migratory
- Arthritis is the second most common systemic presentation

HISTOLOGICAL FEATURES

- Superficial and deep perivascular lymphocytic infiltrate with plasma cells and occasional eosinophils
- Spirochetes may be seen in dermis and/or subcutaneous tissue

OTHER HIGH YIELD POINTS

- The diagnosis can usually be made based on history and presence of characteristic erythema migrans lesion
- Serologic testing for confirmation
- ELISA screening followed by Western blot confirmation
- Because of low sensitivity of serologic testing in early disease and seroconversion may take as long as 68 weeks after a tick bite, patients with typical erythema migrans lesions do not require confirmatory testing and should be treated
- False positive serologies may occur in syphilis, pinta, yaws, leptospirosis, relapsing fever, infectious mononucleosis, and diseases that produce autoantibodies
- Skin biopsy is also helpful
- Silver staining can be performed in search of spirochetes, but sensitivity is low
- Cultures and PCR studies can be performed, but not widely available to clinicians and not practical
- Full history and physical examination with special attention to signs and symptoms of extracutaneous disease
- Patients with extracutaneous involvement may need additional evaluation and studies by other specialists (e.g., lumbar puncture and brain MRI for suspected meningitis/neurologic involvement, EKG, and cardiologic evaluation for Lyme carditis, electrophysiologic tests for suspected neuropathy, ophthalmologic evaluation, rheumatologic evaluation, etc.)

DIFFERENTIAL DIAGNOSIS

- Secondary Syphilis: Clinical presentation and serology are helpful
- Lupus Erythematosus: Vacuolar interface changes and associated periadnexal inflammation
- Drug Eruption: Superficial and deep perivascular lymphocytic infiltrate with admixed eosinophils +/-. epidermal spongiosis with exocytosis and vacuolar change with rare apoptotic keratinocytes

Path Presenter

BACILLARY ANGIOMATOSIS
CLINICAL FEATURES

- These tender pyogenic granuloma-like lesions are due to Bartonella henselae and B. quintana infection, typically in immunosuppressed patients, particularly AIDS
- Reddish friable nodules resembling pyogenic granuloma
- Less commonly plaques or nodules develop
- Multi-system involvement is typical

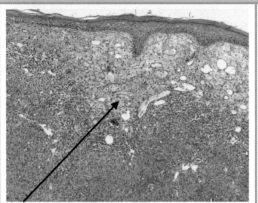

Lobular blood vessel proliferation

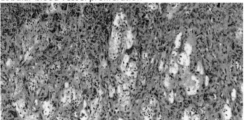

Plump endothelial cells in a background of pale edematous stroma

HISTOLOGICAL FEATURES
- Lobular blood vessel proliferation with plump endothelial cells in a background of pale edematous stroma
- Admixed neutrophilic infiltrate with granulomatous inflammation
- Scattered smudgy amphophilic areas containing Bartonella bacilli in clusters within the proliferation-highlighted by Warthin-Starry

OTHER HIGH YIELD POINTS
- Skin biopsy and visualization of bacilli by Warthin Starry staining
- Culture or PCR for blood and/or tissue for Bartonella species can also be helpful
- Commonly occurs in the setting of immunosuppression, particularly AIDS
- Liver function test shows elevated LDH and alkaline phosphatase levels
- Imaging studies to evaluate for visceral and bone involvement

DIFFERENTIAL DIAGNOSIS
- Kaposi Sarcoma: Spindle cell proliferation with hemorrhage
- Pyogenic Granuloma: No organisms noted with Warthin Starry

Path Presenter

FUNGAL INFECTIONS

Bullous dermatophytosis: Fungal elements

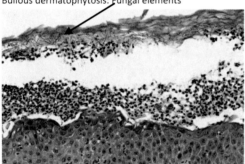

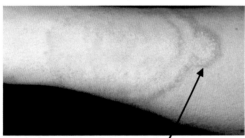

Annular lesion with well demarcated margins

Path Presenter

DERMATOPHYTOSIS

CLINICAL FEATURES
- There are various manifestations of this infection including: atrophic or hyperplastic oral forms, angular cheilitis, moist erythematous areas with pustules at the margin involving the skin folds, and chronic paronychia

HISTOLOGICAL FEATURES
- Hyphae in stratum corneum
- Mild to moderate inflammation usually with some neutrophils
- Sandwich sign-orthokeratosis or parakeratosis in between layers of basket-weave hyperkeratosis

OTHER HIGH YIELD POINTS
- Clinical differentials include Streptococcal Intertrigo, Contact Dermatitis, Intertrigo
- KOH preparation of skin or oral scrapings, Fungal culture for diagnosis
- Biopsy may be helpful to confirm the diagnosis and to rule out alternative possibilities
- Patients with chronic mucocutaneous candidiasis often present with repeated, therapy resistant infections

DIFFERENTIAL DIAGNOSIS
- Tinea Versicolor: Orthokeratosis with hyphae and spores (spaghetti and meat ball appearance), often visible on H&E
- Bullous Impetigo: Subcorneal bulla with few neutrophils and rare acantholytic cells. Gram positive cocci may be seen within the bulla

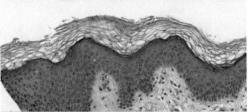
Hyphae and spores in stratum corneum

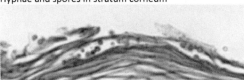

PITYRIASIS VERSICOLOR

CLINICAL FEATURES

- Common superficial fungal infection of skin
- Presents as hyperpigmented or hypopigmented finely scaled macules

HISTOLOGICAL FEATURES

- Epidermis with mild acanthosis and hyperkeratosis
- Fungal elements seen in stratum corneum-hyphae and budding yeast (spaghetti and meat balls) on H&E and with PAS and GMS

DIFFERENTIAL DIAGNOSIS

- Acanthosis nigricans: Papillated epidermal hyperplasia with basilar hyperpigmentation

Path Presenter

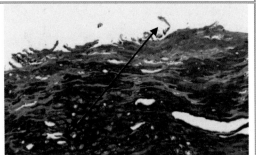
Brown hyphae in stratum corneum on acral skin

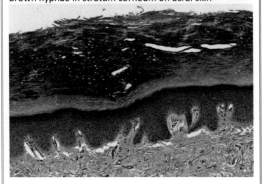

TINEA NIGRA

CLINICAL FEATURES

- This irregular brown macule with minimal scale is often confused with a melanocytic lesion
- It is noted on the palms and soles, mainly in the tropics

HISTOLOGICAL FEATURES

- Brown to black septate hyphae in stratum corneum on acral skin

OTHER HIGH YIELD POINTS

- Clinical differentials include Melanoma in Situ, Talon Noir, Post-Inflammatory Hyperpigmentation, Dye, Fixed Drug Eruption, Addison Disease, Pinta
- Examination of KOH preparations of skin scrapings
- Skin biopsy PCR can rapidly identify Phaeoannellomyces Werneckii
- Dermoscopy may also be helpful to distinguish from melanocytic lesions

DIFFERENTIAL DIAGNOSIS

- Candidosis: Epidermal hyperplasia, with parakeratosis and neutrophils in the cornified layer. Hyphae often in vertical orientation, with spores
- Melanoma-atypical melanocytic proliferation
- Onychomycosis: Fungal hyphae and spores within nail plate

Path Presenter

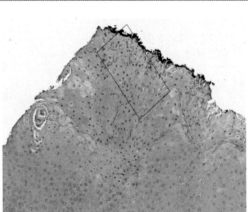
Involvement of stratum corneum

CANDIDOSIS

CLINICAL FEATURES

- There are various manifestations of this infection including: atrophic or hyperplastic oral forms, angular cheilitis, moist erythematous areas with pustules at the margin involving the skin folds, and chronic paronychia

HISTOLOGICAL FEATURES

- Subcorneal pustules with mild to moderate dermal infiltrate, predominantly neutrophils
- Pseudohyphae in stratum corneum, often vertically oriented, admixed yeasts may be seen

OTHER HIGH YIELD POINTS

- Clinical differentials include Streptococcal Intertrigo, Contact Dermatitis, Intertrigo
- KOH preparation of skin or oral scrapings and fungal culture for diagnosis
- Biopsy may be helpful to confirm the diagnosis

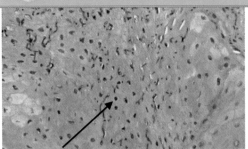

Vertically oriented pseudohyphae in stratum corneum
Erythematous macules: Disseminated Candidiasis

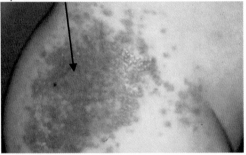

Pustules

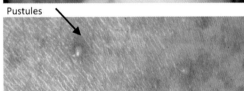

Path Presenter

- Patients with chronic mucocutaneous candidiasis often present with repeated, therapy resistant infections
- **Disseminated Candidosis:** This is frequently associated with multiple organ infections, but blood cultures can be negative. Patients present with fever and associated sepsis and septic shock. Cutaneous lesions include erythematous macules that become papular, pustular, hemorrhagic, or ulcerative, involving the trunk and extremities. Microscopy shows perivascular infiltrate with/without vasculitis. Pseudo hyphae, hyphae and spores in dermis in close apposition to vessels (The hyphae needs to be differentiated from Aspergillus, Histoplasma Capsulatum and Mucor) for the diagnosis. Blood culture and culture of other affected tissue, aspirates and culture of indwelling catheters can be useful for diagnosis
    1. Histologic evaluation of tissue specimen with the aid of special stains for fungi (e.g., PAS, GMS)
    2. Microscopic examination of tissue scrapings with the aid of KOH may also allow quicker diagnosis than H&E evaluation
    3. Urinalysis and urine culture
    4. Serum (1,3)-β-d-glucan (BDG) detection assay
    5. Imaging tests to determine extent of disease and evaluate suspected organ involvement (e.g., chest Xray, echocardiogram, ultrasonography, CT/MRI scans)
    6. Evaluation of cerebrospinal fluid may be indicated for suspected central nervous system involvement
    7. Bronchoscopy may be needed to rule out respiratory tract candidiasis
    8. Ophthalmologic examination

DIFFERENTIAL DIAGNOSIS
- Dermatophytosis: hyphae in stratum corneum
- Tinea Versicolor: Orthokeratosis with small round basophilic spores in the stratum corneum and pseudohyphae. Mild superficial perivascular infiltrate of mainly lymphocytes; histiocytes and plasma cells may be evident
- Bullous Impetigo: Subcorneal bulla with few neutrophils and rare acantholytic cells. Gram positive cocci may be seen within the bulla

Yeast forms within hair follicle
Path Presenter

PITYROSPORUM FOLLICULITIS
CLINICAL FEATURES
- This pruritic disease presents as follicular papules and pustules, particularly involving the chest and upper back
HISTOLOGICAL FEATURES
- Yeast forms within hair follicle, Mild to moderate inflammation
OTHER HIGH YIELD POINTS
- Clinical differentials include, Acne Vulgaris, Candidiasis, Eosinophilic Folliculitis, Steroid Acne, Pseudomonas Folliculitis
- Clinical appearance may highly suggest the diagnosis
- Microscopic evaluation of KOH preparations from pustules, Wood's light exam demonstrates yellow green fluorescence of the papules
- Skin biopsy if there is question about the diagnosis
DIFFERENTIAL DIAGNOSIS
- Fungal Folliculitis: Intra and perifollicular neutrophilic infiltrate with or without eosinophils. Hyphae within follicle and overlying stratum corneum
- Bacterial Folliculitis: Spongiosis of the follicular epithelium with neutrophil accumulation and pustule formation. Bacterial colonies within follicular orifice. May have follicular rupture with dermal abscess formation or granulomatous inflammation
- Suppurative Folliculitis: Acute and chronic inflammatory infiltrate in association with a hair follicle

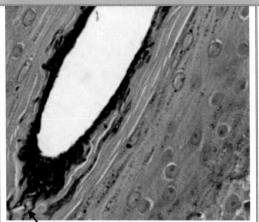

Fungal hyphae
<u>Path Presenter</u>

FUNGAL FOLLICULITIS

HISTOLOGICAL FEATURES

- Intra and perifollicular neutrophilic infiltrate with/without eosinophils
- Hyphae within follicle and overlying stratum corneum
- Majocchi Granuloma: Hyphae and spores within hair follicle and surrounding dermis, with rupture of follicular epithelium. Dermatophyte hyphae can be large and bizarre and can mimic disseminated fungal infection. Clinical correlation and correlation with microbiologic studies is important to distinguish these diagnoses. Dense suppurative and granulomatous mixed inflammatory infiltrate within the surrounding dermis

CLINICAL FEATURES

- Majocchi granuloma presents as circumscribed oval patches of perifollicular papulo-pustules and nodules with or without background erythema and scale
- The extremities are the most common site

OTHER HIGH YIELD POINTS

- Workup includes KOH preparation, Fungal culture and Skin biopsy

DIFFERENTIAL DIAGNOSIS

- Pityrosporum Folliculitis: Only spores
- Suppurative Folliculitis: Acute and chronic inflammatory infiltrate in association with a hair follicle

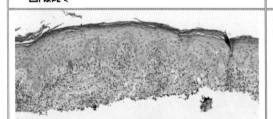

Pseudoepitheliomatous hyperplasia

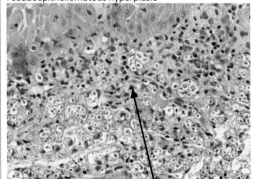

Round yeasts 2-10 microns in size

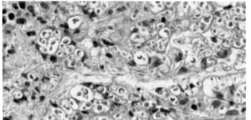

<u>Path Presenter</u>

CRYPTOCOCCUS

CLINICAL FEATURES

- This fungus (Cryptococcus neoformans) is common in soil, pigeon droppings
- Infection can rarely be due to primary inoculation as ulcerated lesions or cellulitis
- More common is dissemination from the lungs presenting as papules, pustules, nodules, herpetiform lesions, or subcutaneous nodules
- In AIDS, head and neck lesions are most common, often resembling molluscum contagiosum

HISTOLOGICAL FEATURES

- Histologically can show granulomatous inflammation or a gelatinous pattern
- Pseudoepitheliomatous hyperplasia with/without ulceration
- Gelatinous form may show very little inflammation, vacuolated gelatinous appearance and scattered organisms in dermis
- Suppurative and granulomatous inflammation with round yeasts (2-10 microns), free and within giant cells

OTHER HIGH YIELD POINTS

- Clinical differentials include, Cryptococcus, Coccidioidomycosis, Penicillium Marneffei, Molluscum Contagiosum, Cytomegalovirus
- Mucicarmine will stain organisms. PAS, GMS positive

DIFFERENTIAL DIAGNOSIS

- Histoplasma Capsulatum: Granulomatous dermatitis with admixed macrophages, lymphocytes, neutrophils, and plasma cells. Intracellular organisms with round, basophilic nuclei and rod-like kinetoplast scattered haphazardly and filling the macrophages
- Blastomycosis: Pseudoepitheliomatous hyperplasia with intraepidermal pustules overlying suppurative granulomatous inflammation in the dermis. Yeasts are few in number, usually found adjacent to or within giant cells. Monomorphic circular yeast forms with thick, asymmetrical, retractile wall may be seen on H&E. If budding is seen, it is broad based. Yeast best visualized with GMS or PAS. Yeast measures approximately 8-15 microns (1-2 times the size of a lymphocyte)
- Lobomycosis: Granulomatous dermatitis. Numerous large yeasts present in chains (pop-beads or "kissing lemons"), often within histiocytes and multinucleated giant cells

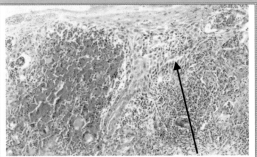
Pseudoepitheliomatous hyperplasia with intraepidermal pustules

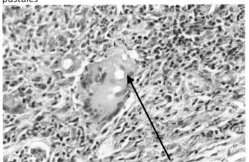
Organisms seen within giant cells 5-15 microns

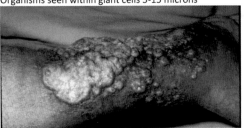
Ulcerated or crusted papules

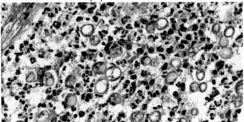
Broad based budding

Path Presenter

Path Presenter

BLASTOMYCOSIS

CLINICAL FEATURES

- Blastomycosis is a pyogranulomatous fungal infection caused by Blastomyces dermatitidis
  Infection occurs by inhalation of aerosolized conidial forms of the fungus from its natural soil habitat
- The inhaled conidia transform at body temperature in lungs and tissues to the yeast phase (thermal dimorphism)
- Pulmonary infection asymptomatic in ~50% of patients. Cutaneous lesions occur as a result of dissemination from the lungs, usually in immunocompetent patients. Skin (20%) > bone (5%) > prostate (2%) > GU (2%) most common sites
- Disease is endemic in the central and southeastern parts of the country (near Mississippi River, Ohio River, Great Lakes)
- Skin lesions are more common on the face, neck, extremities
- The classic lesions are ulcerated or crusted papules or plaques with an erythematous edematous border and central clearing
- The sharply demarcated papules or subcutaneous nodules can transform to ulcerated or verrucous lesions with small pustules or irregular borders at the margins and finally show central healing with atrophic scar studded with telangiectasia
- Chancriform lesions may be accompanied by nodular lymphangitis

HISTOLOGICAL FEATURES

- Suppurative and granulomatous dermatitis
- Overlying pseudoepitheliomatous hyperplasia with intraepidermal pustules
  Uniform shaped organisms (5-15 microns in diameter) with thick refractile walls and broad-based budding
- Organisms seen both extracellularly and within giant cells
- Yeast forms are best visualized with PAS or GMS

OTHER HIGH YIELD POINTS

- Clinical differentials include, Other Deep Fungal, Mycobacterial Infection, Pyoderma Vegetans, Pemphigus Vegetans, Keratoacanthoma
- Histologic evaluation of affected tissue with the assistance of special stains, tissue culture
- Antigen detection assays (serum or urine) available
- Serologic assays measuring antibodies to B. dermatitidis antigen available
- PCR can be performed for molecular identification of B. dermatitidis
- Imaging studies to determine extent of infection

DIFFERENTIAL DIAGNOSIS

- Halogenoderma: Pseudoepitheliomatous hyperplasia and granulomatous inflammation; no organisms
- Coccidioidomycosis: Pseudoepitheliomatous hyperplasia. Spherules with blue-gray granular cytoplasm measuring 10-80 μm in diameter are found in the center of micro abscesses, granulomas or in the cytoplasm of multinucleated giant cells
- Paracoccidioidomycosis: Small thick-walled yeasts (4-40 microns) with narrow based budding, mariner's wheel pattern of budding may be seen

COCCIDIOIDOMYCOSIS

CLINICAL FEATURES

- Caused by Coccidioides immitis, a dimorphic soil fungus native to: San Joaquin Valley of California, Southern portions of Arizona, Northern portions of Mexico and scattered areas in Central America and South America
- The arthroconidia inhaled via dust particles to lung
- Cutaneous lesions are almost always due to dissemination from the lung
- There is an increased incidence in immunosuppressed males

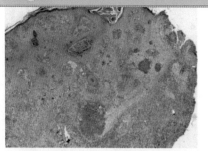

Pseudoepitheliomatous hyperplasia

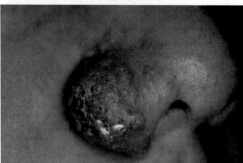

Papulonodular lesion

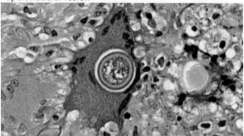

Sporangia in giant cell

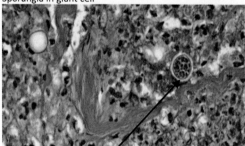

Uniform shaped sporangia

- Clinically patients have papulonodules, pustules, and granulomatous plaques most often on the face, especially the nasolabial folds
- Immunosuppressed states (HIV infection, cancer, prednisone, pregnancy) predispose to dissemination
- Triad of fever, Erythema Nodosum and arthralgias = desert rheumatism; more common in females

HISTOLOGICAL FEATURES
- Background of granulomatous and suppurative dermatitis
- Overlying pseudoepitheliomatous hyperplasia with intraepidermal pustules
- Uniform shaped sporangia (10-80 microns) with multiple endospores (1-4 microns) present both extracellularly and within giant cells

OTHER HIGH YIELD POINTS
- Clinical differentials include: Actinomycosis, Chromoblastomycosis, Erysipelas, Aspergillosis
- Skin biopsy and sampling of other affected tissue, pus, or body fluids
- Culture studies
- Because the organism is highly infectious, culture should not be attempted in in-office setting and laboratory personnel must be made aware if this diagnosis is suspected clinically
- Serologic testing for antibodies against coccidioidal antigens (e.g. tube precipitin, latex agglutination, enzyme immunoassay, immunodiffusion, complement fixation) and urine antigen testing are helpful
- PCR assays and in situ hybridization can be performed
- Chest Xray should be performed in app patients and additional imaging studies if clinically indicated
- Bronchoscopy if clinically indicated
- Lumbar puncture if meningitis is suspected
- May be associated with immunosuppressed states (e.g. HIV, pregnancy), especially in cases of disseminated disease

DIFFERENTIAL DIAGNOSIS
- Blastomycosis: Pseudoepitheliomatous hyperplasia with intraepidermal pustules overlying suppurative granulomatous inflammation in the dermis. Yeasts are few in number, usually found adjacent to or within giant cells. Monomorphic circular yeast forms with thick, asymmetrical, retractile wall may be seen on H&E. If budding is seen, it is broad based. Yeast best visualized with GMS or PAS. Yeast measures approximately 8-15 microns (1-2 times the size of a lymphocyte)
- Paracoccidioidomycosis: Pseudoepitheliomatous hyperplasia with/without ulceration. Suppurative and granulomatous inflammation. Small thick-walled yeasts (4-40 microns) with narrow based budding. Mariner's wheel pattern of budding may be seen
- Pemphigus Vegetans: Epidermal hyperplasia with papillomatosis. Acantholysis. Dense infiltrate of eosinophils in epidermis and in papillary dermis with admixed lymphocytes. DIF- intercellular IgG and C3 in epidermis

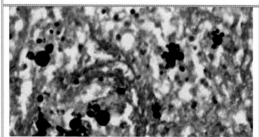

GMS: Mariner's wheel pattern of budding

PARACOCCIDIOIDOMYCOSIS
CLINICAL FEATURES
- Also known as South American blastomycosis, this fungal infection (Paracoccidioides brasiliensis) presents as ulcerative, verrucous, or crusted nodules, most often on the face with pulmonary involvement

HISTOLOGICAL FEATURES
- Pseudoepitheliomatous hyperplasia with/without ulceration
- Suppurative and granulomatous inflammation
- Small thick-walled yeasts (4-40 microns) with narrow based budding
- Mariner's wheel pattern of budding may be seen

CHAPTER 21: INFECTIONS AND INFESTATIONS

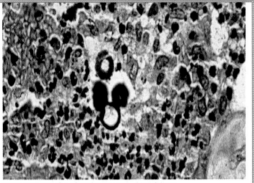

PAS: Mariner's wheel pattern of budding
Mariner's wheel pattern of budding

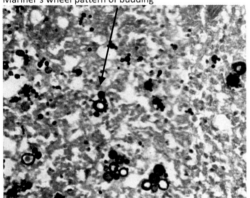

Path Presenter

OTHER HIGH YIELD POINTS

- Clinical differentials include, Actinomycosis, Blastomycosis, Coccidioidomycosis, Histoplasmosis, Mucocutaneous Leishmaniasis, NK T Cell Lymphoma, Sporotrichosis
- Histologic examination of skin biopsy, skin scraping or sputum with the aid of special stains. Culture studies. Imaging to evaluate extent of disease and lymph node involvement
- Biopsy or aspiration of involved lymph nodes or tissue may be performed. Serologic testing is also available, but is not unequivocally diagnostic
- Complete history and physical examination, including evaluation of mucosa, airways, lymph nodes
- Evaluation for adrenal dysfunction: early morning serum cortisol level and ACTH stimulation test
- Patient's immune status is important to consider, as immunocompromised patients (e.g. HIV) may present with more disseminated disease

DIFFERENTIAL DIAGNOSIS

- Blastomycosis: Pseudoepitheliomatous hyperplasia with intraepidermal pustules overlying suppurative granulomatous inflammation in the dermis. Yeasts are few in number, usually found adjacent to or within giant cells. Monomorphic circular yeast forms with thick, asymmetrical, retractile wall may be seen on H&E. If budding is seen, it is broad based. Yeast best visualized with GMS or PAS- measures approximately 8-15 microns (1-2 times the size of a lymphocyte)
- Coccidioidomycosis: Pseudoepitheliomatous hyperplasia. Spherules with blue-gray granular cytoplasm measuring 10-80 μm in diameter are found in the center of micro abscesses, granulomas or in the cytoplasm of multinucleated giant cells
- Lobomycosis: Granulomatous dermatitis. Numerous large yeasts present in chains (pop-beads or "kissing lemons"), often within histiocytes and multinucleated giant cells

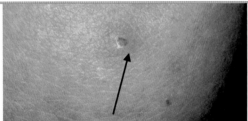

Superficial cutaneous lesions

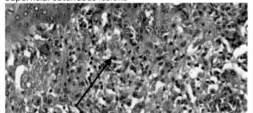

Intracellular organisms (2-4 microns) in histiocytes

Path Presenter

HISTOPLASMOSIS
CLINICAL FEATURES

- Common in Central eastern US
- Commonly affects lungs. Skin lesions present with ulcers, papules, nodules
- In Africa (African Histoplasmosis) solitary or disseminated superficial cutaneous lesions, subcutaneous granulomas or abscesses, or as osteomyelitis with overlying cutaneous extension

HISTOLOGICAL FEATURES

- Intracellular organisms (2-4 microns), surrounded by halo, in histiocytes and multinucleated giant cells in a background of granulomatous and suppurative dermatitis. Better seen with PAS, GMS

OTHER HIGH YIELD POINTS

- African Histoplasmosis presents with larger organisms-similar in size to cryptococcus (8-15 microns)
- Histologic examination and culture of involved tissue (skin, blood, sputum, bronchial washings, spinal fluid, bone marrow, lymph node aspirate, urine, etc.)
- Serum and urine antigen tests (useful in detecting disseminated disease)
- Serologic assays to quantify antibody responses (complement fixation, immunodiffusion)
- PCR can also be performed. Imaging to evaluate extent of disease
- Evaluate for underlying causes of immunosuppression, including HIV testing

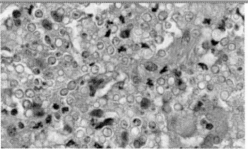

Large intracellular organisms (8-15 microns) in histiocytes in African Histoplasmosis

DIFFERENTIAL DIAGNOSIS
- Leishmaniasis: Granulomatous dermatitis with admixed macrophages, lymphocytes, neutrophils, and plasma cells
- Intracellular organisms with round, basophilic nuclei and rod-like kinetoplast scattered haphazardly and filling the macrophages
- Rhinoscleroma: Dense infiltrate of macrophages with admixed plasma cells. Some of the larger macrophages (Mikulicz cells) contain a large number of Gram-negative bacilli. Bacilli visible on H&E, PAS and Giemsa stains. Pseudoepitheliomatous hyperplasia and fibrosis in older lesions
- Cryptococcus: Pseudoepitheliomatous hyperplasia with/without ulceration. Suppurative and granulomatous inflammation with round yeasts with capsule (4-10 microns), free and within giant cells In immunocompromised patients, inflammation is scarce and yeast form confluent sheets (gelatinous form)

PHAEOHYPHOMYCOSIS
CLINICAL FEATURES
- Various dematiaceous fungi can cause this infection
- Cutaneous lesions can vary from macules, papules, plaques, nodules, or verrucous lesions, with or without ulceration

HISTOLOGICAL FEATURES
- Pigmented hyphae in a background of granulomatous and suppurative dermatitis. Can present as a walled off cystic space

OTHER HIGH YIELD POINTS
- Clinical differentials include, Atypical Mycobacterial Infection, Leishmaniasis, Chromoblastomycosis, Aspergillosis
- Skin biopsy and tissue cultures
- Blood cultures and imaging studies if disseminated disease suspected
- Microscopic examination and cultures of abscess aspirates or tissue of affected extracutaneous organ
- May be associated with immunosuppression, especially in cases of disseminated disease

DIFFERENTIAL DIAGNOSIS
- Chromoblastomycosis: pigmented spores in granulomatous background
- Eumycetoma: White grain eumycetoma, Pseudoepitheliomatous hyperplasia with dense mixed inflammatory infiltrate in dermis with fibrosis around tightly packed grains. These grains are PAS positive and are colonies of fungal hyphae
- Disseminated Candidosis: Epidermal hyperplasia, with parakeratosis and neutrophils in the cornified layer. Hyphae often in vertical orientation, with spores

Pigmented hyphae in a background of granulomatous dermatitis(low power above; high power below)

Path Presenter

SPOROTRICHOSIS
CLINICAL FEATURES
- This fungal infection (Sporothrix schenckii) occurs mostly from inoculation
- A crusted verrucous plaque or ulcerated nodule classically occurs at the site of inoculation with subsequent development of secondary nodules along the draining lymphatics
- Rarely cutaneous lesions can be fixed

HISTOLOGICAL FEATURES
- Granulomatous and suppurative inflammation, sometimes with overlying pseudoepitheliomatous hyperplasia
- Stellate neutrophilic abscesses surrounded by granulomatous inflammation. Cigar shaped (2-8 microns) or round (4-6 microns) yeast forms
- Asteroid bodies may be noted

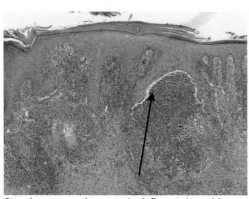

Granulomatous and suppurative inflammation, with overlying Pseudoepitheliomatous hyperplasia

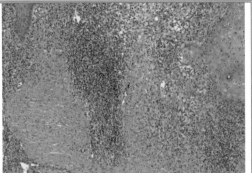

Granulomatous inflammation

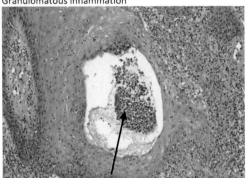

Stellate neutrophilic abscesses

OTHER HIGH YIELD POINTS

- Clinical differentials include: Nocardia, Mycobacteria, Leishmaniasis, Deep Fungal, 'Pasteurella, Tularemia, Cowpox, Anthrax, Pseudomonas pseudomallei
- Clinical appearance may suggest the diagnosis
- Tissue culture to confirm the diagnosis
- Histologic evaluation of skin biopsy specimen with the aid of special stains may reveal the organisms
- Fluorescent labeled antibodies can also help identify the organism
- PCR assay can also be helpful
- Imaging studies and additional evaluation may be indicated if extracutaneous involvement suspected

DIFFERENTIAL DIAGNOSIS

- Atypical Mycobacterial Infection: Histologic findings are variable, ranging from acute suppurative poorly formed granulomas to chronic well-formed tuberculoid granulomas, typically located within the dermis. Epidermal changes range from acanthosis, pseudoepitheliomatous hyperplasia to ulceration. AFB stain will reveal rare organisms in immunocompetent hosts

Path Presenter

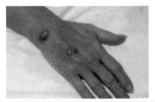

MYCETOMA (EUMYCETOMA/ACTINOMYCETOMA)

White Grain Mycetoma

CLINICAL FEATURES

- This infection is characterized by multiple sinus tracts that drain granules composed of non-dematiaceous fungal hyphae, most commonly on the feet in tropical areas

HISTOLOGICAL FEATURES

- Pseudoepitheliomatous hyperplasia with dense mixed inflammatory infiltrate in dermis with fibrosis around tightly packed grains
- These grains are PAS positive and are colonies of fungal hyphae

OTHER HIGH YIELD POINTS

- Histologic evaluation of grains or skin biopsy of affected area with the assistance of special stains (e.g., GMS, PAS, Gram)
- Tissue culture for further speciation Imaging studies to determine extent of infection

DIFFERENTIAL DIAGNOSIS

- Botryomycosis: Grains surrounded by neutrophilic abscesses and chronic inflammation with fibrosis and foreign body giant cells. Grains have basophilic center composed of bacteria and debris. Splendor-Hoeppli phenomenon describes the eosinophilic hyalinized periphery of the grains composed of IgG and C3 deposits. Grains stain positively for PAS, Giemsa, and Gram
- Actinomycosis: Dense dermal neutrophilic infiltrate (early), Granulomatous inflammation with giant cells (late). Colonies of organisms are seen as "sulfur granules" with basophilic center and acidophilic rim

Dark Grain Mycetoma

CLINICAL FEATURES

- This infection is characterized by multiple sinus tracks that drain granules composed of dematiaceous fungal hyphae, most commonly on the feet in tropical areas

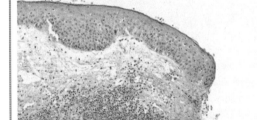

Eumycetoma

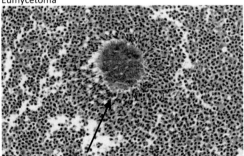

Dark Grain Mycetoma

Neutrophilic abscess in dermis around grains

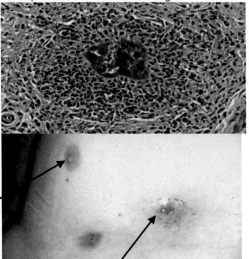
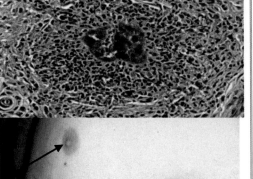
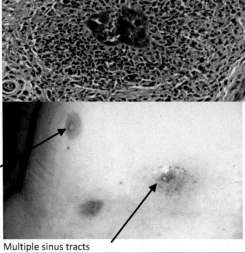

Multiple sinus tracts

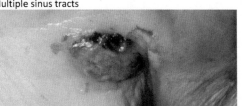

HISTOLOGICAL FEATURES

- Neutrophilic abscess in dermis around grains, surrounded by lymphohistiocytic and granulomatous inflammation
- Grains are composed of broad, 2-5 microns thick, septate hyphae, which frequently form chlamydospores at the periphery of the grain
- They stain with PAS, Giemsa and GMS stains

OTHER HIGH YIELD POINTS

- Histologic evaluation of grains or skin biopsy of affected area with the assistance of special stains (e.g., GMS, PAS, Gram)
- Tissue culture for further speciation
- Imaging studies to determine extent of infection

DIFFERENTIAL DIAGNOSIS

- Botryomycosis: Grains surrounded by neutrophilic abscesses and chronic inflammation with fibrosis and foreign body giant cells. Grains have basophilic center composed of bacteria and debris. Splendor-Hoeppli phenomenon describes the eosinophilic hyalinized periphery of the grains composed of IgG and C3 deposits. Grains stain positively for PAS, Giemsa, and Gram
- Actinomycosis: Dense dermal neutrophilic infiltrate (early), Granulomatous inflammation with giant cells (late). Colonies of organisms are seen as "sulfur granules" with basophilic center and acidophilic rim

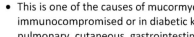

Path Presenter

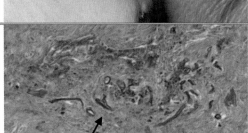

Fungal hyphae

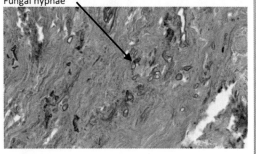

Path Presenter

MUCORMYCOSIS

CLINICAL FEATURES

- This is one of the causes of mucormycosis, an infection seen in immunocompromised or in diabetic ketoacidosis with rhinocerebral, pulmonary, cutaneous, gastrointestinal, and/or central nervous system involvement
- In the skin, erythematous macules enlarge and form a black eschar

HISTOLOGICAL FEATURES

- Epidermal and/or dermal ulceration and necrosis
- Granulation tissue with sparse inflammation in dermis, often with thrombosis
- Broad, hollow appearing hyphae with 90-degree branching

OTHER HIGH YIELD POINTS

- Clinical differentials include Rhinoscleroma, Wegener's Granulomatosis, Paracoccidioidomycosis, Lethal Midline Granuloma, Anthrax, Ecthyma Gangrenosum, Fusariosis, Pseudallescheria boydii Infection
- Histologic evaluation of tissue specimen with the aid of special stains for fungi (e.g., PAS, GMS)
- Part of the specimen can be submitted for frozen tissue processing for more rapid diagnosis
- Microscopic examination of tissue scrapings with the aid of KOH or calcofluor may also allow quicker diagnosis than H&E evaluation. Tissue culture studies as well as blood culture
- If rhinocerebral disease is suspected, immediate CT scan of paranasal sinuses and endoscopic evaluation of nasal passages should take place
- Bronchoalveolar lavage ± biopsy indicated in suspected pulmonary disease. Evaluation of cerebrospinal fluid may be indicated for suspected central nervous system involvement

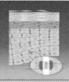
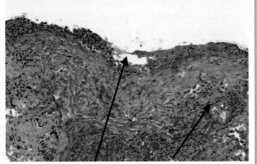

Dermal ulceration   Fungal hyphae

- CT scan should be done before lumbar puncture to minimize risk of brain herniation due to procedure
- Additional imaging of areas of suspected involvement recommended
- Imaging of brain, sinuses, chest, abdomen, and pelvis recommended to evaluate for subclinical disease

DIFFERENTIAL DIAGNOSIS

- Fusarium: Diffuse, mixed infiltrate of neutrophils, lymphocytes, histiocytes and multinucleated giant cells. Narrow, septate non-pigmented hyphae with acute angle branching. Background of necrosis with foci of vessel invasion. May see vascular thrombi, leading to epidermal necrosis
- Aspergillus: Diffuse, mixed infiltrate of neutrophils, lymphocytes, histiocytes and multinucleated giant cells. Narrow, septate non-pigmented hyphae with acute angle branching. Background of necrosis with foci of vessel invasion and thrombosis. In immunocompromised patients, there may be no inflammation
- Candidosis: Epidermal hyperplasia, with parakeratosis and neutrophils in the cornified layer. Hyphae often in vertical orientation, with spores

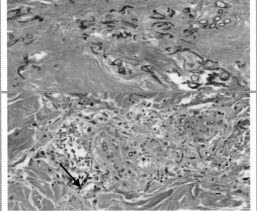

septate hyphae acute angle branching

Path Presenter

FUSARIOSIS

CLINICAL FEATURES

- This fungal infection can be localized or disseminated. Presentation can include nail infection, pustules, subcutaneous nodules, or vasculotropism can result in red macules and papules with central necrosis/infarct/eschar

HISTOLOGICAL FEATURES

- Diffuse, mixed infiltrate of neutrophils, lymphocytes, histiocytes and multinucleated giant cells
- Narrow, septate hyphae with irregular (45 to 90 degrees) acute angle branching. Background of necrosis with foci of vessel invasion. Yeast forms may also be seen

OTHER HIGH YIELD POINTS

- Microscopic examination of Wright stain of skin scrapings or scrapings of other affected tissue
- Biopsy of skin and other affected tissues
- Tissue and blood cultures

DIFFERENTIAL DIAGNOSIS

- Aspergillus: Diffuse, mixed infiltrate of neutrophils, lymphocytes, histiocytes and multinucleated giant cells. Narrow, septate non-pigmented hyphae with acute angle branching. Background of necrosis with foci of vessel invasion and thrombosis. In immunocompromised patients, there may be no inflammation
- Mucor: Epidermal and/or dermal ulceration and necrosis. Granulation tissue with sparse inflammation in dermis, often with thrombosis (angioinvasion). Broad ribbon-like hollow hyphae with rare septations and branching at 90-degree angles

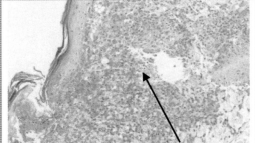

Suppurative and granulomatous dermatitis

PENICILLIOSIS

CLINICAL FEATURES

- This is a systemic fungal (Penicillium Marneffei) infection most often in HIV positive patients
- The skin lesions are umbilicated or ulcerated papules or nodules

HISTOLOGICAL FEATURES

- Suppurative and granulomatous dermatitis
- Intracellular yeasts (3-8 microns), elongated and with septations
- Divide by binary fission

OTHER HIGH YIELD POINTS

- Clinical differentials include Cryptococcus, Coccidioidomycosis, Histoplasmosis, Cytomegalovirus

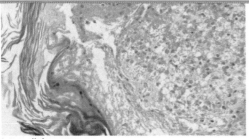

Intracellular yeasts
Path Presenter

- Microscopic examination of Wright stain of skin scrapings or scrapings of other affected tissue
- Biopsy of skin and other affected tissues
- Tissue and blood cultures
- HIV test

DIFFERENTIAL DIAGNOSIS

- Leishmaniasis: Intracellular organisms in a background of mixed inflammation
- Histoplasma Capsulatum: Intracellular yeasts with pseudo capsule (2-4 microns) inside macrophages, evenly distributed and surrounded by pseudo capsule in a background of suppurative and granulomatous inflammation

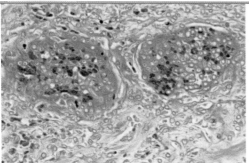

Foci of vessel invasion

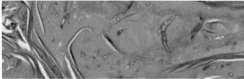

septate hyphae with acute angle branching

ASPERGILLOSIS

CLINICAL FEATURES

- Cutaneous involvement is typically from inoculation or dissemination from the lung in neutropenic patients
- The vasculotropism results in red macules and papules with central necrosis/infarct/eschar

HISTOLOGICAL FEATURES

- Diffuse, mixed infiltrate of neutrophils, lymphocytes, histiocytes and multinucleated giant cells
- Narrow, septate hyphae with acute angle branching. Background of necrosis with foci of vessel invasion

OTHER HIGH YIELD POINTS

- Clinical differentials include Deep Fungal, Opportunistic Fungal, Ecthyma Gangrenosum
- Microscopic examination of Wright stain of skin scrapings or scrapings of other affected tissue
- Biopsy of skin and other affected tissues
- Tissue and blood cultures

DIFFERENTIAL DIAGNOSIS

- Fusarium: Diffuse, mixed infiltrate of neutrophils, lymphocytes, histiocytes and multinucleated giant cells. Narrow, septate non-pigmented hyphae with acute angle branching. Background of necrosis with foci of vessel invasion. May see vascular thrombi, leading to epidermal necrosis
- Mucor: Thick hollow hyphae with wide angle branching

Path Presenter

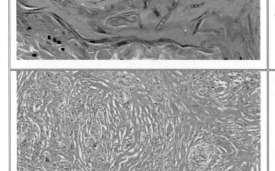

Granulomatous dermatitis and prominent fibrosis

LOBOMYCOSIS

CLINICAL FEATURES

- Infection is generally noted in tropical forest areas on exposed areas, likely as a result of a remote history or inoculation
- The lesions resemble keloids

HISTOLOGICAL FEATURES

- Granulomatous dermatitis and prominent fibrosis
- Numerous organisms (6-12 microns) present in chains(pop-beads), often within histiocytes and multinucleated giant cells

OTHER HIGH YIELD POINTS

- Clinical differentials include Keloid, Scar, Chromoblastomycosis, Leishmaniasis, Xanthoma

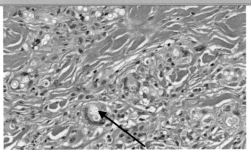
Organisms within multinucleated giant cells

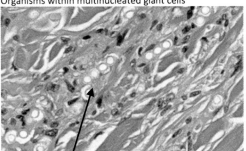
Organisms in chains

- Skin biopsy, microscopic evaluation of skin scrapings or tissue obtained by vinyl adhesive tape technique may also be helpful

DIFFERENTIAL DIAGNOSIS

- Cryptococcus: Pseudoepitheliomatous hyperplasia with/without ulceration. Suppurative and granulomatous inflammation with round yeasts with capsule (4-10 microns), free and within giant cells. In immunocompromised patients, inflammation is scarce and yeast form confluent sheets (gelatinous form)
- Histoplasma Duboisii: Large intracellular organisms (8-15 microns) in histiocytes and multinucleated giant cells in a background of granulomatous dermatitis
- Blastomycosis: Pseudoepitheliomatous hyperplasia with intraepidermal pustules overlying suppurative granulomatous inflammation in the dermis. Yeasts are few in number, usually found adjacent to or within giant cells. Monomorphic circular yeast forms with thick, asymmetrical, retractile wall may be seen on H&E. If budding is seen, it is broad based. Yeast best visualized with GMS or PAS. Yeast measures approximately 8-15 microns (1-2 times the size of a lymphocyte)

Path Presenter

RHINOSPORIDIOSIS

CLINICAL FEATURES

- The lesions of involvement in this condition vary depending on the site affected, but they are commonly observed in the nasal cavity and nasopharynx. These lesions typically present as reddish, polypoidal masses with a bulky and friable mucosal appearance. While rare, other sites of involvement may include the conjunctiva, mouth, larynx, genitalia, and skin
- In the nasal cavity, the lesions initially appear as sessile masses and gradually progress to become fleshy, pedunculated polypoid masses

HISTOLOGICAL FEATURES

- The characteristic morphology of this condition involves the presence of sporangia (up to 500 microns in size) within the stroma of the polyp
- These sporangia vary in size and are typically found within the tissue layers of the polyp. Additionally, the overlying mucosa, which refers to the surface lining of the polyp, may exhibit squamous metaplastic changes
- Mature sporangia in this condition have a thick chitinous wall and contain sporangiospores in various developmental stages. These sporangiospores are basophilic, measuring around 7 to 9 microns in diameter. Rupture of sporangia within the stroma can lead to a pronounced granulomatous response, characterized by the formation of granulomas
- Stroma shows moderate to abundant chronic inflammatory cell infiltrates (lymphocytes, plasma cells and macrophages)

OTHER HIGH YIELD POINTS

- Treatment: Excision of the lesion

DIFFERENTIAL DIAGNOSIS

- Coccidioides immitis: Fungal infection characterized by smaller spherules measuring approximately 30 to 60 microns in diameter. These spherules contain smaller endospores, which range in size from 2 to 5 microns
- Myospherulosis: Condition characterized by the presence of large tissue spaces filled with saclike structures. These structures contain brown spherules that may resemble Prototheca, a type of algae, but are actually clumped red blood cells

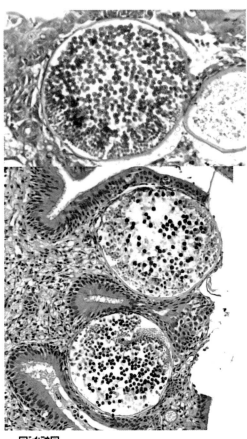

Path Presenter

__ Picture credits: Hina Maqbool

CHAPTER 21: INFECTIONS AND INFESTATIONS

VIRAL INFECTIONS

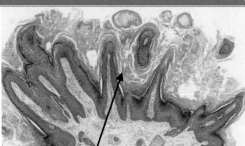

Papillomatous exophytic epidermal proliferation

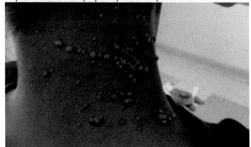

Keratotic papules

Path Presenter

VERRUCA VULGARIS

CLINICAL FEATURES
- These lesions are common in children but also occur in adults, most often on the hands, fingers, and knees as firm keratotic papules
- Filiform lesions are seen around the nose

HISTOLOGICAL FEATURES
- Papillomatous exophytic epidermal proliferation
- Compact hyperkeratosis with vertical columns of round parakeratosis ending with hemorrhagic crust above peaks
- Hypergranulosis with scattered koilocytes-vacuolated superficial keratinocytes with raisin like nuclei
- Infolding of elongated rete ridges towards base. Granulation tissue like stroma

OTHER HIGH YIELD POINTS
- Clinical differentials include, Seborrheic Keratosis, Inflammatory Linear Verrucous Epidermal Nevus, Verrucous Carcinoma, Squamous Cell Carcinoma, Acquired Digital Fibrokeratoma, Acrokeratosis Verruciformis, Angiokeratoma, Poroma, Prurigo Nodularis
- Diagnosis can usually be made on clinical grounds. Skin biopsy can be performed if there is any question about the diagnosis

DIFFERENTIAL DIAGNOSIS
- Seborrheic Keratosis: Epidermal acanthosis, pseudohorn cysts and monotonous nuclei
- Verrucous Squamous Cell Carcinoma: Atypia of keratinocytes, high Ki67
- Epidermal Nevus: Papillated epidermal hyperplasia, can look like SK

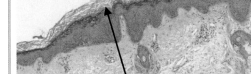

Basket-weave hyperkeratosis

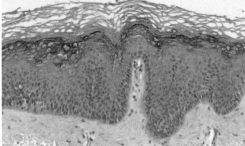

Hyperkeratosis and hypergranulosis

Path Presenter

VERRUCA PLANA

CLINICAL FEATURES
- These warts are typically small, flat, smooth and skin-colored or pink
- The face, dorsal hands, and shins are common sites-usually multiple, small papules
- A linear arrangement can occur from shaving or scratching

HISTOLOGICAL FEATURES
- Basket-weave hyperkeratosis overlying flat topped epidermis with hypergranulosis
- Vacuolated keratinocytes (bird's eye cells) in malpighian layer

OTHER HIGH YIELD POINTS
- Diagnosis can usually be made on clinical grounds
- Skin biopsy can be performed if there is any question about the diagnosis

DIFFERENTIAL DIAGNOSIS
- Epidermodysplasia Verruciformis: Epidermal acanthosis and parakeratosis. Steel-grey cytoplasm of keratinocytes and perinuclear halo. Cytological atypia may be present within the keratinocytes
- Seborrheic Keratosis: There is epidermal acanthosis, papillomatosis with overlying hyperkeratosis. The cells are basaloid, small to medium size with squamoid differentiation are separated with pseudohorn cysts

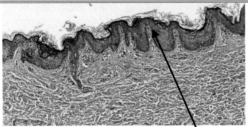

Epidermal acanthosis and parakeratosis

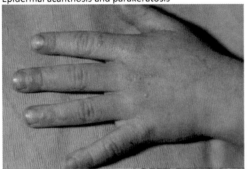

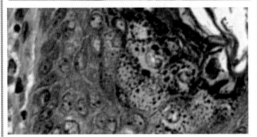

Steel-grey cytoplasm of keratinocyte

EPIDERMODYSPLASIA VERRUCIFORMIS
CLINICAL FEATURES

- This inherited disorder presents with infection by numerous types of HPV (5 &8)
- Flat warts occur on the extremities and face and red to brown scaly flat papules present on the trunk that can resemble tinea versicolor
- There is an increased risk of squamous cell carcinoma in sun exposed areas

HISTOLOGICAL FEATURES

- Epidermal acanthosis and parakeratosis
- Steel-grey cytoplasm of keratinocytes
- Cytological atypia may be present within the keratinocytes

OTHER HIGH YIELD POINTS

- Clinical differentials include Acrokeratosis Verruciformis of Hopf, Actinic Keratosis, Basal Cell Carcinoma, Papular Mucinosis, Verruca Plana
- Work up includes Skin biopsy, HPV typing and molecular genetic testing (EVER1 and EVER2)

DIFFERENTIAL DIAGNOSIS

- Verruca Plana: Alternating "basket-weave" hyperkeratosis with parakeratosis and hypergranulosis; Papillomatosis is minimal; Prominent vacuolated keratinocytes (bird's eye cells) in malpighian layer
- Seborrheic Keratosis: There is epidermal acanthosis, papillomatosis with overlying hyperkeratosis. The cells are basaloid, small to medium size with squamoid differentiation are separated with pseudohorn cysts
- Bowen's Disease: Full thickness atypia of keratinocytes in epidermis

Path Presenter

CONDYLOMA ACUMINATUM
CLINICAL FEATURES

- These warts are typically found in the genital area of sexually active adults
- The lesions are usually numerous, soft filiform papules and plaques
- Commonly HPV 6 &11 (low grade), sometimes 16/18/31 (high grade)

HISTOLOGICAL FEATURES

- Acanthotic epidermis with overlying compact hyperkeratosis and hypergranulosis
- Vacuolated keratinocytes with large grey nuclei
- Streaming of keratinocytes is a helpful feature
- Ki67 positive in scattered keratinocytes in upper one-third of epidermis

OTHER HIGH YIELD POINTS

- Diagnosis can usually be made by visual inspection
- Skin biopsy can be performed to confirm the diagnosis and to rule out alternative possibilities
- Chromogenic in situ hybridization test in search of low and high-risk HPV types can be performed on biopsy specimen
- If clinically indicated, extent of involvement should be documented by anoscopy, sigmoidoscopy, colposcopy, vaginal speculum
- Application of 5% acetic acid can help with identification of lesions
- Women should have routine cervical Pap smears
- In HIV positive males who have sex with males, anal Pap smears should be considered

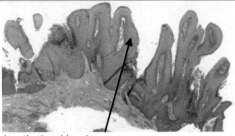

Acanthotic epidermis

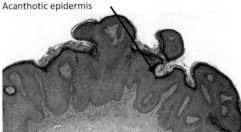

Path Presenter

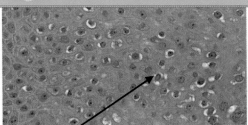
Vacuolated keratinocytes

DIFFERENTIAL DIAGNOSIS
- Bowen's Papulosis: Acanthotic epidermis with full thickness atypia of keratinocytes. Atypical keratinocytes may involve entire epidermis or show scattered cells throughout the epidermis
- Verrucous Squamous Cell Carcinoma: Exo/endophytic verrucous proliferation of well-differentiated keratinocytes with bulbous rete ridges. Squamous epithelial cells have bland appearance with very little atypia. Fibrous stroma with mixed inflammatory infiltrate. Intraepidermal neutrophils as well as within the dermis are an important clue
- Pearly Penile Papule: Scattered dilated vessels and admixed stellate fibroblasts

BOWENOID PAPULOSIS
CLINICAL FEATURES
- This presents as multiple red to brown papules in the genital area of young sexually active adults

HISTOLOGICAL FEATURES
- Acanthotic epidermis with full thickness atypia of keratinocytes
- Atypical keratinocytes may involve entire epidermis or show scattered cells throughout the epidermis

OTHER HIGH YIELD POINTS
- Usually due to high grade HPV subtypes (16/18/31)
- Clinical differentials include Condyloma Acuminata, Condyloma Lata, Molluscum Contagiosum, Extramammary Paget's Disease
- Work up includes skin biopsy, full examination, including anogenital exam for all patients, as well as for sexual partners of patients, cervical exam for female sexual partners of male patients and for female patients
- Coexistence of other sexually transmitted diseases should be considered

DIFFERENTIAL DIAGNOSIS
- Bowen's Disease: Full thickness atypia not related to virus, usually middle-aged to older patients
- Condyloma Acuminatum: no keratinolytic atypia noted
- Seborrheic Keratosis: Acanthotic epidermis with scattered pseudohorn cysts

Acanthotic epidermis with full thickness atypia of keratinocytes   Mitosis and atypia

Path Presenter

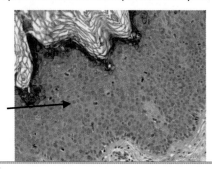
full thickness atypia of keratinocytes

HAND, FOOT, AND MOUTH DISEASE
CLINICAL FEATURES
- This viral infection is due to Coxsackie A16 and less often enterovirus 71
- Young children present with fever, malaise, oral ulcers, and erythematous papules that evolve to gray vesicles on the ventral hands and feet, perineum and buttocks

HISTOLOGICAL FEATURES
- Spongiosis and epidermal necrosis with reticular degeneration
- Ballooning degeneration of individual keratinocytes
- No inclusions
- Papillary dermal edema with superficial perivascular lymphocytic inflammation

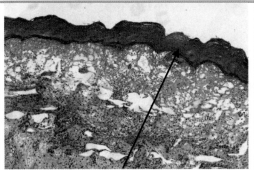
Spongiosis and epidermal necrosis

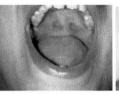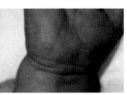

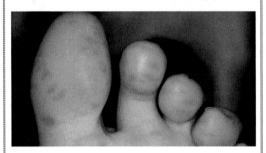

OTHER HIGH YIELD POINTS
- Clinical differentials include Herpangina, Erythema Multiforme, Herpes
- This is a primarily clinical diagnosis
- Viral culture can be performed on skin vesicles
- Skin biopsy may be performed if there is a question about the diagnosis

DIFFERENTIAL DIAGNOSIS
- Orf: Epidermal necrosis and parakeratotic crust and acanthosis; Reticular degeneration. Dermal edema. Cytoplasmic and nuclear inclusions. Perivascular lymphocytic infiltrate +/- eosinophils
- Herpes: Dermal edema with ballooning degeneration of keratinocytes with acantholysis followed by intradermal vesicle formation; Multinucleation of keratinocytes (fusing of adjacent cells), molding and margination of nuclear chromatin; Intranuclear and cytoplasmic basophilic and/or pale ground-glass inclusions; Background of neutrophilic inflammation

Path Presenter

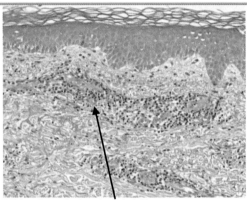

Mild perivascular lymphocytic infiltrate

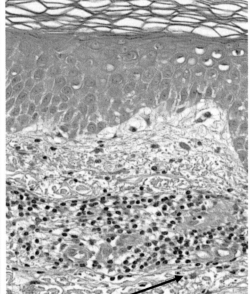

Extravasation of RBC

PARVOVIRUS B19

CLINICAL FEATURES
- This group of viruses causes a variety of clinical syndromes
- The most common cutaneous infections include erythema infectiosum (Fifth disease) and Papular purpuric gloves and sock syndrome (PPGSS)
- Fifth disease occurs in children as erythema of the cheeks with rhinorrhea and later more diffuse erythematous macules and papules with a reticulate, lace like pattern
- PPGSS occurs in teens and young adults with pruritus, edema, and erythema of the hands and feet with fever
- Over a few days the lesions become purpuric

HISTOLOGICAL FEATURES
- Mild vacuolar alteration at DEJ with lymphocytic exocytosis and scattered dyskeratotic cells
- Mild perivascular lymphocytic infiltrate with admixed eosinophils and neutrophils
- Extravasation of red blood cells

OTHER HIGH YIELD POINTS
- Clinical differentials include, Other Viral Exanthem, Rheumatological Disorder, Drug Eruption
- In most cases, diagnosis can be made clinically without additional confirmatory studies
- Skin biopsy is usually nonspecific but may help rule out alternative possibilities
- Endothelial cells and epidermal keratinocytes from biopsies of papular purpuric gloves and socks syndrome have demonstrate positive immunoreactivity with antiB19 antibodies
- Laboratory testing may be helpful if there is any question about the diagnosis or if there is contact with pregnant individual
- Lab work includes parvovirus serology and PCR testing
- CBC with differential with reticulocyte count to screen for aplastic crisis, which occurs more often in patients with underlying hematologic abnormalities
- Fetal ultrasound to detect hydrops
- Parvovirus B19 infection may also trigger a hemophagocytic syndrome, presenting with cytopenia, liver dysfunction, coagulopathy, hemophagocytosis and elevated ferritin

Path Presenter

DIFFERENTIAL DIAGNOSIS
- Drug Eruption: Superficial and deep perivascular lymphocytic infiltrate with admixed eosinophils +/-. Epidermal spongiosis with exocytosis and vacuolar change with rare apoptotic keratinocytes admixed eosinophils.
- Lupus Erythematosus: Vacuolar or lichenoid interface dermatitis. Perivascular and periadnexal lymphocytic infiltrate Increased dermal mucin

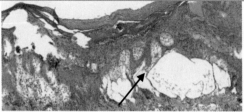

Epidermal necrosis and reticular degeneration

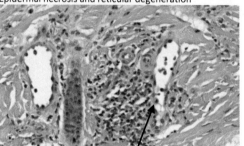

Perivascular lymphocytic infiltrate

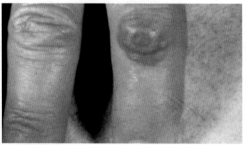

Path Presenter

ORF
CLINICAL FEATURES
- Ecthyma contagiosum (Orf) is due to exposure to infected sheep and goats
- This presents most on the hands as papules at the site of inoculation
- The lesions go through six 1-week stages (maculopapular, targetoid, nodular and weeping, regenerative, papillomatous, and regressive) before resolving

HISTOLOGICAL FEATURES
- Epidermal necrosis and reticular degeneration
- Dermal edema
- Predominantly cytoplasmic and occasional nuclear inclusions
- Perivascular lymphocytic infiltrate

OTHER HIGH YIELD POINTS
- Clinical differentials include, Cowpox, Milker's Nodule, Anthrax, Erysipeloid, Keratoacanthoma, Pyogenic Granuloma
- Diagnosis can usually be made by correlating clinical appearance with history of contact with goats or sheep
- Histologic examination of skin biopsy is useful. Electron microscopy or PCR can be performed on tissue
- May be associated with erythema multiforme

DIFFERENTIAL DIAGNOSIS
- Erythema Multiforme: Preserved basket-weave stratum corneum. Necrotic/dyskeratotic keratinocytes at all levels. Interface vacuolar dermatitis. Superficial perivascular lymphocytic infiltrate +/- eosinophils
- Hand Foot And Mouth Disease: Spongiosis and epidermal necrosis with reticular degeneration; Ballooning degeneration of individual keratinocytes; No viral inclusions; Superficial perivascular lymphocytic inflammation
- Molluscum Contagiosum: Epidermal acanthosis with cup-shaped lesion. Reticular degeneration and vesiculation are not features in comparison to other pox-related lesions; Molluscum bodies – large intracytoplasmic inclusion bodies (Henderson–Patterson bodies) within epidermal keratinocytes; Low power: lobulated, well-circumscribed, somewhat crateriform intradermal pseudotumor-like lesion; Ruptured lesions may show exuberant inflammatory response

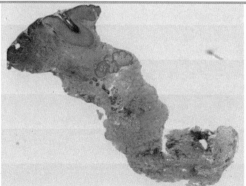

inflammatory destructive process involving epidermis and papillary dermis and extending down to the eccrine adnexal unit

MONKEYPOX
CLINICAL FEATURES
- Fever starts 10 to 14 days after exposure
- Rash usually develops 1 to 3 days after the fever
- Conjunctivitis is reported in 30% of patients without the smallpox vaccine
- Normally, the disease lasts from 2 to 4 weeks, but time and severity may increase in young, malnourished, and immunocompromised patients
- Generally, the clinical presentation resembles that of smallpox, but Mpox has a specific distinguishing feature: the lymphadenitis, especially in submental, submandibular, cervical, and inguinal regions
- Every person is considered infectious from the onset of symptoms with macular, papular, vesicular, and pustular phases until the disappearance of skin lesions and complete re-epithelization

HISTOLOGICAL FEATURES
- Ballooning degeneration of basal keratinocytes

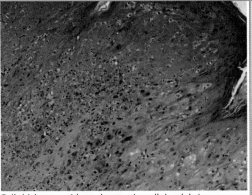

Full thickness epidermal necrosis, cellular debris

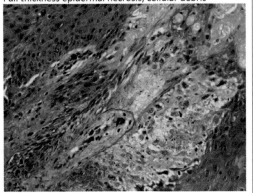

Epidermal necrosis with ballooning degeneration
Text and images contributed by Turcios Escobar, Saul
MD, University of Illinois at Chicago

- Spongiosis of a mildly acanthotic epidermis that may worsen up to full thickness necrosis of a markedly acanthotic epidermis containing few viable keratinocytes
- A lichenoid-mixed inflammatory cell infiltrate may be found showing progressive exocytosis
- One can see inflammation of the superficial and deep vascular plexus, eccrine units and follicles
- Karyorrhexis accompanied by scattered eosinophils
- Eccrine ducts necrosis
- Viral cytopathic effect is evidenced by multinucleated syncytial keratinocytes
    - Type B inclusion bodies are described in some cases

OTHER HIGH YIELD POINTS
- Clinical history of the lesions is key in guiding clinicopathological correlation
- Accurate diagnosis of Mpox by RT-PCR is important for guiding patient management and proper isolation
- When clinical presentation and histology with herpetic changes, we should consider Mpox in the differential diagnosis and think on possible coinfections

DIFFERENTIAL DIAGNOSIS
- Syphilis: Lymphohistiocytic inflammation admixed with plasma cells. IHC may highlight treponemal spirochetes in the vascular endothelium
- Disseminated histoplasmosis: Papules, pustules, and nodules throughout the body. GMS and PAS reveal the fungus
- Disseminated blastomycosis: Papules, pustules, and subcutaneous nodules developing into ulcers within weeks to months. PAS and GMS highlight organisms
- Herpes Simplex Virus/Varicella Zoster Virus: Multinucleated keratinocytes, epidermal necrosis, and full-thickness necrosis can be found. PCR or IHC are confirmatory

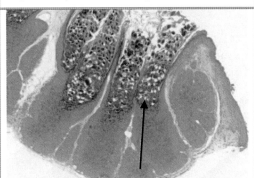

Epidermal acanthosis with cup-shaped lesion

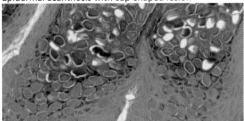

Eosinophilic cytoplasmic inclusions
Path Presenter

MOLLUSCUM CONTAGIOSUM
CLINICAL FEATURES
- These viral papules are common on the face, trunk and extremities of young children, particularly those with atopic eczema
- The lesions are small shiny umbilicated papules
- They can also be seen in the genital area of sexually active young adults

HISTOLOGICAL FEATURES
- Epidermal acanthosis with cup-shaped lesion
- Eosinophilic cytoplasmic inclusions that push the nucleus and granules to the side (Henderson-Patterson bodies)
- Ruptured lesions may show exuberant inflammatory response

OTHER HIGH YIELD POINTS
- Clinical differentials include, Cryptococcus, Coccidioidomycosis, Penicillium Marneffei, Cytomegalovirus, Basal Cell Carcinoma, Benign Cephalic Histiocytosis, Condyloma Acuminatum, Elastosis Perforans Serpiginosa, Lichen Nitidus
- Skin biopsy for diagnosis
- Full examination, including anogenital exam for all patients, as well as for sexual partners of patients
- Cervical exam for female sexual partners of male patients and for female patients, coexistence of other sexually transmitted diseases should be considered

DIFFERENTIAL DIAGNOSIS
- Herpes: Dermal edema with ballooning degeneration of keratinocytes with acantholysis followed by intradermal vesicle formation; Multinucleation of keratinocytes (fusing of adjacent cells), molding and margination of nuclear

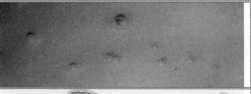

chromatin; Intranuclear and cytoplasmic basophilic and/or pale ground-glass inclusions; Background of neutrophilic inflammation
- Hand Foot And Mouth Disease: Spongiosis and epidermal necrosis with reticular degeneration; Ballooning degeneration of individual keratinocytes; No viral inclusions; Superficial perivascular lymphocytic inflammation

HERPES SIMPLEX/HERPES ZOSTER

CLINICAL FEATURES
- These viruses (HSV I, HSV II, and VZV) cause tender grouped blisters on an erythematous base with variable recurrences
- HSV I is most common around the mouth while HSV II is most commonly a genital infection
- VZV primarily causes chickenpox, but recurrence occurs dermatomally
- VZV also tends to present as folliculitis with focal necrosis

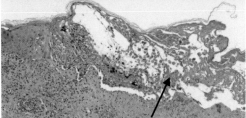
Ballooning degeneration of keratinocytes with acantholysis

HISTOLOGICAL FEATURES
- Intraepidermal vesiculation, acantholysis with or without ulceration
- Ballooning degeneration of keratinocytes with acantholysis. Multinucleation, molding and margination of nuclear chromatin. Background of neutrophilic inflammation

OTHER HIGH YIELD POINTS
- Aphthous Ulcers, Primary Syphilis, Granuloma Inguinale, Lymphogranuloma Venereum, Chancroid, Behcet's Disease
- Diagnosis can usually be made on clinical grounds. Additional workup to confirm the diagnosis include: Tzanck smear, direct fluorescence antigen studies, viral culture, PCR studies
- Skin biopsy is also helpful to confirm the diagnosis and to rule out alternative possibilities
- Serologic testing available for HSV, but a positive test does not necessarily indicate that the viral infection is the cause of the current lesion
- Brain imaging in herpes encephalitis. Lumbar puncture may be considered in this setting as well
- Chest Xray for possible pneumonitis
- HIV testing if clinically indicated
- Refer to other specialists for further evaluation depending on organ system involved

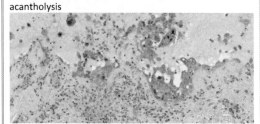
Margination, molding, multi-nucleation

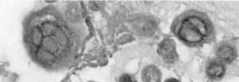
Tender grouped blisters in an erythematous base

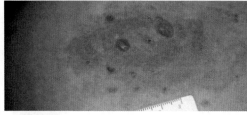

DIFFERENTIAL DIAGNOSIS
- Erythema Multiforme: Vacuolar interface changes with dyskeratosis at all levels of epidermis
- Drug Eruption: Superficial and deep perivascular lymphocytic infiltrate with admixed eosinophils +/-. Epidermal spongiosis with exocytosis and vacuolar change with rare apoptotic keratinocytes
- Viral Exanthem: Superficial and deep perivascular lymphocytic infiltrate with admixed eosinophils. Dermal fibrosis and changes suggestive of necrobiosis may be seen

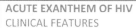
Path Presenter

ACUTE EXANTHEM OF HIV

CLINICAL FEATURES
- This is a collective term for the pruritus of HIV and can be follicular or non-follicular

HISTOLOGICAL FEATURES
- Superficial and deep perivascular lymphocytic infiltrate with admixed eosinophils
- Dermal fibrosis and changes suggestive of necrobiosis may be seen

OTHER HIGH YIELD POINTS
- Skin biopsy. Cultures of skin lesions to rule out infectious etiology
- Skin scrapings to evaluate for scabies infestation

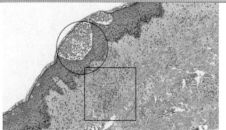
Superficial perivascular dermatitis, spongiosis, and necrotic keratinocytes; Can be pustular in superficial lesions

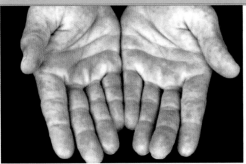

Acute exanthem of HIV

Path Presenter

- Workup includes but is not limited to: CBC with differential, serum IgE levels, HIV test and CD4 count.
- Rule out other causes of pruritus, such as renal disease, liver disease, non-Hodgkin lymphoma, etc.

DIFFERENTIAL DIAGNOSIS

- Eosinophilic Folliculitis: Peri and intrafollicular eosinophils with admixed lymphocytes
- Cytomegalovirus: Hallmark here are intranuclear large mostly eosinophilic inclusions with halo – "owl-eye inclusions;" Inclusions maybe seen in skin fibroblasts, macrophages, endothelial cells, histiocytes, and ductal cells; Occasional multinucleate giant cells with or without inclusions; Background of neutrophilic inflammation in dermis; Leukocytoclastic vasculitis/perineuritis with spongiosis – for ulcerative and bullous lesions
- Infectious Mononucleosis: Mild spongiosis with focal parakeratosis. Superficial perivascular lymphocytic infiltrate. Scattered atypical lymphocytes in infiltrate

---

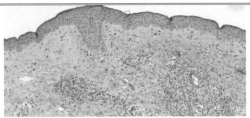

Perifollicular inflammation with admixed eosinophils

Path Presenter

HIV-ASSOCIATED EOSINOPHILIC FOLLICULITIS

CLINICAL FEATURES

- This is a pruritic eruption that occurs in HIV patients with CD4 counts around 200
- Edematous follicular papules far outnumber pustules and most are excoriated. The upper trunk, head, neck, and midline back are most affected

HISTOLOGICAL FEATURES

- Spongiosis of follicular infundibulum with predominant eosinophilic infiltrate both intrafollicular and within the dermis

OTHER HIGH YIELD POINTS

- Biopsy to confirm diagnosis and to exclude alternative possibilities
- Correlation with clinical features, patient's ethnicity, and social history is also helpful
- Detection of HPV from lesional tissue (e.g., Southern blot, PCR)

DIFFERENTIAL DIAGNOSIS

- Ofuji Disease: Common in Asian patients
- Eosinophilic Pustular Folliculitis of Infancy: Seen in infants

---

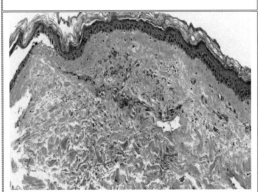

Perivascular lymphocytic infiltrate in dermis associated with microthrombi in vessels

Path Presenter

COVID-19

CLINICAL FEATURES

- Variable clinical presentations-maculopapular/morbilliform rash, urticarial rash, bullous lesions, petechia/purpura, chilblain like rash and rarely EM like presentation

HISTOLOGICAL FEATURES

- Variable depending on clinical presentation
- Maculopapular lesions show epidermal spongiosis associated with perivascular lymphocytic infiltrate in dermis and admixed eosinophils
- Urticarial Lesions show papillary dermal edema and mild perivascular lymphocytic infiltrate and few eosinophils
- Chilblain like lesions show focal vacuolar changes at DEJ with perivascular lymphocytic infiltrate in dermis associated with microthrombi in vessels
- Vesicular lesions show intraepidermal bulla with acantholysis, dyskeratosis and ballooned keratinocytes. Dermis shows edema and perivascular lymphocytic infiltrate
- Petechial lesions show perivascular and interstitial neutrophils with leukocytoclasia

OTHER HIGH YIELD POINTS

- Patients die mainly due to lung infection and early detection by skin rash could be helpful to initiate early treatment

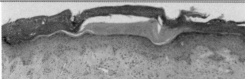
Intraepidermal bulla

DIFFERENTIAL DIAGNOSIS
- Drug Eruption: Usually shows more eosinophils. Clinical history can be helpful
- Vasculopathy associated disorders: Less likely history of fever, respiratory infections

PARASITIC AND MISCELLANEOUS INFECTIONS

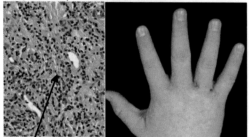
Mite, ova or scybala in stratum corneum

Perivascular inflammation with prominent eosinophils

Path Presenter

SCABIES
CLINICAL FEATURES
- Severe generalized pruritus that spares the head in adults
- Burrows on or between the fingers, the soles, or the sides of the feet
- Nodules may develop particularly in the genital area or axilla

HISTOLOGICAL FEATURES
- Mite, ova or scybala in stratum corneum
- Perivascular and interstitial inflammation with prominent eosinophils

OTHER HIGH YIELD POINTS
- Clinical differentials include Eczema, Prurigo, Drug Eruption, Eosinophilic Folliculitis, Gianotti-Crosti Syndrome, Langerhans Cell Histiocytosis, Urticaria, Pityriasis Rubra Pilaris
- Clinical findings may highly suggest the diagnosis
- Microscopic examination of mineral oil preparation of skin scrapings Dermoscopy may be helpful
- Skin biopsy can also be helpful in diagnosis

DIFFERENTIAL DIAGNOSIS
- Drug Eruption: Superficial and deep perivascular lymphocytic infiltrate with admixed eosinophils +/-. epidermal spongiosis with exocytosis and vacuolar change with rare apoptotic keratinocytes

Path Presenter

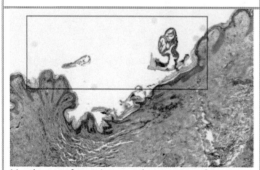
Mouth parts of organisms may be seen on surface or within the dermis

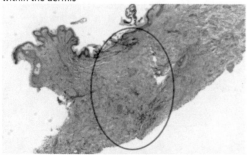
Wedge-shaped perivascular and interstitial inflammation

TICK BITE
CLINICAL FEATURES
- The blood meal extracted by ticks through the skin is typically painless but can result in eventual nodules
- The most important tick born infections in the United States are Lyme disease and Rocky Mountain Spotted Fever

HISTOLOGICAL FEATURES
- Wedge-shaped perivascular and interstitial inflammation with prominent eosinophils
- Mouth parts of organisms may be seen on surface or within the dermis

OTHER HIGH YIELD POINTS
- The diagnosis can usually be made based on history or identification of attached tick
- Tick identification services available through local departments of health and other institutions

DIFFERENTIAL DIAGNOSIS
- Spider Bite: Histological findings in arthropod bite reaction are highly variable. Classically, a dense, wedge-shaped superficial and deep perivascular and interstitial inflammatory infiltrate is present. Eosinophils are a prominent finding and are a useful clue when seen away from the vessels (interposed between collagen bundles) and in the deeper dermis. The epidermis is variably spongiotic; this is typically more prominent at the center where the arthropod mouth parts pierce the skin. Mouth parts may be present at the

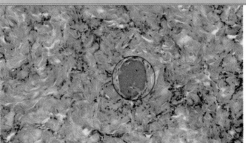

Vascular thrombosis can be seen, which can mimic cryoglobulinemia

center of the lesion which aids in diagnosis. Less often, secondary vasculitis and atypical lymphocytes can be identified
- Drug Eruption: Superficial and deep perivascular lymphocytic infiltrate with admixed eosinophils +/-. Epidermal spongiosis with exocytosis and vacuolar change with rare apoptotic keratinocytes
- Scabies: On H&E, scabies infestations are diagnosed when a scabies mite, ova or scybala is found within the stratum corneum. Spongiosis and eosinophilic spongiosis may be present to varying degrees within the epidermis. In the dermis, a superficial and deep perivascular and interstitial inflammatory infiltrate is present with prominent numbers of eosinophils

Path Presenter

epidermal and dermal necrosis

Mixed perivascular and interstitial infiltrate

Path Presenter

SPIDER BITE
CLINICAL FEATURES
- Spiders generally produce either neurotoxic or cytotoxic venom
- The symptoms associated with a spider bite varies depending on the species of spider and the type of venom
- Black widow spiders produce neurotoxins while brown recluse spiders produce a cytotoxic venom that results in pain and swelling a few hours after the bite
- In the case of brown recluse spiders this typically eventuates in necrosis
HISTOLOGICAL FEATURES
- Wedge shaped areas of epidermal and dermal necrosis
- Mixed perivascular and interstitial infiltrate of eosinophils and neutrophils with variable vasculitis
OTHER HIGH YIELD POINTS
- Clinical differentials include, other Arthropod Assault, Venomous Bite
- This is primarily a clinical diagnosis based on history and clinical presentation
- If safely feasible, collection and identification of the spider
- If systemic toxicity is a clinical concern (particularly in brown recluse or black widow spider bites), patient should be hospitalized and should be closely monitored
- Evaluation for hemolysis, rhabdomyolysis, renal failure, and coagulopathy should be performed
DIFFERENTIAL DIAGNOSIS
- Pyoderma Gangrenosum: Findings are variable depending on the site biopsied and the stage of the lesion. Lesions show dense neutrophilic infiltrate; the advancing edge of the ulcer may demonstrate leukocytoclastic lymphocytic vasculitis with endothelial cell swelling and extravasated erythrocytes
- Arthropod Bite: Histological findings in arthropod bite reaction are highly variable. Classically, a dense, wedge-shaped superficial and deep perivascular inflammatory infiltrate with admixed eosinophils is noted

Acral skin with flea beneath stratum corneum

TUNGIASIS
CLINICAL FEATURES
- This disorder results in severe generalized pruritus that spares the head
- It can result in burrows on or between the fingers, the soles or the sides of the feet, Nodules may develop particularly in the genital area or axilla
HISTOLOGICAL FEATURES
- Acral skin with flea beneath stratum corneum (Tunga Penetrans)
- Often gravid female with eggs
- Mixed inflammatory infiltrate

Gravid female flea

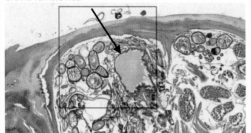

OTHER HIGH YIELD POINTS

- Clinical differentials include, Eczema, Prurigo, Drug Eruption, Eosinophilic Folliculitis, Gianotti-Crosti Syndrome, Langerhans Cell Histiocytosis, Urticaria, Pityriasis Rubra Pilaris
- Clinical findings may highly suggest the diagnosis
- Microscopic examination of mineral oil preparation of skin scrapings
- Dermoscopy and skin biopsy may be helpful

DIFFERENTIAL DIAGNOSIS

- Arthropod Bite: Histological findings in arthropod bite reaction are highly variable. Classically, a dense, wedge-shaped superficial and deep perivascular and interstitial inflammatory infiltrate is present. Eosinophils are a prominent finding and are a useful clue when seen away from the vessels and in the deeper dermis

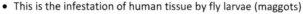

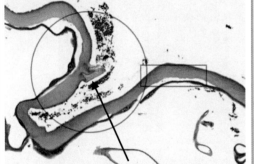

Pigmented setae and chitinous wall

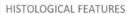

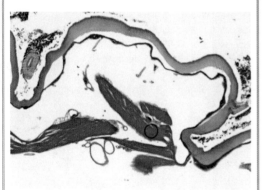

Skeletal muscle of worm (low power above, high power below)

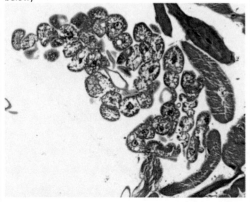

MYIASIS

CLINICAL FEATURES

- This is the infestation of human tissue by fly larvae (maggots)
- This can occur on an open wound or can be furuncular
- The furuncular form is most commonly caused by Dermatobia hominis and occurs in Central and South America
- Furuncular myiasis occurs when the botfly eggs that were deposited on a mosquito enter the skin during the mosquito bite
- The maturing lesion has a central pore through which the breathing tube can often be observed

HISTOLOGICAL FEATURES

- Maggots in dermis or subcutaneous tissue
- Diffuse mixed infiltrate of lymphocytes, histiocytes and eosinophils
- Histology shows pigmented setae, chitinous wall and skeletal muscle of worm

OTHER HIGH YIELD POINTS

- Diagnosis can be done by extraction of larva and submission of larva for further speciation
- Skin biopsy can be performed to exclude alternative possibilities
- Additional imaging studies (e.g. MRI, ultrasound) may be helpful, especially in the evaluation of deeper infestation, including cerebral myiasis

DIFFERENTIAL DIAGNOSIS

- Arthropod Bite: Histological findings in arthropod bite reaction are highly variable. Classically, a dense, wedge-shaped superficial and deep perivascular and interstitial inflammatory infiltrate is present. Eosinophils are a prominent finding and are a useful clue when seen away from the vessels and in the deeper dermis
- Tungiasis: Acral skin with flea beneath stratum corneum. Often gravid female with eggs. Mixed inflammatory infiltrate
- Spider Bite: Histological findings in arthropod bite reaction are highly variable. Classically, a dense, wedge-shaped superficial and deep perivascular and interstitial inflammatory infiltrate is present. Eosinophils are a prominent finding and are a useful clue when seen away from the vessels (interposed between collagen bundles) and in the deeper dermis. The epidermis is variably spongiotic; this is typically more prominent at the center where the arthropod mouth parts pierce the skin. Mouth parts may be present at the center of the lesion which aids in diagnosis. Less often, secondary vasculitis and atypical lymphocytes can be identified

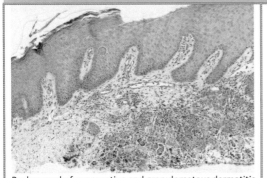

Background of suppurative and granulomatous dermatitis

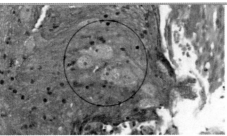

Organisms with septations showing morula and daisy forms seen both free and within macrophages

PROTOTHECOSIS
CLINICAL FEATURES
- This achloric algae (Prototheca) is found in stagnant water, tree slime, and soil
- Verrucous or ulcerated papulonodules or umbilicated crusted papules occur at the site of inoculation

HISTOLOGICAL FEATURES
- Background of suppurative and granulomatous dermatitis
- Organisms with septations showing morula and daisy forms seen both free and within macrophages (2-10 microns)

OTHER HIGH YIELD POINTS
- Clinical differentials include, Tinea, Pyoderma Gangrenosum, Deep Fungal Infection, Anthrax, Mycobacterium Marinum Infection, Olecranon Bursitis, Blastomycosis like Pyoderma
- Cultures on Sabouraud agar fluorescent antibody reagents on culture and tissue
- May occur in patients with immunosuppression

DIFFERENTIAL DIAGNOSIS
- Deep Fungal Infection: Granulomatous and suppurative inflammation, often with overlying pseudoepitheliomatous hyperplasia. Fungal elements highlighted by PAS and GMS stains within the infiltrate

Path Presenter

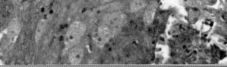

Trophozoites (15-25 microns) with ample cytoplasm, eccentric nuclei, and prominent nucleoli, some showing phagocytized RBC (high power below)

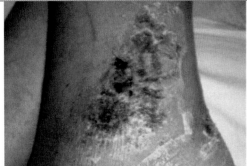

AMEBIASIS
CLINICAL FEATURES
- This is caused by fecal-oral or sexual transmission of Entamoeba histolytica
- Cutaneous lesions are most common on the trunk, abdomen, buttock or perineum and result from ulceration of an underlying abscess

HISTOLOGICAL FEATURES
- Ulceration with underlying acute and chronic inflammation, sometimes with granulomatous component
- Trophozoites (15-40 microns) with ample cytoplasm, eccentric nuclei and prominent nucleoli; some showing phagocytized RBC

Path Presenter

TRYPANOSOMIASIS
CLINICAL FEATURES
- American trypanosomiasis, known as Chagas disease, is due to protozoal transmission by the reduviid bug with development of an erythematous nodule at the bite site, usually on the face
- If near the eye this is called Romana sign
- Acutely, fever and adenopathy can occur with a morbilliform or urticarial eruption
- Cardiac and gastrointestinal involvement are the biggest chronic concerns.
- African trypanosomiasis, known as sleeping sickness, is due to the bite of a tsetse fly with resultant chancre and adenopathy

CHAPTER 21: INFECTIONS AND INFESTATIONS

HISTOLOGICAL FEATURES
- Epidermal acanthosis with ulceration. Perivascular lymphocytic infiltrate with admixed plasma cells and histiocytes
- Dermal edema with/without vasculitis

OTHER HIGH YIELD POINTS
- Clinical differentials include, Malaria, HIV Disease, Brucellosis, Borreliosis, Cryptococcal Meningitis, Visceral Leishmaniasis, Periorbital Cellulitis, Angioedema
- **African trypanosomiasis**
- Detection of parasites in skin, blood, lymph node, cerebrospinal fluid, skin chancre aspirates, or bone marrow
- Lumbar puncture should be performed whenever the diagnosis is suspected
- Skin biopsy may be helpful
- Serologic antibody detection test is available for T.gambiense, but not unequivocally diagnostic
- Molecular testing (e.g., PCR, loop mediated isothermal amplification, etc.)
- Additional workup includes but are not limited to: CBC with differential, ESR, CRP, albumin levels, complement levels, quantitation of serum immunoglobulins
- Imaging studies (e.g., head CT, MRI) to determine extent of disease American trypanosomiasis (Chagas disease)

- Identification of parasites in the blood, especially in acute disease
- Diagnosis of chronic disease is usually based on serologic testing (indirect immunofluorescence, ELISA, indirect hemagglutination, etc.), as there are too few circulating parasites at this stage of disease for microscopic detection and on hemoculture
- There may be a role for PCR assays in the diagnosis of acute Chagas disease
- Imaging studies to evaluate for various organ manifestations (e.g., cardiac, esophageal, colon)
- EKG (including 24-hour continuous EKG)
- Additional procedures as clinically indicated (e.g., endoscopy, esophageal manometry)

DIFFERENTIAL DIAGNOSIS
- Histoplasma Capsulatum: Intracellular yeasts with pseudocapsule (2-4 microns) inside macrophages, evenly distributed and surrounded by pseudocapsule in a background of suppurative and granulomatous inflammation
- Rhinoscleroma: Dense infiltrate of macrophages with admixed plasma cells. Some of the larger macrophages (Mikulicz cells) contain large number of Gram-negative bacilli. Bacilli visible on H&E, PAS and Giemsa stains

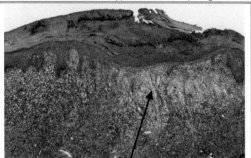
Granulomatous dermatitis and admixed macrophages, lymphocytes, neutrophils, plasma cells

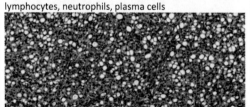
Organisms within macrophages

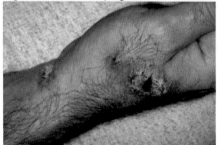
Ulcerated crusted nodule

LEISHMANIASIS
CLINICAL FEATURES
- This protozoal infection is transmitted by the sand fly and presents as erythematous papules that enlarge into an ulcerated crusted nodule
- Diffuse cutaneous, mucocutaneous, and visceral disease can occur

HISTOLOGICAL FEATURES
- Granulomatous dermatitis with admixed macrophages, lymphocytes, neutrophils, and plasma cells
- Intracellular organisms (2-3 microns) with round, basophilic nuclei and rod-like kinetoplast scattered haphazardly and filling the macrophages

OTHER HIGH YIELD POINTS
- Skin biopsy and biopsy of other affected tissue
- Culture using Novy-MacNeal-Nicolle medium or chick embryo media
- PCR study is the most sensitive and specific test
- In the United States, the Centers for Disease Control and Prevention offer diagnostic services
- They should be contacted before specimen for diagnosis is collected, in order to receive instructions and transport media
- Serologic tests for visceral leishmaniasis, such as rK39 antibody test
- Full history and physical examination, including evaluation of oral and respiratory mucosa and checking for organomegaly
- Laboratory tests are unremarkable in cutaneous or mucocutaneous disease
- In visceral leishmaniasis, laboratory evaluation to be considered include CBC with differential, complete metabolic panel including liver function test, SPEP
- Bone marrow aspiration (and splenic aspiration in diagnostically difficult cases) may be indicated in cases of visceral leishmaniasis
- HIV test should also be considered in cases of leishmaniasis
- Clinical differentials include NK-T Cell Lymphoma, Basal Cell Carcinoma, Blastomycosis, Chromboblastomycosis, Histoplasmosis, Rhinoscleroma, Pyoderma Gengrenosum

DIFFERENTIAL DIAGNOSIS
- Histoplasma Capsulatum: Intracellular yeasts with pseudocapsule (2-4

Path Presenter

microns) inside macrophages, evenly distributed and surrounded by pseudocapsule in a background of suppurative and granulomatous inflammation
- Rhinoscleroma: Dense infiltrate of macrophages with admixed plasma cells. Some of the larger macrophages (Mikulicz cells) contain a large number of Gram-negative bacilli. Bacilli visible on H&E, PAS and Giemsa stains

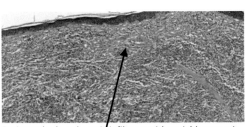

Perivascular lymphocytic infiltrate with variable necrosis and hemorrhage

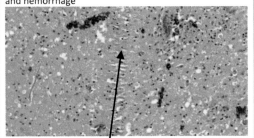

Trophozoites within macrophages seen in brain tissue

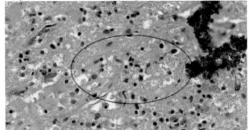

Trophozoites (2-8 microns) or cysts (8-30 microns) containing numerous bradyzoites are seen free or within macrophages

Path Presenter

TOXOPLASMOSIS
CLINICAL FEATURES
- This protozoal infection is transmitted by the sand fly and presents as erythematous papules that enlarge into an ulcerated crusted nodule
- Diffuse cutaneous, mucocutaneous, and visceral disease can occur

HISTOLOGICAL FEATURES
- Perivascular lymphocytic infiltrate with variable necrosis and hemorrhage
- Trophozoites (2-8 microns) or cysts (8-30 microns) containing numerous bradyzoites are seen free or within macrophages
- PAS positive

OTHER HIGH YIELD POINTS
- Direct identification of organism from affected tissue, body fluids or blood
- Immunoperoxidase stain available
- Additional procedures may be necessary if clinically necessary: lumbar puncture, lymph node biopsy, amniocentesis, bronchoalveolar lavage, brain biopsy, ocular aspiration, etc. Serologic testing (IgM capture ELISA, avidity testing, agglutination testing)
- Imaging studies to determine extent of disease (e.g., CT, MRI, PET, fetal ultrasound)
- Neuroimaging should be performed on patients with neurologic symptoms
- PCR assay can be performed
- Cultures can be done by inoculation of human cell lines or inoculating mice

DIFFERENTIAL DIAGNOSIS
- Infectious Mononucleosis: Mild spongiosis with focal parakeratosis. Superficial perivascular lymphocytic infiltrate. Scattered atypical lymphocytic infiltrate
- Cytomegalovirus: Hallmark here are intranuclear large mostly eosinophilic inclusions with halo – "owl-eye inclusions;" Inclusions maybe seen in skin fibroblasts, macrophages, endothelial cells, histiocytes, and ductal cells; Occasional multinucleate giant cells with or without inclusions; Background of neutrophilic inflammation in dermis; Leukocytoclastic vasculitis/perineuritis with spongiosis – for ulcerative and bullous lesions
- Drug Eruption: Superficial and deep perivascular lymphocytic infiltrate with admixed eosinophils +/-. Epidermal spongiosis with exocytosis and vacuolar change with rare apoptotic keratinocytes

Calcified ova with granulomatous dermatitis

SCHISTOSOMIASIS
CLINICAL FEATURES
- **Schistosoma Haematobium:** This trematode is found in the Middle East, India, and Africa. The larval cercariae burrow through the skin when exposed to contaminated water. This may result in pruritus and papules at the site of penetration and fever, hepatosplenomegaly, lymphadenopathy, and pneumonitis. There is eventual migration of the adult to the bladder. Cutaneous granulomas of the genitalia and perineum present as vegetating, soft, fistulous masses
- **Schistosoma Mansoni:** The larval cercariae of this trematode burrow through the skin when exposed to contaminated water. They may develop pruritus and papules at the site of penetration and have fever, hepatosplenomegaly,

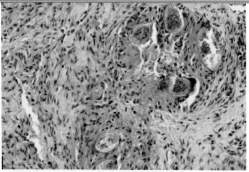
Calcified ova with granulomatous dermatitis

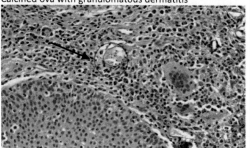
Background of granulomatous dermatitis. Scattered rare ova with stippled contents and vertical spine

Path Presenter

lymphadenopathy, and pneumonitis. There is eventual migration of the adult to the mesenteric blood vessels. Cutaneous granulomas of the buttocks and perineum present as vegetating, soft, fistulous masses

- **Schistosoma Japonicum:** This trematode is found in the Far East. The larval cercariae burrow through the skin when exposed to contaminated water. This may result in pruritus and papules at the site of penetration and fever, hepatosplenomegaly, lymphadenopathy, and pneumonitis. There is eventual migration of the adult to the mesenteric blood vessels. Cutaneous granulomas of the buttocks and perineum present as vegetating, soft, fistulous masses

HISTOLOGICAL FEATURES

- Background of granulomatous dermatitis
- Scattered rare ova with stippled contents and spine. Location of spine varies with species
- Rarely adult worm seen in blood vessels

OTHER HIGH YIELD POINTS

- Clinical differentials include Swimmer's Itch, Sea bather's Eruption, Jellyfish Sting
- Detection of eggs in urine and less commonly, in feces
- ELISA detecting antischistosomal antibodies is available
- Circulating parasite antigens and antigens in stool/urine can also be detected
- Biopsy of involved organs, including skin, may reveal eggs
- Additional workup and imaging may be indicated to investigate involvement of other organs

DIFFERENTIAL DIAGNOSIS

- Arthropod Bite: Histological findings in arthropod bite reaction are highly variable. Classically, a dense, wedge-shaped superficial and deep perivascular and interstitial inflammatory infiltrate is present. Eosinophils are a prominent finding and are a useful clue when seen away from the vessels and in the deeper dermis
- Drug Eruption: Superficial and deep perivascular lymphocytic infiltrate with admixed eosinophils +/-. Epidermal spongiosis with exocytosis and vacuolar change with rare apoptotic keratinocytes

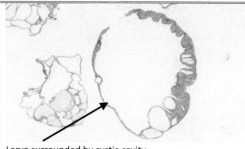
Larva surrounded by cystic cavity

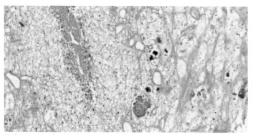
Calcareous bodies

CYSTICERCOSIS

CLINICAL FEATURES

- This is caused by the pork tapeworm (Taenia Solium)
- Rarely infection can manifest as a solitary painless cutaneous nodule

HISTOLOGICAL FEATURES

- Larva (6-18 mm long) with cystic cavity & fibrosis in dermis/ subcutaneous fat
- Scolex with hooklets and two pairs of sucker cups must be seen
- Surrounding mild inflammation, intense if the larva dies
- Calcareous bodies-purplish oval calcified concretions- may be seen

OTHER HIGH YIELD POINTS

- Clinical differentials include Subcutaneous Masses, Cysts, Trichinosis
- Radiographs of affected areas (e.g., head, extremities) reveal calcified cyst.
- Lesions can be demonstrated via other imaging tests (CT, MRI)
- Enzyme linked immunoblot assay is serologic test of choice. Serum ELISA and hemagglutination tests can also be performed
- Biopsy of cutaneous lesion may demonstrate the organism
- CBC with differential. Stool for ova and parasite
- Lumbar puncture for cerebrospinal fluid analysis if clinically indicated

DIFFERENTIAL DIAGNOSIS

- Dirofilaria: Granulomatous inflammation with/without neutrophils. Tightly coiled worm with thick muscular layer interrupted by lateral cords, usually in subcutaneous tissue

Path Presenter

- Wuchereria bancrofti: Filarial roundworm in lymphatic channels. Surrounding mild inflammation
- Tungiasis: Acral skin with flea beneath stratum corneum. Often gravid female with eggs. Mixed inflammatory infiltrate

ONCHOCERCIASIS
CLINICAL FEATURES
- This nematode disorder is seen in tropical Africa and Central and South America where it is known as river blindness. It is transmitted in the larval stage (Onchocerca volvulus) by the bite of the black fly
- The adult worm develops in the dermis as a large nodule and produces microfilaria that migrate through the host causing loose redundant skin in the groin, scaling and depigmentation of the skin (leopard skin), and blindness
HISTOLOGICAL FEATURES
- Adult female (100-500 microns) with paired uteri seen within subcutaneous tissue surrounded by dense fibrosis and foreign body reaction
- Microfilariae (5-10 microns) may be seen freely within dermis
OTHER HIGH YIELD POINTS
- Clinical differentials include, Acquired ichthyosis, Allergic Contact Dermatitis, Chemical Leukoderma, Dermatophytosis, Arthropod Bites, Lichen Planus, Post inflammatory Pigment Alteration
- Skin snip test. Identification of microfilariae or adult worms in skin biopsy or nodule excisions would also be helpful and would also rule out alternative possibilities
- Slit lamp examination of eyes. Mazzotti reaction test or patch test
- Onchocerca volvulus antigen test in urine or tears can also be performed
- PCR testing from skin specimens can also be performed
DIFFERENTIAL DIAGNOSIS
- Wuchereria Bancrofti: Filarial roundworm in lymphatic channels. Surrounding mild inflammation
- Dirofilaria: Granulomatous inflammation with/without neutrophils. Tightly coiled worm with thick muscular layer interrupted by lateral cords, usually in subcutaneous tissue
- Sparganum Proliferum: Larva with longitudinal and horizontal muscle bundles and a longitudinal excretory duct seen in subcutaneous tissue. Cavity surrounded by fibrosis and a granulomatous response with admixed lymphocytes, plasma cells and eosinophils

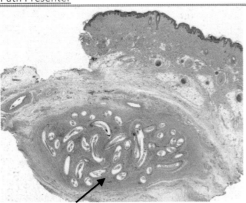

Parasite within subcutaneous tissue surrounded by dense fibrosis

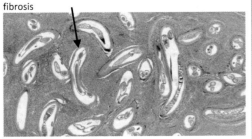

Path Presenter

DIROFILARIASIS
CLINICAL FEATURES
- Typically manifests as subcutaneous nodules or lung disease
HISTOLOGICAL FEATURES
- Granulomatous inflammation with/without neutrophils
- Tightly coiled worm (Dirofilaria immitis) with thick muscular layer interrupted by lateral cords, usually in subcutaneous tissue
OTHER HIGH YIELD POINTS
- This nematode disorder is transmitted to humans by a mosquito vector
- Biopsy of involved tissue
- Full history and physical examination to initiate evaluation for extent of disease
- Evaluation by ophthalmologist to exclude ocular involvement
- Workup may also include but are not limited to: CBC with diff, PCR studies, imaging studies (e.g. chest Xray, CT, MRI, ultrasound) to determine extent of disease and organs involved
- Serologic tests exist, but are not routinely available or routinely used in clinical practice

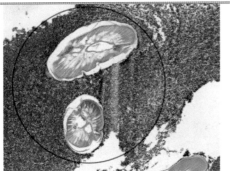

Coiled worm with granulomatous inflammation

Path Presenter

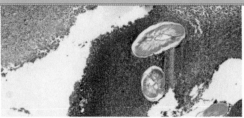

Parasite within subcutaneous tissue

DIFFERENTIAL DIAGNOSIS

- Onchocerciasis: Adult female with paired uteri seen within subcutaneous tissue surrounded by dense fibrosis and foreign body reaction
- Tungiasis: Acral skin with flea beneath stratum corneum. Often gravid female with eggs. Mixed inflammatory infiltrate
- Sparganum Proliferum: Larva with longitudinal and horizontal muscle bundles and a longitudinal excretory duct seen in subcutaneous tissue. Cavity surrounded by fibrosis and a granulomatous response with admixed lymphocytes, plasma cells and eosinophils

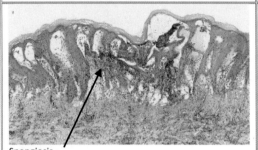

Spongiosis

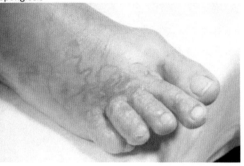

Path Presenter

CUTANEOUS LARVA MIGRANS

CLINICAL FEATURES

- This results from penetration of nematode larva through the skin, usually on the feet, buttocks, or abdomen forming pruritic erythematous papules or vesicles with extending erythematous serpiginous tracts

HISTOLOGICAL FEATURES

- Spongiosis with overlying scale crust
- Perivascular inflammation with many eosinophils
- Sometimes larva seen (up to 1 cm) in deep epidermis, more often cavities left by organism are seen in the epidermis

OTHER HIGH YIELD POINTS

- Clinical differentials include, Allergic Contact Dermatitis, Arthropod Bite Reaction, Dermatophytosis, Dirofilariasis, Erythema Annulare Centrifugum, Jellyfish Sting
- This is a primarily clinical diagnosis
- Dermoscopy may be helpful
- Skin biopsy may demonstrate the larva and may exclude alternate possibilities
- May be complicated by Loeffler syndrome, which consists of pulmonary infiltrates and eosinophilia in the blood and sputum

DIFFERENTIAL DIAGNOSIS

- Allergic Contact Dermatitis: The acute stage shows spongiosis with/without vesiculation. Lymphocytic exocytosis and a superficial perivascular lymphocytic infiltrate, often with eosinophils are identified
- Arthropod Bite: Histological findings in arthropod bite reaction are highly variable. Classically, a dense, wedge-shaped superficial and deep perivascular and interstitial inflammatory infiltrate is present. Eosinophils are a prominent finding and are a useful clue when seen away from the vessels and in the deeper dermis

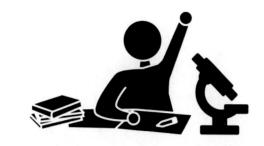

ACE MY PATH
Come Ace With Us!

CHAPTER 22: DISORDERS OF
COLLAGEN AND ELASTIC TISSUES

TERRANCE LYNN, MD

DISORDERS OF COLLAGEN AND ELASTIC TISSUES

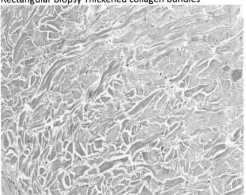
Rectangular biopsy Thickened collagen bundles

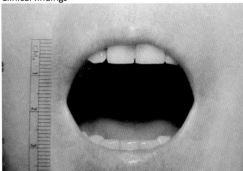
Clinical findings

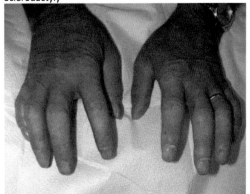
Sclerodactyly

MORPHEA AND SCLERODERMA

CLINICAL FEATURES

- These group of disorders are characterized by deposition of collagen in skin and sometimes other organs. Localized scleroderma is referred to as morphea. Systemic scleroderma includes limited forms and diffuse forms (also called progressive systemic sclerosis)
- Seen in both **adults and children.** Adults are usually **females** in the 4th decade of age while children are in the 1st decade of lif

  Limited Scleroderma:
  - Includes **CREST Syndrome**
  - Thickening of skin of distal **elbows** and **knees**, Raynaud phenomenon, and pulmonary hypertension
    Anticentromere antibody in about **80%** of cases

  Diffuse Scleroderma:
  - Includes CREST Syndrome
  - Thickening of skin proximal to elbows and knees, Raynaud phenomenon, and interstitial lung disease, renal failure, or myocardial involvement
  - **Antitopoisomerase1 (anti-Scl-70)** in about 30% of cases

  Morphea
  - Localized to the skin, typically presents on trunk and extremities as indurated plaque(s) with a violaceous border like ring
  - Has different clinical presentations: Circumscribed, linear, generalized, pansclerotic, mixed, systemic (Scleroderma)
  - Linear morphea involves the frontoparietal area and is referred to as "en coup de sabre"

HISTOLOGIC FEATURES

Early lesional findings:
- Mild lymphocytic inflammation that surrounds the superficial and deep vessels, adnexal structures, and nerves
- **Eosinophils** and plasma cells can be seen in reticular dermis or dermal-subcutis interface
- **Edematous** changes in the upper dermis
- Endothelial cells may be plump
- **Collagen** may be "darker" in appearance and **slightly thickened**
- Mucin may be seen in dermis

Developed (late) lesional findings:
- Rectangular biopsy
- Sclerosis of dermis with thickened collagen bundles with atrophy of adnexa
- Loss of perieccrine fat
- Elastic fibers are present but compressed and sometimes clumped
- Early lesions may show mucin
- Thickened small blood vessels with narrowing of lumen
- Mild perivascular lymphocytic infiltrate with some scattered plasma cells and macrophages. Can be rarely moderate to dense infiltrate
- Subcutaneous morphea (morphea profundus) shows hyalinization in deep dermis and subcutaneous septa and fascia

OTHER HIGH YIELD POINTS

- **Colloidal iron** (or other mucin stain) highlights the extracellular mucin
- **Loss of CD34** staining in the dermis

DIFFERENTIAL DIAGNOSIS

- **Scleredema:** hypertrophic collagen bundles, mucin intervening between

Path Presenter

- **Sclerodermoid GVHD:** Reticular and papillary dermis involved with associated changes of GVHD
- **Scleromyxedema:** upper and mid-reticular dermis with prominent mucin and scattered spindle cells
- **Radiation-induced dermatitis:** atypical cells, elastosis, ectatic vessels
- **Nephrogenic systemic fibrosis:** upper and mid-reticular dermis with prominent mucin
- **Lichen sclerosus et atrophicus:** sclerosis of papillary dermis only

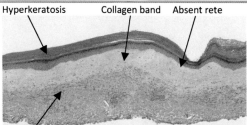

Hyperkeratosis   Collagen band   Absent rete

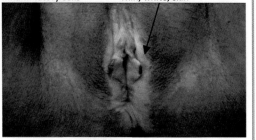

Inflammatory cells   Thin, white, skin

Path Presenter

LICHEN SCLEROSUS
CLINICAL FEATURES

- Seen in **elderly females (post-menopausal) individuals**
- Thin, white-gray "cigarette paper" skin, intense pruritis and excoriation
- Usually affects the labia majora, minora, clitoris, and anus
- As disease progresses, clitoris often is "buried" under clitoral hood
- Can have overlying scale/crust

HISTOLOGIC FEATURES

- **Hyperkeratosis,** loss of rete ridges, basement membrane thickening
- **Sclerosis** of papillary dermis
- **Vacuolar interface reaction** with band-like inflammatory response
- **Homogenous hyalinized collagen bundles**
- Can have erosion and ulceration
- Lymphocytes and plasma cells, can have some eosinophils

DIFFERENTIAL DIAGNOSIS

- **Scleredema:** hypertrophic collagen bundles, mucin intervening between
- **Sclerodermoid GVHD:** Reticular and papillary dermis involved with associated changes of GVHD
- **Scleromyxedema:** upper and mid-reticular dermis with prominent mucin and scattered spindle cells
- **Radiation-induced dermatitis:** atypical cells, elastosis, ectatic vessels

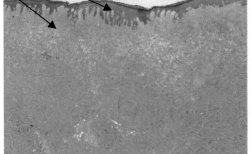

Sclerosis   Acanthosis

Bizzare fibroblasts   Ectatic vessels

RADIATION DERMATITIS
CLINICAL FEATURES

- Seen in **exposure to radiation (treatment, occupation, accidental)**
- Erythema, variable blisters, and telangiectasia
- Atrophic and/or shiny skin, variable hyper- and hypopigmentation

HISTOLOGIC FEATURES

- **Hyperkeratosis, variable acanthosis,** epidermal atrophy
- **Sclerosis** of **superficial dermis** but can be full thickness
- **Multinucleated** and **stellate fibroblasts with nuclear inclusions, nuclear irregularities**
- **Ectatic blood vessels** with or without fibrin thrombi

DIFFERENTIAL DIAGNOSIS

- **Lichen sclerosus:** Hyperkeratosis, loss of rete, sclerosis of papillary dermis, band-like inflammatory infiltrate, no atypical fibroblasts
- **Morphea:** thick collagen bundles, lacks sclerosis and bizarre fibroblasts

Path Presenter

CHAPTER 22: DISORDERS OF COLLAGEN AND ELASTIC TISSUES

Acral skin

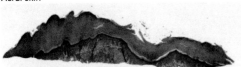

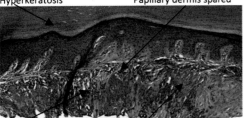

Hyperkeratosis   Papillary dermis spared

Acellular   Elastotic material

Path Presenter

COLLAGENOUS AND ELASTOTIC MARGINAL PLAQUES OF HANDS (CEMPH)
CLINICAL FEATURES
- Seen in **elderly individuals** with **extensive sun exposure**
- Radial and ulnar aspects of hands have **discrete, translucent papules** that coalesce and **form linear plaques**
- Can have overlying scale/crust
HISTOLOGIC FEATURES
- **Acanthotic** and **hyperkeratotic epidermis**
- Globs of **gray-blue elastotic material** with/without calcifications but papillary dermis is spared
- **Collagen** bundles are **haphazardly arranged**
- **Matrix is acellular** and there is **limited vascularity**
DIFFERENTIAL DIAGNOSIS
- **Acrokeratoelastoidosis of Costa:** hyperkeratosis, epidermal hyperplasia, fragmented elastic fibers, collagen degeneration
- **Nodular solar elastosis:** No collagen degeneration or calcified elastic fibers
- **Colloid milium:** No calcifications, has gray-blue elastotic material
- **Acquired elastotic hemangioma:** band-like aggregation of capillaries that are parallel to dermis
- **Acrokeratosis verruciformis:** no dermal elastotic mass

Thickened interlobular septa   Thickened adipose

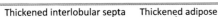

Eosinophils   Lymphocytes

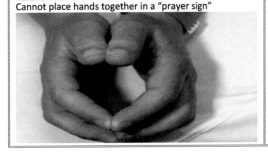

Cannot place hands together in a "prayer sign"

EOSINOPHILIC FASCIITIS (Shulman's Disease)
CLINICAL FEATURES
- **Women** are **most affected**, presenting with **painful, erythematous**, and **indurated skin** which **mimics scleroderma. "Dry Riverbed" appearance**
- Patients are often **unable to put hands together in a "prayer sign"**
- Acute onset after vigorous exercise
- Various associations: **Malignancy** (especially **cutaneous T-cell lymphoma**), **Borrelia burgdorferi**, arthropod assaults, **medications**, or **vigorous workouts**
- May spontaneously convalesce or require treatment
- May progress to scleroderma with about 30% of cases having comorbid morphea
HISTOLOGIC FEATURES
- Deep dermis has sclerosis and atrophic adnexal structures
- Adipose tissue is thickened and has **septal and interlobular fascial thickening**
- Infiltrate of inflammatory cells with **eosinophils** (may or may not be very prominent), histiocytes, lymphocytes, and plasma cells
- **Fascia is edematous** and **thickened**
IMMUNOFLUORESCENCE
- May have C3 and immunoglobulins in vessel walls
OTHER HIGH YIELD POINTS
- **Hypergammaglobulinemia** and increased circulating immune complexes
- Positive **antinuclear antibody (ANA)**
- **Peripheral eosinophilia** on the complete blood count
DIFFERENTIAL DIAGNOSIS
- **Scleroderma:** Septal and fascial thickening, lacks inflammation
- **Linear scleroderma:** dermal fibrosis
- **Morphea profunda:** Hyalinization and thickened fascia and septa

Path Presenter

Epidermal flattening

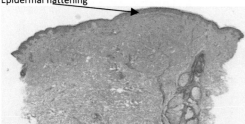

Mucin and admixed hypocellular spindle cells

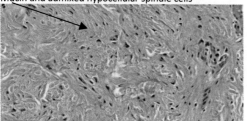

Waxy papules

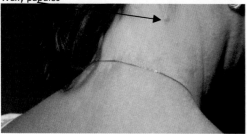

Induration of Skin

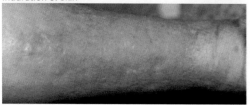

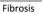

PAPULAR MUCINOSIS (SCLEROMYXEDEMA)
CLINICAL FEATURES

- Has **3 major clinical forms**: Generalized papular, sclerodermoid, localized (lichen myxedematosus), and atypical

  Generalized papular and sclerodermoid:
  - Skin is **thickened, indurated**, but **flesh colored pebbled skin** involving the face, head, neck, and eventually majority of the skin
  - Patients will note **pruritis** and also **leonine facies**
  - **Decreased mobility** of fingers, extremities, and face over the years
  - May have other **systemic symptoms**: Raynaud disease, myopathy, neurologic defects, and restrictive lung disease

  Localized (Lichen myxedematosus):
  - **Numerous waxy papules** on face, neck, hands, and trunk but **lacks any progressive skin sclerosis**

  Atypical:
  - Overlapping features of the above

HISTOLOGIC FEATURES

  Scleromyxedema:
  - Abundant **mucin deposition, increased** production of **collagen**, and **irregular fibroblasts** in the mid to upper dermis
  - Older lesions have **atrophy of pilosebaceous units** and **epidermal flattening**
  - May have **perivascular lymphocytic infiltrate**

  Lichen myxedematosus:
  - **Diffuse mucin deposition** and **few irregular fibroblasts**
  - **No increased collagen** production or **fibrosis**
  - **Increased mast cells**

DIFFERENTIAL DIAGNOSIS

- **Nephrogenic systemic fibrosis:** often has deeper involvement
- **Pretibial myxedema:** no increase in fibroblasts or collagen
- **Scleredema:** mucin deposition more prominent in deeper dermis, no increase in fibroblasts, swollen collagen fibers
- **Interstitial granuloma annulare:** granulomatous inflammation and interstitial mucin

Path Presenter

Fibrosis

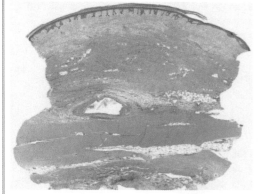

Path Presenter

NEPHROGENIC FIBROSING DERMOPATHY (NEPHROGENIC SYSTEMIC FIBROSIS)
CLINICAL FEATURES

- Can **present at any age** but is most common in **older patients** with **renal failure** (more commonly seen in patients on dialysis, few reports on non-dialysis patients)
- Patients report **papules and plaques on skin;** lesions commonly distributed symmetrically and initially involve lower extremities. Subsequently spread proximally to involve the upper extremities and trunk is usually involved and may have muscle weakness, pruritus, or pain
- May have sclerodactyly or contractures
- Over time they become hard and "woody" sometimes assuming a "cobblestone" appearance

HISTOLOGIC FEATURES

- **Dermal fibrosis** with **increased number of fibroblasts** which frequently **orient parallel** to the epidermis, Fibroblasts are positive for CD34 and Procollagen 1
- **Increased mucin deposition** that surrounds the fibroblasts
- **Haphazard collagen** arrangement

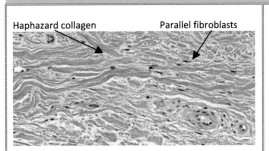

Haphazard collagen · Parallel fibroblasts

- May have osseous sclerotic bodies, multinucleated giant cells, and crossing elastic fibers
- Mucin is stained by **Colloidal iron**

DIFFERENTIAL DIAGNOSIS

- **Scleromyxedema:** Increased mucin deposition and fibrosis
- **Scleroderma:** lacks mucin and will have increased dermal fibrosis
- **Reticular erythematous mucinosis:** increased mucin in upper and mid-dermis, perivascular inflammation

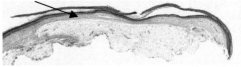

Dermal collagen replaced by adipose

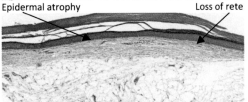

Epidermal atrophy · Loss of rete

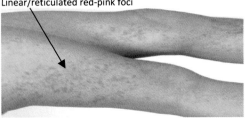

Linear/reticulated red-pink foci

Path Presenter

FOCAL DERMAL HYPOPLASIA (GOLTZ SYNDROME)

CLINICAL FEATURES

- **Genodermatosis** presenting at birth involving the eyes, teeth, skeleton, skin, genitourinary, gastrointestinal, cardiovascular, and central nervous system
- Cutaneous lesions present as **linear or reticulated red-pink foci** of **atrophic skin** and are distributed **along lines of Blaschko**
- Other clinical findings include coloboma, osteopathia striata, and ectrodactyly
- Inheritance is **X-linked dominant, found mostly in females**
- Mutation in PORCN gene

HISTOLOGIC FEATURES

- **Dermal atrophy, causing replacement** of collagen with **adipose** and new formation of **fat around vessels**
- Subcutaneous **fat extends to the epidermis** and cause **atrophy of epidermis**

OTHER HIGH YIELD POINTS

- Inheritance is **X-linked dominant**
- Mutation in PORCN gene

DIFFERENTIAL DIAGNOSIS

- **Scleromyxedema:** Increased mucin deposition and fibrosis
- **Scleroderma:** lacks mucin and will have increased dermal fibrosis
- **Reticular erythematous mucinosis:** increased mucin in upper and mid-dermis, perivascular inflammation

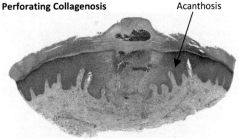

Perforating Collagenosis · Acanthosis

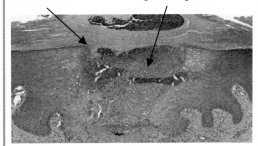

Dilated follicle · Degenerating debris

PERFORATING DERMATOSES

CLINICAL FEATURES

Kyrle Disease:
- Usually young to older adults with **bilateral**, widespread **eruption of verrucous** or **hyperkeratotic nodules** and papules with central **keratotic craters** occurring on legs, **trunk**, head, neck
- Lacks involvement of mucosal membranes, palms, and soles

Perforating Folliculitis:
- Young to middle-aged female **adults** with erythematous, **follicular-based papules** and **nodules** on **buttocks** and **extensor surfaces** of extremities

Reactive Perforating Collagenosis:
- Inherited form occurs in **infants and young children** and has recurrent **skin-colored papules (usually appear after superficial trauma)** that **progressively enlarge** over a period of weeks, **develop umbilication**, and then **regress** and leaves **hypopigmentation** or **cicatrix**
- Acquired form in adults with similar symptoms

Elastosis Perforans Serpiginosa
- Usually seen in **wide age range** and presents as **keratotic papules** that **form a ring** and have an **atrophic central aspect**
- Most often seen on the **neck**

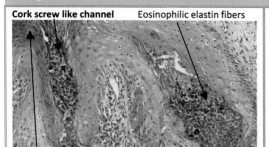
Cork screw like channel   Eosinophilic elastin fibers

Hyperkeratosis
Follicular based papules on exensor surfaces

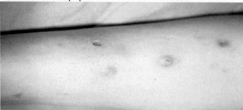

Elastosis Perforans Serpiginosa

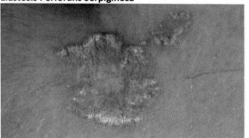

Path Presenter

- Commonly associated with **Down's Syndrome, Ehlers-Danlos syndrome, Marfan Syndrome, PXE and Acrogeria**

Acquired Perforating Dermatosis
- Seen in middle-aged adults and presents as any of the above lesions and occurs on the **extensor surfaces** of **lower extremities**
- Usually is seen in patients with **renal disease or diabetes**

HISTOLOGIC FEATURES
- All entities have the **transepidermal elimination** of **amorphous debris**

Kyrle Disease:
- Keratin and degenerating inflammatory debris filling an epidermal invagination
- Epidermal hyperplasia around invagination

Perforating Folliculitis:
- **Dilated hair follicle** with degenerating cellular or **basophilic debris**
- May have granulomatous inflammation or curled up hair shafts

Reactive Perforating Collagenosis:
- **Early lesions**: broad-based degenerating collagen layer overlying a thin epidermis with thin parakeratosis
- **Old lesions**: **central umbilication** with a plug entrapping parakeratotic debris, degenerating inflammatory debris, and **collagen**
- Adjacent **collagen fibers** are **vertically oriented** and **involve plug**
- Peripheral epidermis has **acanthosis** and **hyperkeratosis**
- **Trichrome stain sometimes used**

Elastosis Perforans Serpiginosa:
- **Corkscrew like channel** which is filled with **eosinophilic elastin fibers** and acellular degenerating debris
- Epidermis surrounding the channel has **hyperkeratosis** and **acanthosis**
- Increased elastic fibers in dermis at base of perforation
- Base of lesion has **granulomatous inflammation** and **multinucleated giant cells**
- Bramble bush lumpy bumpy elastic fibers with lateral buds in dermis seen in penicillamine induced EPS

Acquired Perforating Dermatosis: May have features of any of the above
- **Verhoeff/Elastic van Gieson** stains elastic fibers
- **Trichrome** stains collagen

DIFFERENTIAL DIAGNOSIS
- **Periumbilical perforating pseudoxanthoma elasticum:** calcified elastic fibers in clumps that undergo transepidermal elimination
- **Perforating granuloma annulare:** palisading granulomas, necrobiotic collagen, inflammatory cells, fibrin deposition

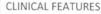

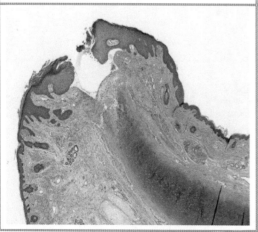

CHONDRODERMATITIS NODULARIS HELICIS (CNH)
CLINICAL FEATURES
- Presents as **tender erythematous nodule, typically at an area on the ear helix that undergoes pressure during sleep "Pressure ulcer"**
- Often has overlying **scale** or is **ulcerated**
- Clinically, it may mimic basal cell carcinoma or squamous cell carcinoma

HISTOLOGIC FEATURES
- **Crateriform ulcer** with **hyperkeratosis, parakeratosis,** and **acanthosis**
- **Fibrinoid degeneration** of dermal collagen and necrosis under the ulcer
- Underlying granulation tissue like stroma and mixed inflammatory infiltrate
- Cartilage is not typically involved; however, degeneration of cartilage sometimes noted Trans-epidermal elimination also described

DIFFERENTIAL DIAGNOSIS
- **Relapsing polychondritis:** Perichondrial inflammation, pyknotic nuclei, mixed inflammation, destruction of chondrocytes

Ulcer with scale

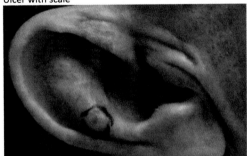

- **Ulcer/Excoriation:** lack of fibrin and telangiectatic vessels

Path Presenter

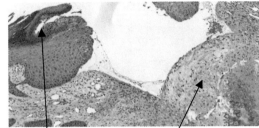

Parakeratosis   Fibrinoid degeneration

Clumped elastic fibers

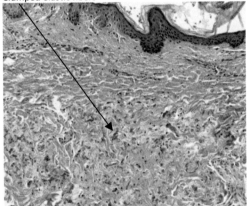

PSEUDOXANTHOMA ELASTICUM
CLINICAL FEATURES
- Usually has an onset in **childhood** or **early adolescence-gene defect on chromosome 16**
- **Females** twice as affected as males
- Presents as **multiple small, yellow papules** that are arranged in a **linear** or **reticular pattern**. Can **coalesce** and form a **cobblestone-like appearance**
- Often on neck and axillary region. "Plucked chicken skin" look. Groin may be affected
- **Ocular manifestations** include **retinal angioid streaks**
- **Cardiac manifestations** are due to vascular fragility and mitral valve prolapse

HISTOLOGIC FEATURES
- Reticular dermis has **clumped, fragmented**, and/or **calcified elastic fibers**
- May have basophilic appearance due to the calcium deposition
- **Verhoeff-van Gieson stain** highlights the abnormal elastic fibers
- **Von Kossa** highlights the calcium deposition
- **Perforating PXE may show transepidermal elimination**

OTHER HIGH YIELD POINTS
- **Autosomal recessive** inheritance of a **mutation** in the **ABCC6 gene**

DIFFERENTIAL DIAGNOSIS
- **Fibroelastolytic papulosis:** atrophy of epidermis, melanophages, clumped elastic fibers
- **Calciphylaxis:** clumped elastic fibers and calcifications in reticular dermis
- **Focal dermal elastosis:** no fragmentation of elastic fibers
- **Periumbilical perforating calcific elastosis**-histology similar. Not associated with PXE

Cobblestone-like appearance

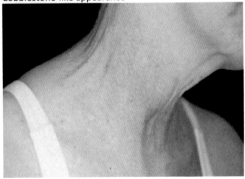

Path Presenter

Reticulated erythema

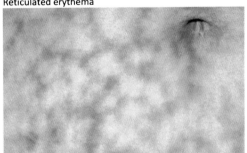

ERYTHEMA AB IGNE
CLINICAL FEATURES
- Usually **asymptomatic** and believed to be due to **chronic thermal radiation (e.g. laptop computer on a lap) usually thighs, shins, lower back**
- Presents as **erythematous macules** or **patches**
- Older lesions show **reticulate hyperpigmentation, scaling, atrophy,** dusky **erythema**, and **telangiectasia**

HISTOLOGIC FEATURES
- **Atrophy of the epidermis** and **rete flattening** with **atypical keratinocytes** and **maturation dysfunction**
- **Pigment incontinence**, degenerated collagen, and **increased elastosis**

CHAPTER 22: DISORDERS OF COLLAGEN AND ELASTIC TISSUES

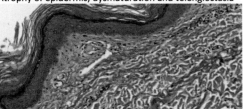

Atrophy of epidermis, dysmaturation and telengiectasia

- Telangiectasias are present
- **Verhoeff-van Gieson stain** shows the dense, curled or branched elastic fibers

DIFFERENTIAL DIAGNOSIS

- **Livedo reticularis:** aggregates of RBCs in superficial vessels, vascular wall thickening, thrombi, no elastosis, or epidermal atypia
- **Thermal burn injury:** Cytolysis and necrosis of all cells
- **Poikiloderma:** telangiectasia, vacuolar change, elastosis, lacks atypia in keratinocytes, no dysmaturation or dyskeratosis

Path Presenter

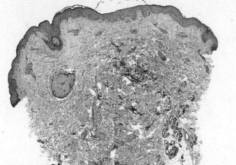

Normal appearing epidermis

Flaccid skin with bulging appearance

ANETODERMA
CLINICAL FEATURES

- Usually in **young adults** that have **numerous areas of flaccid skin, may show herniated or sometimes** bulging appearance
- Most common location is on the **upper extremities** and **trunk**
- **Primary Anetoderma:** associated with positive anticardiolipin antibodies, lupus anticoagulant, and anti-β2-glycoprotein 1 antibody
- **Secondary anetoderma:** associated with infectious etiologies and lymphoma

HISTOLOGIC FEATURES

- **Absence or near absence** of **elastic fibers** in papillary and reticular dermis
- May have inflammatory infiltrate of lymphocytes, histiocytes, or plasma cells
- **Normal appearing epidermis** and dermis on H&E
- **Verhoeff-van Gieson stain** shows loss of elastic fibers

DIFFERENTIAL DIAGNOSIS

- **Cutis laxa:** decrease in elastic fibers in reticular and papillary dermis
- **Mid-dermal elastolysis:** loss of elastic fibers in the mid-dermis
- **Fibroelastolytic papulosis:** loss of elastic fibers only in the papillary dermis
- **Perifollicular elastolysis:** loss of elastic fibers surrounding hair follicles

Path Presenter

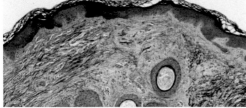

Variable degree of elastic fiber abnormalaities

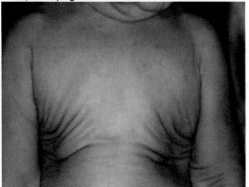

Loose, droooping and inelastic skin

CUTIS LAXA
CLINICAL FEATURES

- Usually noticed in **children** due to the loose and inelastic skin drooping around the eyelids (bloodhound appearance), cheeks, neck, and abdomen
- May have ectropion
- Multiple subtypes and various additional systemic manifestations
- **Generalized adult acquired cutis laxa:** may occur after eczema, erythema multiforme, dermatitis herpetiformis, or angiocentric T-cell lymphoma
- **Localized adult cutis laxa:** seen in patients with sarcoidosis, syphilis, vasculitides, multiple myeloma, and rheumatoid arthritis

HISTOLOGIC FEATURES

- "Normal" appearance on H&E, needs special stains
- Depending on severity and inheritance pattern, **variable degree of elastic fiber abnormalities** including globular **deposits, shortened,** or may have **hazy borders**
- **Verhoeff-van Gieson, orcein, or Weigert** shows the abnormal elastic fibers

OTHER HIGH YIELD POINTS

- Autosomal recessive, autosomal dominant, or x-linked recessive
- Mutations in *FBLN4, FBLN5, ATP6V0A2, PYCR1, ATP7A*

DIFFERENTIAL DIAGNOSIS

- **Ehlers-Danlos syndrome:** large and irregular collagen fibers, normal elastic
- **Pseudoxanthoma elasticum:** fragmented and clumped elastic fibers

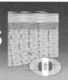
- **Anetoderma:** complete loss of elastic fibers
- **Mid-dermal elastolysis:** loss of elastic fibers but retained in papillary and reticular dermis

MID-DERMAL ELASTOLYSIS

CLINICAL FEATURES

- Majority of cases occur in **females** and the **median age is 40**
- Most commonly affects the **shoulders**, **upper extremities**, **trunk**, and back
- Has three distinct clinical presentations: Type1-3
- **Type 1 (Classic):** Large symmetrical areas of skin with fine wrinkling that are along the Langer lines
- **Type 2:** Smaller papular lesions that leave the hair follicle indented in the central aspect
- **Type 3:** Erythematous and reticular pattern

HISTOLOGIC FEATURES

- **Minimal, if any, findings on H&E**, may have minute lymphocytic inflammation around the vessels
- **Absence of elastic fibers in the mid-dermis**, but retained in deep dermis
- **Verhoeff-van Gieson** shows loss of mid-dermal elastic fibers

DIFFERENTIAL DIAGNOSIS

- **Anetoderma:** complete loss of elastic fibers
- **Cutis laxa:** decrease in elastic fibers in reticular and papillary dermis
- Normal skin

Path Presenter

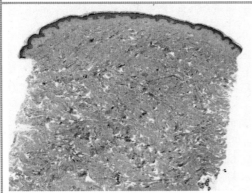

Loss of elastic fibers

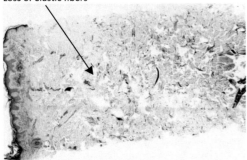

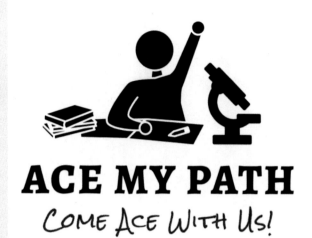

ACE MY PATH
Come Ace With Us!

CHAPTER 23: ALOPECIA

ANGELA JIANG, MD, NATHAN BOWERS, MD
JESUS ALBERTO CARDENAS DEL LA GARZA, MD

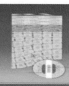

ALOPECIA

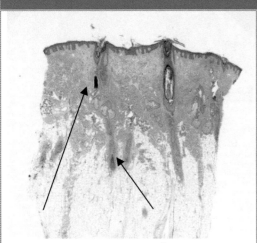

Pigment cast   Catagen/Telogen hair

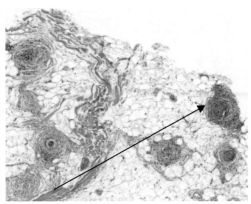

Peribulbar lymphocytic infiltrate

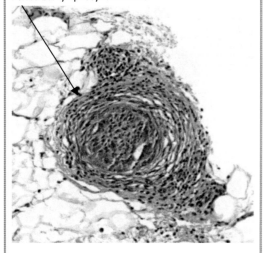

ALOPECIA AREATA

CLINICAL FEATURES

- Common **autoimmune non-scarring alopecia** in children and young adults
- Presents as single or multiple **round, bald patches**
- Infrequently, it may involve the entire scalp (alopecia totalis) or entire body (alopecia universalis)
- Nail abnormalities (particularly pitting) are present in 1/5 of cases
- Pull test is positive on the edges of active patches
- Trichoscopy - **Exclamation point hairs** (broken short hairs with proximal thinner portion and thicker distal end), black dots, yellow dots, broken hairs, and vellus hairs

HISTOLOGIC FEATURES

- Varies depending on stage of lesion biopsied
- **Acute: Intense peribulbar lymphocytic infiltrate (swarm of bees)** and increase in catagen and telogen hair follicles
- Subacute: Terminal hairs decrease, catagen/telogen shift
- **Chronic: Miniaturized hair follicles**, most hair follicles are in telogen phase, nanogen follicles may be present
- Other findings: **Fibrous tracts** with lymphocytes or **eosinophils**, **pigment casts**, abnormal hair follicles with features of both anagen and catagen/telogen, dilated follicular infundibula

OTHER HIGH YIELD POINTS

- Alopecia areata has **more miniaturized hairs than androgenetic alopecia**, also has small dystrophic anagen follicles and melanin within fibrous tracts
- **Trichotillomania lacks miniaturized hairs** and inflammation
- Androgenetic alopecia and telogen effluvium lack inflammation
- Syphilis usually has more plasma cells, but the histological presentation may be identical, and special stains and serology may be necessary

DIFFERENTIAL DIAGNOSIS

Acute/subacute:

- LICHEN PLANOPILARIS - dense lichenoid infiltrate composed of mainly lymphocytes that involves basal keratinocytes of infundibular portion of hair follicle
- SYPHILIS - usually has more plasma cells but the histological presentation may be identical
- TINEA CAPITIS - mixed inflammatory infiltrate, fungal spores within or surrounding hair shaft

Chronic:

- ANDROGENTIC ALOPECIA - miniaturization of hair follicles, no nanogen follicles
- TELOGEN EFFLUVIUM - not as many telogen hairs compared to alopecia areata (AA can be >50% telogen hairs)

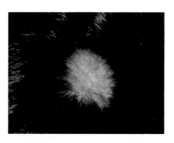

Alopecia areata solitary patch

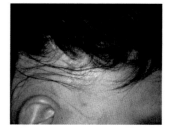

Ophiasis alopecia areata

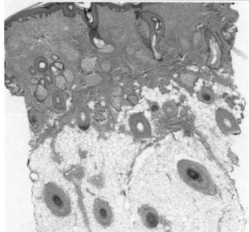

Miniaturized hair

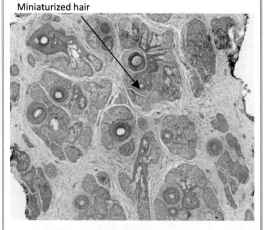

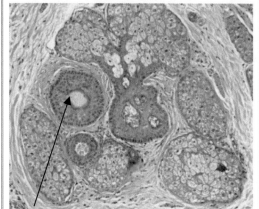

Catagen hair

ANDROGENETIC ALOPECIA (MALE PATTERN HAIR LOSS / FEMALE PATTERN HAIR LOSS)

CLINICAL FEATURES

- **Most common alopecia worldwide**
- Family history is common
- Male pattern usually affects the temporal, frontal, and vertex areas
- **Female pattern** may be diffuse or affect the vertex or frontoparietal area while the **frontal hairline is usually spared**
- In both patterns, the **occipital region is not affected**
- **Trichoscopy - variability in hair shaft diameter**, follicular units with 1-2 hairs, yellow dots, brown peripilar sign (brown halo around hair shaft)

HISTOLOGIC FEATURES

- **Miniaturization of hair follicles (reduction of diameter, size, and depth)**
- Number of hair follicles is normal
- **Increase** number of hairs in **catagen and telogen**
- Decreased anagen to telogen ratio
- **Increase** number of **vellus hairs**
- A mild to moderate lymphocytic infiltrate may be present around the infundibulum
- Presence of **follicular streamers (stellae)** below miniaturized hairs
- Preservation but miniaturization of sebaceous glands and arrector pili

OTHER HIGH YIELD POINTS

- **Telogen effluvium lack miniaturization**
- **Inflammation** in androgenetic alopecia **may resemble lichen planopilaris**

DIFFERENTIAL DIAGNOSIS

- TELOGEN EFFLUVIUM – increased number to telogen hairs compared to androgenetic alopecia and no miniaturization of follicles
- TRACTION ALOPECIA – pigment casts, increased catagen/telogen hairs, and trichomalacia
- ALOPECIA AREATA - Peribulbar lymphocytic infiltrate (swarm of bees), chronic alopecia areata will have significantly higher telogen shift

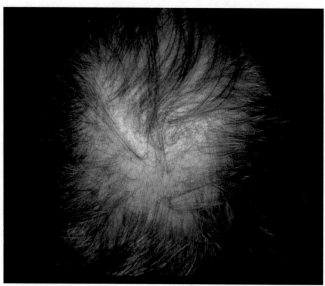

Vertex male pattern hair loss

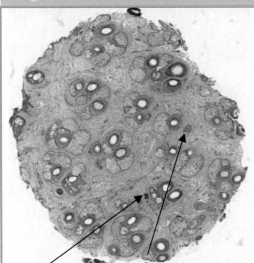

Telogen hair   Telogen hair

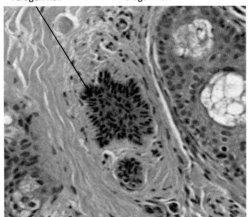

TELOGEN EFFLUVIUM
CLINICAL FEATURES
- **Non-scarring and non-inflammatory alopecia**
- Many different triggers including infections, drugs, hormonal changes, emotional stress, surgery, thyroid disorders, iron deficiency, or weight changes
- Occurs **2-3 months after trigger** event
- Pull test is positive
- Hair loss may be diffuse or more accentuated on the **bitemporal region**
- Divided into acute or chronic (>6 months)
- **Daily hair loss >100-150**
- Trichoscopy - **No specific findings (diagnosis of exclusion)**, empty follicles, decreased hair density, no diameter variability
HISTOLOGIC FEATURES
- **Findings depend on the time of the biopsy**
- Late cases may have normal histology
- **Increase in telogen hair >20-25% but typically <50%**
- No increased vellus hairs, miniaturization, or inflammation
- **Ratio of terminal: vellus hair >7:1**
OTHER HIGH YIELD POINTS
- Telogen effluvium lacks inflammation and miniaturization
DIFFERENTIAL DIAGNOSIS
- ANDROGENETIC ALOPECIA - miniaturization of hair follicles
- TRACTION ALOPECIA - pigment casts and trichomalacia
- ALOPECIA AREATA - Peribulbar lymphocytic infiltrate (swarm of bees), >50% telogen hairs in chronic alopecia areata with nanogen follicles and miniaturized follicles
- TRICHOTILLOMANIA - disrupted follicular anatomy

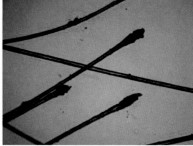

Trichogram showing telogen hairs with classic "club shape" at hair root

TRICHOTILLOMANIA
CLINICAL FEATURES
- Hair disorder secondary to the **habit of pulling hairs**
- May be accompanied by additional **psychiatric disorders**
- Friar Tuck Sign - round patch of incomplete alopecia on the central crown or vertex, surrounded by a rim of unaffected hair
- May affect any area of the scalp or body
- **Diagnosis is mostly clinical**
Trichoscopy
- **Irregularly broken hairs** at different levels, hook/coiled hairs **V-sign** (pulled hairs emerging from the same follicular cut at the same level forming a V), flame hairs (wavy, thin residue after hair pulling), trichoptilosis (distal hair split)
HISTOLOGIC FEATURES
- **Pigment casts**
- **Distorted follicles**

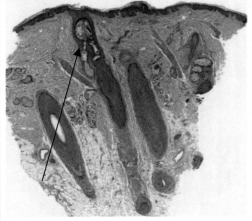

Trichomalacia

Pigment cast

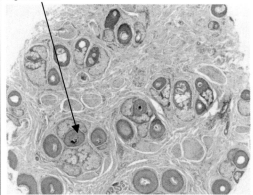

Pigment cast

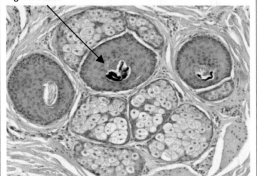

Path Presenter

- High percentage of hairs in catagen or telogen phases
- Empty follicular ducts
- **Absence of inflammation**
- Trichomalacia (distortion of the hair shaft with irregular pigmentation)
- Peri- and intrafollicular hemorrhage may be present secondary to repeated trauma

OTHER HIGH YIELD POINTS

- Histologic findings vary depending on the time of the biopsy
- Findings similar to trichotillomania may be found in alopecia areata or syphilitic alopecia

DIFFERENTIAL DIAGNOSIS

- ALOPECIA AREATA - peribulbar lymphocytic infiltrate (swarm of bees), no follicular distortion
- SYPHILIS - usually has more plasma cells but the histological presentation may be identical
- TELOGEN EFFLUVIUM – similar catagen/telogen shift but no distorted follicular anatomy
- TRACTION ALOPECIA – can appear histologically similar and requires clinical presentation to distinguish

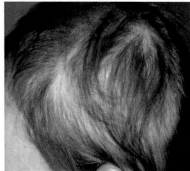

Trichotillomania

LICHEN PLANOPILARIS AND FRONTAL FIBROSING ALOPECIA

CLINICAL FEATURES

- **Scarring/cicatricial alopecia** that presents as pruritic, perifollicular erythema and scale at active sites
- Lichen planopilaris (LPP) classically affects the vertex scalp, but the clinical course and pattern of hair loss is highly variable
- **Frontal fibrosing alopecia (FFA) is considered a variant of LPP** that primarily affects postmenopausal women on the frontal scalp
- **Trichoscopy – Perifollicular erythema and scale**, rarely white dots

HISTOLOGIC FEATURES

- Dense **lichenoid infiltrate** composed of mainly lymphocytes that involves basal keratinocytes of **infundibular and isthmic portion** of hair follicle
- Interfollicular epidermis is usually spared, but in 25% of cases can show features of lichen planus
- **Early findings**: Focal **lymphoid aggregates** and **perifollicular mucinous fibrosis** around infundibulum
- **Late findings**: Dense **lymphoid infiltrates** of lymphocytes with occasional **cytoid** bodies. May lose classic features due to **scarring of dermis.** Loss of follicles and adnexal structures
- Frontal fibrosing alopecia may have less dense inflammation and more apoptotic cells within the hair follicle epithelium

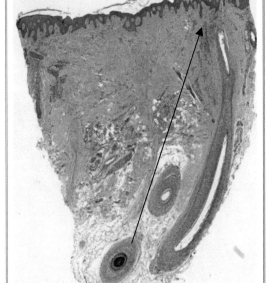

Scarring Lymphoid inflammation at infundibulum

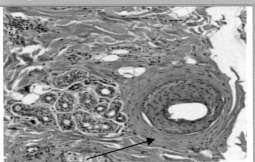

Perifollicular mucinous fibrosis

Path Presenter

OTHER HIGH YIELD POINTS
- Graham-Little syndrome: triad of LPP, nonscarring alopecia in axilla and groin, and follicular papules on trunk, extremities, and face

DIFFERENTIAL DIAGNOSIS
- DISCOID LUPUS – interface dermatitis with pigment incontinence, involvement of the interfollicular epithelium, reduplication of the basement membrane, follicular plugging, dermal mucin deposition, and perivascular/periadnexal lymphoplasmacytic infiltrate
- TRACTION ALOPECIA - pigment casts, increased catagen/telogen hairs, and trichomalacia
- FOLLICULITIS DECALVANS - dense infiltrate, containing neutrophils, that involves the upper part of the follicle and the perifollicular dermis, follicle rupture leading to granulomas and perifollicular fibrosis
- CENTRAL CENTRIFUGAL CICATRICIAL ALOPECIA – can also present with premature desquamation of the inner root sheath which should affect all inflamed follicles (vs LPP is unlikely to have premature desquamation in relatively noninflamed follicles)

ALOPECIA MUCINOSA (FOLLICULAR MUCINOSIS)

CLINICAL FEATURES
- **Two main types: primary benign idiopathic follicular mucinosis and secondary follicular mucinosis**
- Children usually present the benign variety
- Secondary type is usually associated to **hematological malignancies** (particularly cutaneous lymphomas)
- Favors **head and neck** regions
- Diverse presentation including plaques and papules
- Trichoscopy – Limited information, **Brownish-yellow dots**, **red dots**, follicular plugs of amorphous material

HISTOLOGIC FEATURES
- **Abundant mucin in and** around sebaceous gland and hair follicles
- **Mixed infiltrate** that includes lymphocytes, histiocytes, and eosinophils
- In cases of association with lymphoma, **neoplastic lymphocytes** may be observed

OTHER HIGH YIELD POINTS
- **Workup for lymphoma and other hematological malignancies** is recommended

DIFFERENTIAL DIAGNOSIS
- FOLLICULOTROPIC MYCOSIS FUNGOIDES –epidermotropism of atypical lymphocytes in follicular epithelium

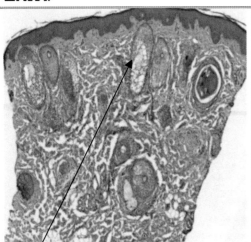

Mucin deposit around hair follicle

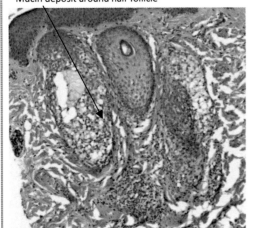

Mixed inflammatory infiltrate

Path Presenter

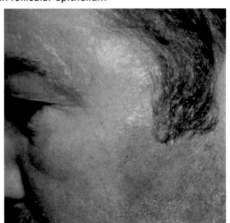

Plaque of follicular mucinosis

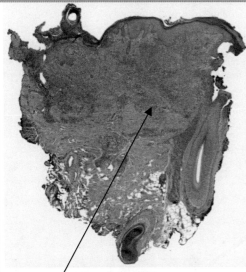

Dense mixed infiltrate in the dermis

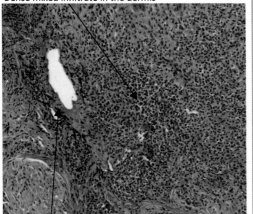

Destruction of hair follicle

Path Presenter

DISSECTING CELLULITIS OF THE SCALP

CLINICAL FEATURES

- Part of the **"follicular occlusion tetrad"**, which includes acne conglobata, hidradenitis suppurativa, and pilonidal sinus
- Presents with deep-seated nodules with a predilection for the **crown, vertex, and upper occipital scalp**
- Nodules coalesce to form **boggy, purulent, and fluctuating nodules and eventually sinus tracts**

HISTOLOGIC FEATURES

- **Early** lesions demonstrate **dense perifollicular mainly lymphocytic infiltrate** affecting the lower dermis and upper subcutis
- Fully developed lesions demonstrate **a mixture of neutrophils, lymphocytes, and plasma cells** with an increase in catagen/telogen follicles
- Late-stage lesions demonstrate destruction of the hair follicle, acneiform **dilatation of the infundibula**, and **deep sinus tracts**

OTHER HIGH YIELD POINTS

- If associated with follicular occlusion triad, patients are at **risk** of developing **HLA-B27 negative spondyloarthropathy**

DIFFERENTIAL DIAGNOSIS

- TINEA CAPITIS - mixed inflammatory infiltrate, fungal spores within or surrounding hair shaft
- FOLLICULITIS DECALVANS - dense infiltrate, containing neutrophils, that involves the upper part of the follicle and the perifollicular dermis, follicle rupture leading to granulomas and perifollicular fibrosis

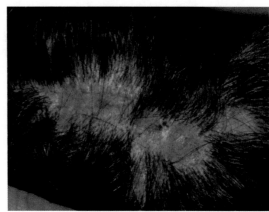

Dissecting cellulitis of the scalp

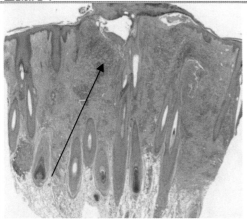

Dense inflammation in upper part of perifollicular dermis

FOLLICULITIS DECALVANS

CLINICAL FEATURES

- Primarily occurs in young adults with both sexes equally affected
- **Single or multiple plaques of alopecia with painful pustules, papules, and crust, staph commonly cultured**
- Has predilection for the **vertex scalp** but can involve any part of the scalp
- **Tufted folliculitis (multiple hairs emerging from single follicle)** may be seen; especially on the occipital scalp

TRICHOSCOPY

- Hallmark of folliculitis decalvans is the presence of multiple hairs emerging from one singe dilated follicular orifice (**polytrichia**) and generally vary from 5-20 hair shafts per follicular orifice

HISTOLOGIC FEATURES

- Dense **infiltrate**, containing **neutrophils**, that involves the upper part of the follicle (especially lower infundibulum) and the perifollicular dermis

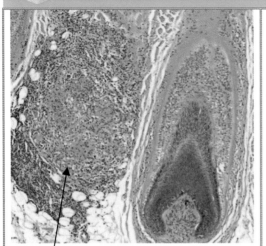
Granulomatous inflammation

- Follicles eventually rupture leading to **granulomas and perifollicular fibrosis**
- Acneiform dilatation of infundibula
- Follicles fused at the infundibulum with perifollicular fibrosis at level of isthmus/infundibulum (polytrichia, **compound hair follicle**)
- Late stage shows wedge-shaped loss of elastic tissue and dermal fibrosis

DIFFERENTIAL DIAGNOSIS
- TINEA CAPITIS - mixed inflammatory infiltrate, fungal spores within or surrounding hair shaft
- DISSECTING CELLULITIS - dense perifollicular mainly lymphocytic infiltrate affecting the lower dermis and upper subcutis, late-stage destruction of the hair follicle, acneiform dilatation of the infundibula, and deep sinus tracts

Path Presenter

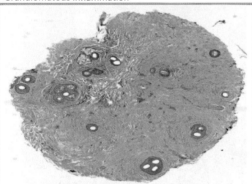
Loss of follicular architecture

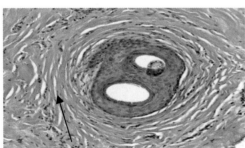
Concentric fibrosis

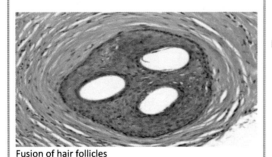
Fusion of hair follicles

CENTRAL CENTRIFUGAL CICATRICIAL ALOPECIA
CLINICAL FEATURES
- Cicatricial alopecia with predilection for the vertex scalp with centrifugal spread
- **Most common form of primary scarring alopecia in Black women in the United States**
- **Inflammation can be discrete clinically** and may **mimic androgenetic alopecia**
- Pustules and small perifollicular papules are sometimes present
- Trichoscopy - **Peripilar white gray halo** Found in majority of patients and has high specificity and sensitivity for CCCA

HISTOLOGIC FEATURES
- Variable **perifollicular lymphocytic infiltrate** around the **lower infundibulum and isthmus**
- **Perifollicular concentric fibrosis**
- **Premature desquamation** of the **inner root sheath below eccrine glands, can even affect follicles without inflammation**
- **Fusion of follicles** including their root sheaths surrounded by concentric fibrosis
- Loss of follicular architecture, naked hair shafts within fibrous streamers, and syringoma like dilatation of eccrine ducts
- If pustular lesion, infiltrate containing neutrophils

OTHER HIGH YIELD POINTS
- Genetics (**PAD13 mutations**), metabolic syndrome (association with type II diabetes), autoimmune factors, bacterial infections, and acne are thought to be possible contributing factors
- CCCA may present with concomitant androgenetic alopecia

DIFFERENTIAL DIAGNOSIS
- LICHEN PLANOPILARIS - dense lichenoid infiltrate composed of mainly lymphocytes that involves basal keratinocytes of infundibular portion of hair follicle, unlikely to have premature desquamation of inner root sheath in noninflamed follicles
- ACNE KELOIDALIS – can show similar histopathologic findings and requires clinical correlation to differentiate
- FOLLICULITIS DECALVANS - dense infiltrate, containing neutrophils, that involves the upper part of the follicle and the perifollicular dermis

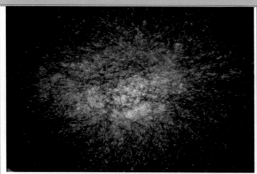

Path Presenter

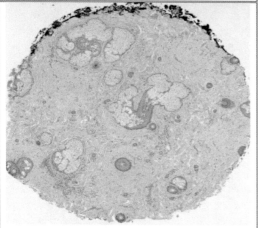

Loss of terminal hair follicles

TRACTION ALOPECIA

CLINICAL FEATURES

- Secondary to **tension of the hair follicle**, usually due to hairstyles
- **Acute** phase: non-inflammatory and **reversible** alopecia
- **Chronic** phase: may lead to **scarring**
- Typically involves **frontotemporal regions**
- **Trichoscopy – black dots, broken hairs, yellow dots, empty hair follicles, vellus hairs**

HISTOLOGIC FEATURES

- **Early** lesions: findings **similar to trichotillomania** with **pigment casts, increased catagen/telogen hairs, and trichomalacia**
- **Late** lesions: appreciated loss of terminal hair follicles or **"follicular drop out," vellus hairs remain intact**
- Terminal hair follicles appear to be replaced by fibrotic fibrous tracts
- **Preservation of the sebaceous glands**
- Absence or mild perifollicular inflammatory infiltrate

OTHER HIGH YIELD POINTS

- Chronic traction alopecia may lead to scarring and irreversible hair loss
- **Fringe sign: retained hairs along the frontal/temporal rim**

DIFFERENTIAL DIAGNOSIS

- LICHEN PLANOPILARIS - dense lichenoid infiltrate composed of mainly lymphocytes that involves basal keratinocytes of infundibular portion
- ALOPECIA AREATA - peribulbar lymphocytic infiltrate (swarm of bees), no follicular distortion
- TRICHOTILLOMANIA - pigment casts, increased catagen/telogen hairs, and trichomalacia; can appear histologically similar and requires clinical correlate

Path Presenter

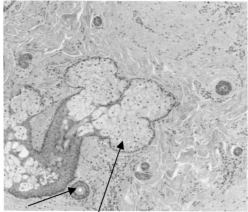

Vellus hairs and sebaceous lobules preserved

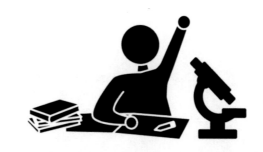

ACE MY PATH
Come Ace With Us!

CHAPTER 24: NAIL DISCORDERS

CHELSEA HUANG, MD

NAIL DISORDERS

Fungal hyphae in the nail plate

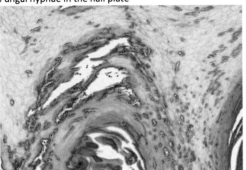

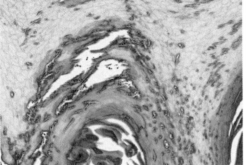

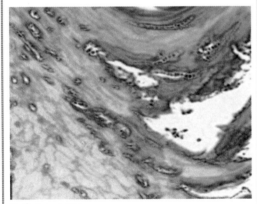

Path Presenter

ONYCHOMYCOSIS
CLINICAL FEATURES
- The most common form presents as **distal, thick subungual keratin.** Can rarely involve the proximal nail fold or presents as white spots on the nail plate
- Clinical DIFFERENTIAL DIAGNOSIS: Nail Psoriasis, Nail Dystrophy, Bacterial Paronychia, Darier Disease, Lichen Planus, Onycholysis, Pachyonychia Congenita, Yellow-nail Syndrome

HISTOLOGIC FEATURES
- Fungal **hyphae and spores** within the nail plate; highlighted by **PAS or GMS**
- May see increased subungual debris and neutrophils within the nail plate

OTHER HIGH YIELD POINTS
- Submit nail clippings or curettings, including dystrophic subungual debris, for histologic evaluation with **PAS or GMS stain,** and/or **fungal culture**
- **Highest yield for KOH preparations is the subungual debris**

DIFFERENTIAL DIAGNOSIS
PARONYCHIA
- Acute cases show purulent exudate. Chronic cases show overlying scale crust with spongiosis and dermal perivascular lymphocytes, histiocytes and plasma cells infiltrate
- Unlike onychomycosis, negative for fungal elements

PSORIASIS
- Nail dystrophy and neutrophils can be seen in the nail bed. Unlike onychomycosis, negative for fungal elements

PSEUDOMONAS
- Nail dystrophy and neutrophils can be seen in the nail bed. Classic pseudomonas nails will have a yellow-green color
- Presence of gram-negative rod (pseudomonas) and absence of fungal elements (negative PAS or GMS)

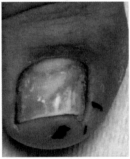
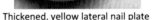
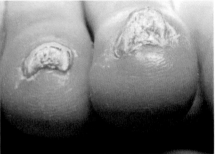

Thickened, yellow lateral nail plate   Thickened, hypertrophic nails from fungal infection

Numerous cysts in the nail bed

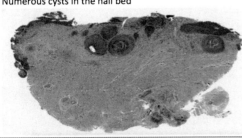

ONYCHOLEMMAL CYST
CLINICAL FEATURES
- Also known as **subungual epidermoid inclusions or cysts**
- **Variable** clinical presentations including **onychodystrophy, ridging, thickening,** or **pigmentation of the nail**

HISTOLOGIC FEATURES
- Cyst(s) in **nail bed** with lining resembling **nail bed epithelium**

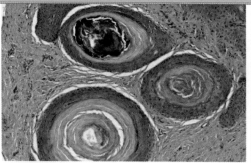

Path Presenter

- Presence of **abrupt keratinization** reminiscent of an isthmus-catagen cyst (pilar cyst) with **intermittent, focal granular layer** surrounding **pink, laminated keratin**

OTHER HIGH YIELD POINTS

- This is a benign diagnosis
- Nail bed biopsy itself may be therapeutic

DIFFERENTIAL DIAGNOSIS

EPIDERMAL INCLUSION CYST

- Cyst lined by squamous epithelium with granular layer containing lamellated keratin. Unlike onycholemmal cyst, site not at the nailbed and with only focal areas of granular layer

ONYCHOLEMMAL CARCINOMA

- Shares features of onycholemmal cysts, but with infiltrating architecture, increased cellularity, necrosis, and cellular atypia

Multiple fibroepithelial projections

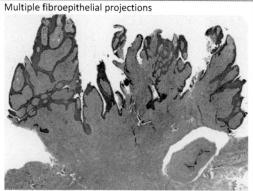

Sharp demarcation peritumoral stroma and dermis

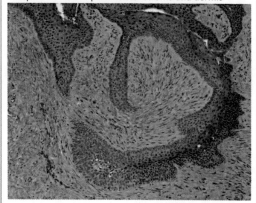

Path Presenter

ONYCHOMATRICOMA

CLINICAL FEATURES

- Benign tumor affecting the finger of middle-aged adults
- Characteristically presents with a **longitudinal, thickened band** and over-curvature of the nail
- **Multiple holes** are visible in the **free margin** of the nail plate, a so-called "wormwood" pattern
- Clinical DIFFERENTIAL DIAGNOSIS: Acquired Digital Fibrokeratoma, Squamous Cell Carcinoma in situ, Subungual Osteochondroma, Onychomycosis, Subungual Exostosis, Subungual Keratoacanthoma, Verruca

HISTOLOGIC FEATURES

- Thickened **papillomatous matrix epithelium** surrounded by basal cells
- The surrounding stroma has a **glove and stocking pattern**
- Appearing as multiple **fibroepithelial projections** extending into thickened nail plate
- **Peritumoral stroma is sharply demarcated** from underlying dermis
- **Pleomorphic, Proliferative and pigmented variants have been described**
- **Fibroblasts are CD34 +**

DIFFERENTIAL DIAGNOSIS

VERRUCA VULGARIS

- Papillomatous exophytic epidermal proliferation with infolding of rete ridges towards base and granulation tissue-like stroma
- Features of viral changes such as koilocytes and rounded parakeratosis are present

ACQUIRED DIGITAL FIBROKERATOMA

- Vertically oriented thick collagen bundles and stromal stellate fibroblasts can help distinguish from onychomatricoma

DIGITAL MUCOUS CYST

- Large myxoid area that contains stellate fibroblasts, sometimes with microcystic spaces. Location at the base of the nail

Proliferation of varying sized, infiltrative nests

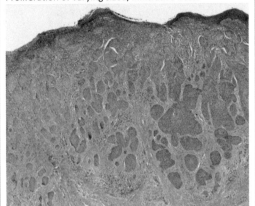

Abrupt onycholemmal keratinization with keratinocyte pleomorphism

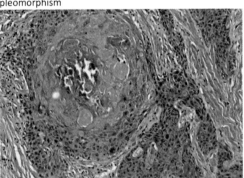

ONYCHOLEMMAL CARCINOMA

CLINICAL FEATURES

- These are **slow growing** tumors in the **elderly**
- Varied clinical presentations: **paronychia**, **onychodystrophy**, and **warty**

HISTOLOGIC FEATURES

- **Infiltrative** growth pattern
- **Lobular** proliferation of **solid nests** and **small keratinous cysts** with foci of **abrupt central keratinization** (onycholemmal keratinization)
- **Keratinocyte atypia** with pleomorphism and atypical mitotic figures

OTHER HIGH YIELD POINTS

<u>Path Presenter</u>

- Rare entity

DIFFERENTIAL DIAGNOSIS

SQUAMOUS CELL CARCINOMA OF NAIL

- **Keratinizing** proliferation of atypical keratinocytes involving epithelium of periungual epidermis, nail bed and matrix. Overlapping histologic features with onycholemmal carcinoma but less marked keratinous cysts with onycholemmal keratinization

ONYCHOLEMMAL CYST

- Cyst with lining resembling epithelium of nail bed (**onycholemmal**) with **only focal** granular layer. Shares features of onycholemmal carcinoma, but without infiltrating architecture, increased cellularity, necrosis, and cellular atypia

VERRUCA VULGARIS OF NAIL

- **Lacks the** infiltrative growth pattern and cellular atypia of onycholemmal carcinoma

---

Acanthotic nail bed epithelium with elongated rete ridges

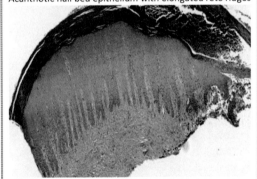

Diminished granular layer, parakeratosis, and thinned suprapapillary plate

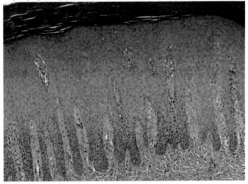

NAIL PSORIASIS

CLINICAL FEATURES

- Nail involvement in psoriasis can present as **pits, onycholysis, subungual hyperkeratosis,** and **salmon patches (oil drops)**
- Clinical DIFFERENTIAL DIAGNOSIS: Acrokeratosis Paraneoplastica, Alopecia Areata, Bazek Syndrome, Allergic Contact Dermatitis, Keratoderma Blennorrhagicum, Lichen Planus, Pityriasis Rubra Pilaris

HISTOLOGIC FEATURES

- **Regularly acanthotic** nail bed epithelium with **elongated rete ridges**
- **Diminished granular laye**r with overlying **parakeratosis** and **neutrophilic scale crust**
- **Thinned suprapapillary plates** with **dilated capillaries** within dermal papillae
- **Nail plate** with collections of **neutrophils. Negative PAS staining**

OTHER HIGH YIELD POINTS

- Diagnosis can usually be made on clinical grounds
- Nail unit biopsy can be performed if there is any doubt about the diagnosis
- Obtain imaging in patients with joint symptoms to workup psoriatic arthritis

DIFFERENTIAL DIAGNOSIS

ONYCHOMYCOSIS

- Nail plate clipping with PAS highlighting fungal hyphae

ALLERGIC CONTACT DERMATITIS

- Histologically, spongiosis is present. The presence of eosinophils and Langerhans microabscesses also point towards a diagnosis of allergic contact dermatitis. Nail plate neutrophils are not present

Dilated capillaries within dermal papillae

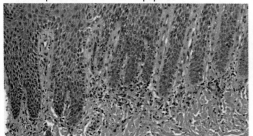

Path Presenter

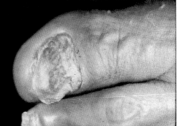

Marked onycholysis of the nails   Yellow, dystrophic nails

Band-like lichenoid inflammation

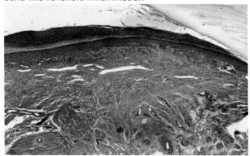

Compact hyperkeratosis overlying a lichenoid interface dermatitis

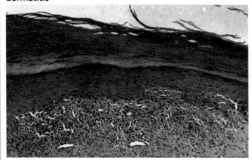

Path Presenter

LICHEN PLANUS INVOLVING THE NAIL

CLINICAL FEATURES

- Nail findings include thinning, fissures, and **dorsal pterygium**
- Nail changes may occur in isolation, without skin or mucosal findings
- Clinical DIFFERENTIAL DIAGNOSIS: Alopecia Areata, Graft Versus Host Disease, Lichen Striatus, Psoriasis, Onychomycosis, Yellow Nail Syndrome

HISTOLOGIC FEATURES

- **Band-like lichenoid infiltrate of lymphocytes** with overlying **compact hyperkeratosis** and **wedge-shaped hypergranulosis**
- **Parakeratosis** typically **absent**
- **Eosinophils** typically **absent**

OTHER HIGH YIELD POINTS

- Clinical appearance may highly suggest the diagnosis. Nail biopsy is diagnostic
- Nail matrix is most frequently involved
- A full mucocutaneous examination is warranted in search of evidence of lichen planus elsewhere

DIFFERENTIAL DIAGNOSIS

ONYCHOMYCOSIS

- Lichenoid inflammation may be present in both onychomycosis and lichen planus. However, **fungal hyphae and spores** highlighted by PAS in onychomycosis

GRAFT VERSUS HOST DISEASE

- Histological overlap with lichen planus
- Lichenoid nail changes can be seen in chronic GVHD. Clinical clues needed with graft versus host disease showing other systemic symptoms that precede nail change

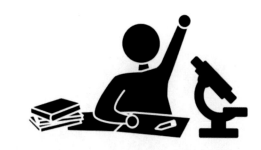

ACE MY PATH
Come Ace With Us!

CHAPTER 25: DISORDERS OF
PIGMENTATION

FRANCHESCA CHOI, MD RPh

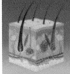

DISORDERS OF PIGMENTATION

Reduced melanin amount in basal keratinocytes

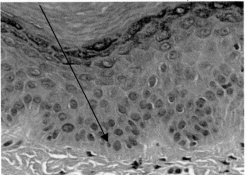

In contrast, normal skin melanocytes, melanophages

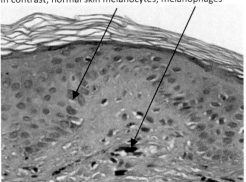

Path Presenter

VITILIGO

CLINICAL FEATURES

- Well-demarcated, asymptomatic, depigmented macules and patches
- Sites of predilection include the fingers, wrists, axillae, groins, genitals, perioral, and periocular areas
- Exhibits the **Koebner phenomenon** whereupon trauma induces new lesions

HISTOLOGIC FEATURES

- **Markedly reduced to absent melanin** around basal keratinocytes
- **Markedly reduced to absent melanocytes**
- Melanocytes may be increased in size with an increased number of dendrites near the advancing border, and lymphocytes may be minimally increased at the dermal-epidermal junction
- Can be difficult to diagnose via histology. The use of SOX-10 or Melan-A and a **control biopsy from adjacent non-affected skin for comparison** is helpful

OTHER HIGH YIELD POINTS

- Melanocyte destruction leads to the absence of functional melanocytes
- Most commonly associated with **thyroid dysfunction,** type 1 diabetes mellitus, Addison's disease, pernicious anemia, halo nevi, alopecia areata, and uveitis

DIFFERENTIAL DIAGNOSIS

IDIOPATHIC GUTTATE HYPOMELANOSIS

- Epidermis may show atrophic changes with overlying basket-weave hyperkeratosis. Decreased (but not absent) melanocytes. May need to stain

PITYRIASIS ALBA

- Melanocytes are normal in number. Mildly reduced basal melanin

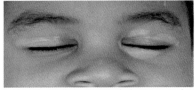
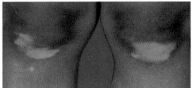

Well-demarcated, depigmented macules on the eyelids and knees

Scattered melanophages, increased amount of melanin

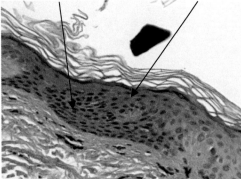

Path Presenter

POST-INFLAMMATORY HYPERPIGMENTATION (PIH)

CLINICAL FEATURES

- Hyperpigmented macules and patches
- The preceding inflammation may be obvious or subclinical

HISTOLOGIC FEATURES

- Scattered **melanophages in the papillary dermis** with a normal or increased amount of melanin in the basal layer of epidermis
- There is a **normal number of melanocytes present**

OTHER HIGH YIELD POINTS

- May take several months to fully resolve. Frequently seen in darker skin
- May be exacerbated by sunlight, and photoprotection is an important part of treatment

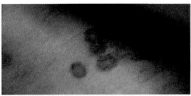

Hyperpigmented dark brown macules and patches on the neck

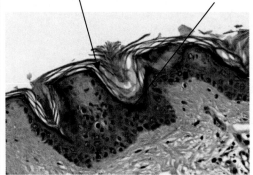

Hyperkeratosis with slight irregular acanthosis

Papillomatosis

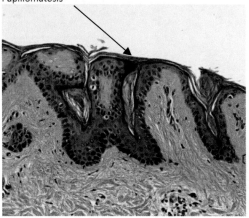

Path Presenter

ACANTHOSIS NIGRICANS
CLINICAL FEATURES
- Velvety, papillomatous hyperpigmented patches, predominant in intertriginous areas but can also occur on the cheeks, neck and hands

HISTOLOGIC FEATURES
- **Hyperkeratosis and papillomatosis but only slight irregular acanthosis**
- Normal or thickened granular cell layer
- Poorly developed rete ridges
- Basal layer hyperpigmentation common
- Dermis shows only sparse perivascular lymphocytes
- No epidermal spongiosis or exocytosis
- **No melanocytic proliferation.** The brown color of lesion caused more by hyperkeratosis than by melanin, although in some instances it may be the result of increased melanosomes in the stratum corneum

OTHER HIGH YIELD POINTS
- Associated with **insulin resistance, obesity**
- Malignant type is associated with abdominal adenocarcinoma (particularly gastric), squamous cell carcinoma, sarcoma, Hodgkin/non-Hodgkin lymphoma, and melanoma
- Can be accompanied by Leser-Trelat sign with the sudden appearance of numerous seborrheic keratoses

DIFFERENTIAL DIAGNOSIS
CONFLUENT AND RETICULATED PAPILLOMATOSIS
- Cannot be distinguished histologically
LINEAR EPIDERMAL NEVI
- More marked acanthosis, more compact orthokeratotic stratum corneum
- Pilosebaceous units are rudimentary

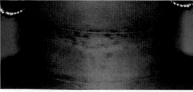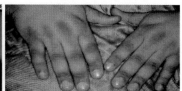

Dark brown papillomatous velvety macules and patches on neck, hands and fingers

Mild hyperkeratosis and papillomatosis

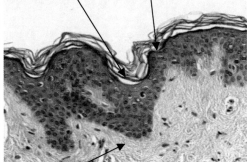

Focal acanthosis, limited largely to the valleys between elongated papillae

Path Presenter

CONFLUENT AND RETICULATED PAPILLOMATOSIS
CLINICAL FEATURES
- Discrete, flat, brown papules that coalesce into plaques at the center with a reticulated periphery; stuck-on scale. Predilection chest and upper back

HISTOLOGIC FEATURES
- Mild **hyperkeratosis** and **papillomatosis**
- Focal acanthosis, limited largely to the valleys between elongated papillae
- Mild dilation of vessels in superficial venous plexus

DIFFERENTIAL DIAGNOSIS
ACANTHOSIS NIGRICANS
- Cannot be distinguished histologically, overlapping features
LINEAR EPIDERMAL NEVI
- More marked acanthosis; more compact orthokeratotic stratum corneum

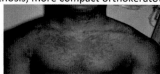

Dark-brown confluent papules and plaques on the central chest and upper back

Psoriasiform epidermal proliferation

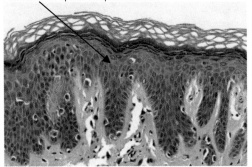

"Reticulated seborrheic keratosis-like" pattern of dilated follicular infundibulum

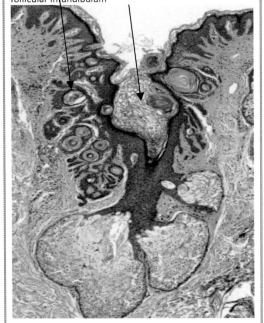

DOWLING-DEGOS DISEASE

CLINICAL FEATURES

- Heavily pigmented macules arranged in a reticulate pattern with a tendency to coalesce on flexural skin, "reticulate pigmented anomaly of the **flexures**"- axilla, groin and antecubital fossa, beginning in adulthood

HISTOLOGIC FEATURES

- **Psoriasiform** epidermal proliferation
- Infiltrate of lymphocytes about dermal vessels
- Hyperpigmentation of the basilar keratinocytes (prominent at rete ridges) with either a normal or slightly increased number of melanocytes
- Club-shaped rete ridges that branch to form **antler horn-like pattern** often at sides of **cystically dilated follicular infundibula (resembling reticulated seborrheic keratosis)**

OTHER HIGH YIELD POINTS

- **Dominantly inherited** dermatosis related to mutations of the **keratin 5 gene**
- In the same spectrum with Reticular Acropigmentation of Kitamura
- Associated with pitted perioral scars, hyperpigmented comedones, hidradenitis suppurativa, multiple cysts and abscesses, and squamous cell carcinomas/keratoacanthomas

DIFFERENTIAL DIAGNOSIS

GALLI-GALLI DISEASE (acantholytic variant of Dowling-Degos Disease)

- Additionally has suprabasilar acantholysis, clinically indistinguishable

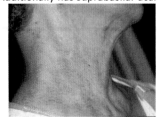 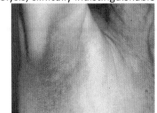

Brown, reticulate, coelescing macules on neck and axilla

Path Presenter

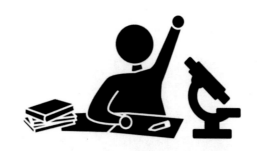

ACE MY PATH
Come Ace With Us!

CHAPTER 26: DISORDERS OF
KERATINIZATION

ANGELA JIANG, MD
POOJA SRIVASTAVA, MD

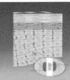
DISORDERS OF KERATINIZATION

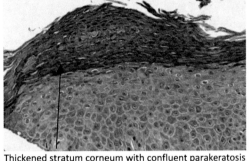

Thickened stratum corneum with confluent parakeratosis and preservation of granular layer

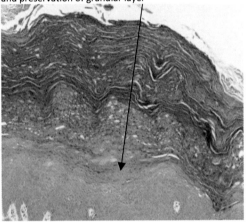

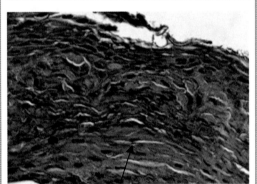

Retained keratohyalin granules within the stratum corneum

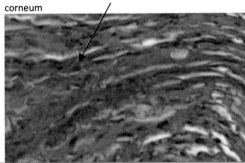

AXILLARY GRANULAR PARAKERATOSIS

CLINICAL FEATURES

- **Pruritic, hyperkeratotic brown-red** papules and plaques, commonly in axilla
- Can occur in other **intertriginous** areas
- Most commonly affects **adult women**

HISTOLOGIC FEATURES

- Thickened stratum corneum with **confluent parakeratosis and increased eosinophilic staining**
- **Retention of keratohyalin granules** in the stratum corneum
- **Preservation of stratum granulosum**
- Minimal superficial perivascular lymphocytic inflammation

OTHER HIGH YIELD POINTS

- Hypothesized to be caused by a defect in **filaggrin** metabolism causing **retention of keratohyalin granules**
- May be associated with an **irritant contact dermatitis**
- Can be treated with keratolytic agents such as topical and systemic retinoids, topical ammonium lactate, topical and systemic antifungals. Destructive therapies such as cryotherapy have been effective
- Spontaneous resolution can occur

DIFFERENTIAL DIAGNOSIS

- Tinea cruris – septate hyphae within the stratum corneum, highlighted by PAS or GMS stains
- Inverse psoriasis – neutrophils within the stratum corneum, hypogranulosis

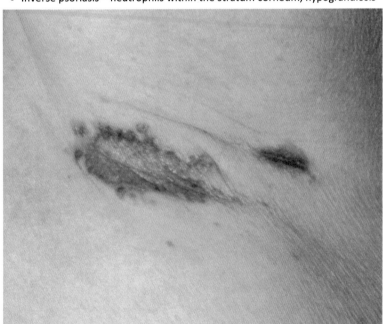

Hyperkeratotic brown-red papules and plaques

Path Presenter

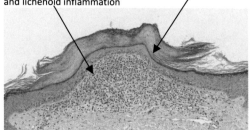

Compact hyperkeratosis overlying an atrophic epidermis and lichenoid inflammation

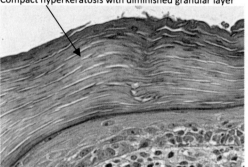

Compact hyperkeratosis with diminished granular layer

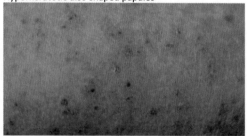

Hyperkeratotic disc-shaped papules

HYPERKERATOSIS LENTICULARIS PERSTANS (FLEGEL'S DISEASE)

CLINICAL FEATURES

- Small (1-5 mm), red-brown, asymptomatic, hyperkeratotic **"disc-shaped"** papules
- Typically presents on the **distal extremities** (dorsal feet and lower legs), including the palms and soles
- Larger papules often have peripheral collarettes of fine scale
- Begins in **adulthood** and persists

HISTOLOGIC FEATURES

- Discrete zones of **compact lamellar hyperkeratosis** and parakeratosis overlying an **atrophic epidermis**
- Underlying superficial **lichenoid** lymphoid infiltrate with occasional dyskeratosis. Infiltrate is CD8 predominant

OTHER HIGH YIELD POINTS

- Autosomal dominant, but can develop sporadically
- Absent or altered **lamellar granules (Odland bodies)** of keratinocytes on electron microscopy. Lamellar granules influence stratum corneum desquamation

DIFFERENTIAL DIAGNOSIS

- Kyrle disease – keratin plug and inflammatory material perforating through the epidermis
- Porokeratosis – cornoid lamellae with underlying dyskeratosis will be present
- Lichen Nitidus – should lack the hyperkeratosis and generally has a collarette of epidermis surrounding the lichenoid inflammation
- Atrophic lichen planus – hyperorthokeratosis with wedge-shaped **hypergranulosis** and epidermal atrophy

Path Presenter

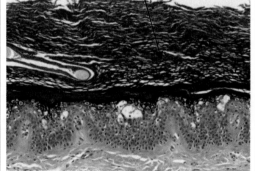

Thickened stratum corneum with confluent parakeratosis

Path Presenter

EPIDERMOLYTIC HYPERKERATOSIS

CLINICAL FEATURES

- **Epidermolytic ichthyosis (bullous ichthyosis, bullous congenital ichthyosiform erythroderma)** initially presents with large erosions, mild scaling, and **erythroderma at birth**
- After several months, the erosions are replaced by hyperkeratosis with **thickened corrugated scale, especially prominent at the flexures**
- Moderate adherent white-brown scale can develop in a generalized distribution or preferentially over frictional areas

HISTOLOGIC FEATURES

- Marked compact to basket-weave hyperkeratosis with variable parakeratosis
- Upper spinous layer with **large keratohyalin granules**
- Increased eosinophilia of the keratinocytes with **epidermolysis**

OTHER HIGH YIELD POINTS

- **Autosomal dominant** disorder
- **Keratin 1 and Keratin 10** gene mutation
- At birth, management is to monitor for sepsis
- In adulthood, therapies are targeted towards managing the hyperkeratosis such as emollients, humectants, oral retinoids

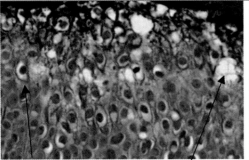
Vacuolization of the granular layer and epidermolysis

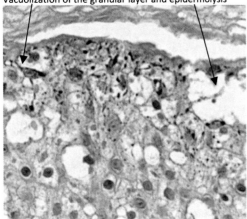
Hyperkeratosis with absent granular layer

- Changes of epidermolytic hyperkeratosis may be observed in other entities, such as an **epidermal nevus**. If this is observed, there is an increased risk of **epidermolytic ichthyosis** in offspring
- **Epidermolytic palmoplantar keratoderma (Vorner syndrome)** will have the same histopathological findings and is associated with **Keratin 1 and Keratin 9** mutations

DIFFERENTIAL DIAGNOSIS

- Warts – papillomatosis and koilocytic change, lacking epidermolysis
- Acantholytic dyskeratotic disorders (Darier's disease, Grover's disease, warty dyskeratoma) – keratinocytes are rounded and lack spinous connections

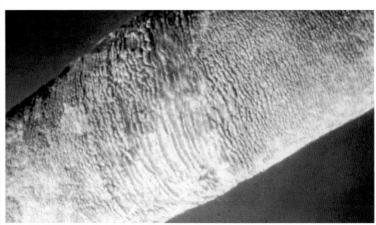
Corrugated scale of the flexural surface

ICHTHYOSIS VULGARIS

CLINICAL FEATURES

- **Onset in infancy**
- **Diffuse dry scale**, most prominently on the extensor extremities and often associated with **accentuated skin lines of the palms**
- Often **spares the flexures**
- Larger scale can be observed on the lower legs

HISTOLOGIC FEATURES

- Mild to moderate **compact hyperkeratosis**
- **Diminished to absent granular layer**
- Follicular plugging
- Diminished adnexa-sebaceous glands and eccrine glands

OTHER HIGH YIELD POINTS

- **Autosomal dominant**
- Associated with loss of function of **filaggrin** mutation
- Associated with **keratosis pilaris and atopic dermatitis**

DIFFERENTIAL DIAGNOSIS

- Tinea corporis – septated hyphae within the lower stratum corneum, often with brisk dermal inflammation
- Tinea versicolor – spores and hyphae in the upper stratum corneum
- Erythrasma – vertical fine filaments within the stratum corneum
- Vitiligo – decreased density of melanocytes along the dermal-epidermal junction
- Amyloid – light pink deposits within the superficial papillary dermis
- Argyria – small black granules in the sweat glands
- Pityriasis rotunda – can present with orthohyperkeratosis and diminished stratum granulosum, typically has increased pigmentation of the basal keratinocytes and mild superficial perivascular lymphocytic inflammation

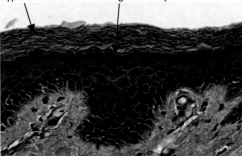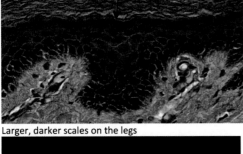
Larger, darker scales on the legs

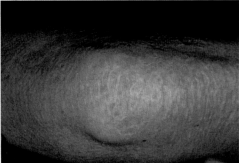
Path Presenter

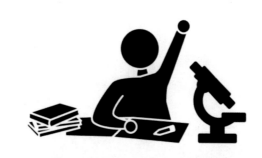

ACE MY PATH
Come Ace With Us!

CHAPTER 27: DEPOSITIONAL
DISORDERS

LORENA MAIA CAMPOS COSTA, MD

CUTANEOUS MUCINOSIS

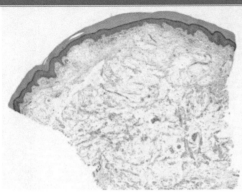
Empty spaces filled with mucin

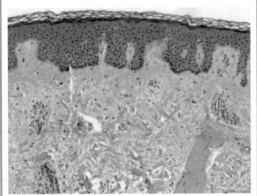
Mucin may appear as wispy, faint blue threads between collagen bundles

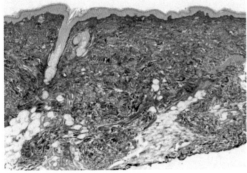
Colloidal iron: mucin deposits involving the full thickness of the dermis

Path Presenter

PRETIBIAL MYXEDEMA

CLINICAL FEATURES

- Localized deposition of mucin in skin of patients with autoimmune thyroid disease, mainly in Grave's disease, especially those with exophthalmos
- Thick, pink, yellow and waxy, sharply circumscribed plaques, and nodules
- Often in pretibial skin, but it could occur in other sites exposed to frequent trauma
- Indurations with prominence of follicles, typically have 'peau d'orange' appearance and secondary hypertrichosis is occasionally present
- Asymptomatic or mildly pruritic
- Typically resolves spontaneously, though in rare patients, lesions may progress to involve legs, feet, or hands completely, resulting in a severe form of elephantiasis with multiple polypoid and fungating nodules

HISTOLOGIC FEATURES

- Large amount of dermal mucin deposits causing separation of collagen bundles
- Mucin appears as wispy, faint blue threads on routine H&E
- Deposit of mucin involves the full thickness of the dermis
- Epidermis is usually hyperkeratotic with follicular plugging and may show papillomatosis and acanthosis in verrucous lesions
- Satellite fibroblasts are evident, but no increase in number except in elephantiasis form
- Increased collagen may be seen in chronic lesions

SPECIAL STAINS

- Hale colloidal iron and Alcian blue demonstrates mucin deposition

DIFFERENTIAL DIAGNOSIS

SCLEROMYXEDEMA

- Mucin deposition in superficial and mid dermis, increased fibroblasts, and fine collagen fibers deposition

SCLEREDEMA

- Thickened dermis with increased spaces filled with mucin between collagen bundles filled with mucin
- Deep dermis mucin deposits with no inflammation and normal fibroblasts

FOCAL CUTANEOUS MUCINOSIS

- Well demarcated, dome shaped papule containing a pool of mucin in the dermis

SUPERFICIAL ANGIOMYXOMA

- Prominent myxoid stroma with hypocellular proliferation of bland spindle fibroblasts
- Multiple thin-walled blood vessels, may have perivascular neutrophils

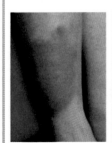
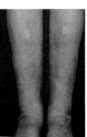
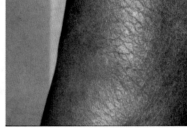

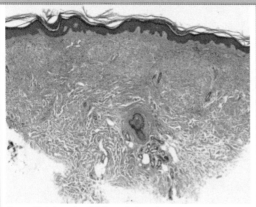

Superficial and mid dermis involvement

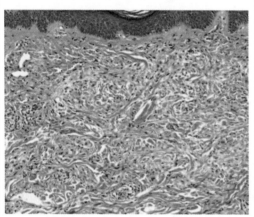

Mucin, spindle fibroblast and fine collagen fibers

Path Presenter

Path Presenter

SCLEROMYXEDEMA

CLINICAL FEATURES

- Small papules that coalesce into plaques with diffuse sclerosis of the skin
- Distribution: face, neck, forearm, hands
- Progressive skin thickening and folds, that can involve almost the entire body
- Localized variant known as Lichen Myxedematosus
- May have spontaneous resolution
- Associated with immunoglobulin (Ig) G lambda gammopathy

HISTOLOGIC FEATURES

- Interstitial mucin deposition in superficial and mid dermis
- Increased disorganized fibroblastic proliferation in papillary dermis
- Fine collagen fibers deposition
- Flat epidermis with atrophic pilosebaceous unit and mild superficial perivascular lymphocytic infiltrate may be seen in chronic lesions

DIFFERENTIAL DIAGNOSIS

NEPHROGENIC SYSTEMIC FIBROSIS

- Occurs in patients with renal failure
- Increased dermal mucin, spindled fibroblasts and nodules of collagen containing entrapped elastic fibers

GENERALIZED MYXEDEMA

- Large amount of mucin deposition involving full thickness dermis causing separation of collagen bundles
- Satellite fibroblasts are evident, but no increase in number

SCLEREDEMA

- Thickened dermis with increased spaces filled with mucin between collagen bundles
- Deep dermis mucin deposits with no inflammation and normal fibroblasts

INTERSTITIAL GRANULOMA ANNULARE

- Granulomatous inflammation surrounded by interstitial mucin

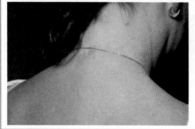 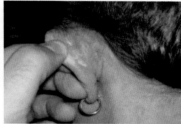

SCLEREDEMA

CLINICAL FEATURES

- Also called Scleredema of Buschke
- Symmetrical, asymptomatic, non-pitting edema with dermal induration
- Most often affects the upper back skin and may involve upper extremities with sparing of hands and feet
- Usually associated with insulin-dependent diabetes mellitus
- Less frequently associated with monoclonal gammopathy, streptococcal pharyngitis, and viral infections

HISTOLOGIC FEATURES

- Normal epidermis
- Thickened reticular dermis, often at expense of subcutaneous fat
- Broadened collagen fibers with interstitial mucin deposits, most prominent in deep dermis
- Normal amount of fibroblast and no inflammatory infiltrate
-

Thick dermis with deep dermal mucin

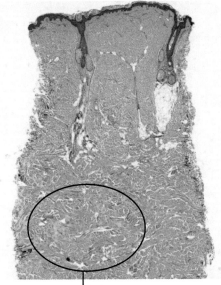

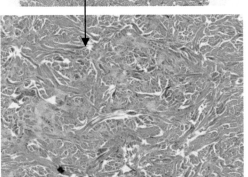

Mucin between normal collagen fibers

OTHER HIGH YIELD POINTS

- Mucin may not be present in all lesions and histologic features may be subtle
- The only clue would be the increased spaces between collagen bundles in deep dermis

DIFFERENTIAL DIAGNOSIS

MORPHEA

- Early lesions with perivascular, periadnexal, and interstitial lymphocytic infiltrate
- Developed lesion showing hypertrophic and crowded collagen bundles with atrophy of adnexal structures

SCLEROMYXEDEMA

- Mucin deposition in superficial and mid dermis, increased fibroblasts, and fine collagen fibers deposition

GENERALIZED MYXEDEMA

- Large amount of mucin deposition involving full thickness dermis causing separation of collagen bundles
- Satellite fibroblasts are evident, but no increase in number

NEPHROGENIC SYSTEMIC FIBROSIS

- Occurs in patients with renal failure
- Increased dermal mucin, spindled fibroblasts and nodules of collagen containing entrapped elastic fibers

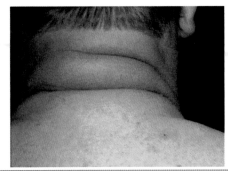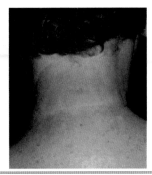

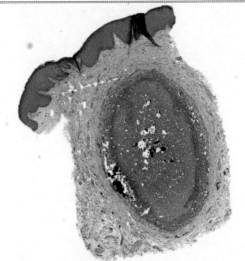

Well-circumscribed, dark blue to purple, amorphous deposit in the dermis

CALCINOSIS CUTIS

CLINICAL FEATURES

- There are four forms of calcinosis cutis; idiopathic, dystrophic, metastatic and iatrogenic
- Subepidermal calcified nodule: idiopathic, single, small nodule usually seen on face of child and commonly around eye
- Scrotal calcinosis: idiopathic, multiple, asymptomatic nodules, older males
- Dystrophic: most common subtype, calcium deposits in previously damaged tissue
- Metastatic: associated with hypercalcemia or hyperphosphatemia
- Calciphylaxis: Ulcerated skin with black eschar, violaceous reticulated plaques on posterior limbs
- Iatrogenic

HISTOLOGIC FEATURES

- Amorphous or crystalline, basophilic, often fractured deposits within the dermis and subcutis
- May be surrounded by granulomatous reaction and/or fibrosis
- Subepidermal calcified nodule: deposits located predominantly in the upper dermis, pseudoepitheliomatous hyperplasia with frequent transepidermal elimination of calcium
- Scrotal calcinosis: acellular, purple, well-circumscribed dermal nodules surrounded by smooth muscle bundles

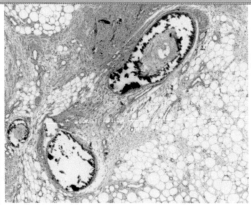

Calciphylaxis: calcification of small-sized vessel in the subcutaneous

Path Presenter

- In metastatic and dystrophic: calcium presents as granules or small deposits in the dermis or massive deposit in the subcutis
- Calciphylaxis: calcium deposits in small vessels of the dermis and subcutis, with thrombosis, panniculitis often with necrosis

SPECIAL STAINS

- Von Kossa' s silver stain calcium black and Alizarin red stain calcium red

DIFFERENTIAL DIAGNOSIS

GOUT

- Crystalline extracellular amphophilic lipid deposits
- Foamy macrophages dispersed through dermis

ERUPTIVE XANTHOMA

- Crystalline extracellular amphophilic lipid deposits
- Foamy macrophages dispersed through dermis

OXALOSIS

- Yellow-brown, birefringent, radially oriented needle shaped crystals deposits in reticular dermis and subcutis

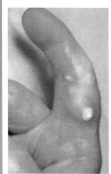 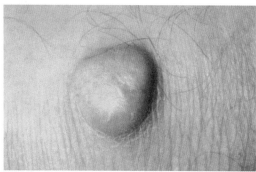

CUTANEOUS OSSIFICATION

CLINICAL FEATURES

- Bone formation in the skin may be primary or secondary within a preexisting lesion such as trauma, neoplastic or inflammatory diseases
- Osteoma cutis: rare primary cutaneous ossification
- Solid, skin-colored subcutaneous nodules of variable sizes and shapes
- Face of females and scalp in males
- May be associated with Albright's hereditary osteodystrophy, progressive osseous heteroplasia, and Gardner's disease

HISTOLOGIC FEATURES

- Dense eosinophilic deposits in the dermis or subcutaneous tissue
- Osteocytes within small lacunae, haversian canals, and osteoclast may be seen
- Transepidermal elimination can occur
- Marrow spaces may be present

DIFFERENTIAL DIAGNOSIS

OSTEOCHONDROMA

- Lamellar bone with mature cartilage

CALCINOSIS CUTIS

- Amorphous or crystalline, basophilic, calcium deposits within the dermis and subcutis

DERMAL OSTEOSARCOMA

- Ill-defined with pleomorphic, hyperchromatic cells
- Osteoid and bone formation produced by tumor cells, without interposition of cartilage

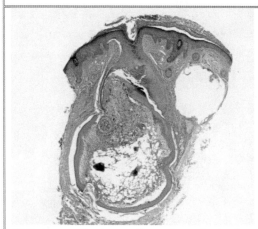

Well-circumscribed area of bone formation in the dermis

Path Presenter

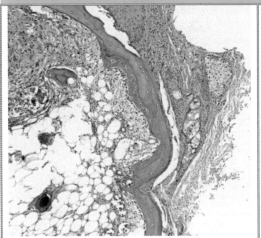

Mature, well-formed bone with central marrow spaces and fatty connective tissue

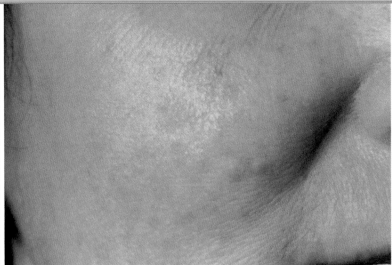

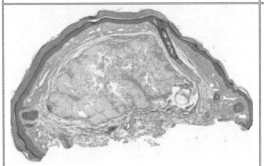

Well circumscribed nodule of amorphous pale eosinophilic deposit within the dermis

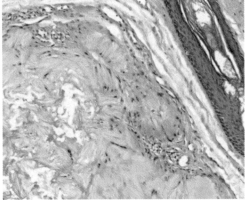

Pale eosinophilic material with palisading histiocytic infiltrate

Path Presenter

GOUT

CLINICAL FEATURES

- Disorder of uric acid metabolism that affects joints, bones, skin, and soft tissues
- Can present as acute or chronic arthritis or tophaceous gout
- Yellow, solitary, or multiple grouped papules and/or nodules
- Typically appears over bony prominences such as fingers joints and elbows
- Other sites: ears, extensor surface of extremities, trunk
- Skin ulceration can be present
- Tophi commonly involve olecranon bursa and Achilles tendon

HISTOLOGIC FEATURES

- Deposits of uric acid crystals composed of amorphous, feathery, weakly eosinophilic material within the dermis and subcutaneous tissue
- Palisading granulomatous infiltrate surrounding amorphous material
- Residual needle-shaped empty spaces of crystals may be seen

OTHER HIGH YIELD POINTS

- Uric acid crystals show negative birefringence under polarizing light microscopy if tissue is fixed in ethanol and processed without water-soluble chemicals
- Positive with Von Kossa; DeGalantha is more specific

DIFFERENTIAL DIAGNOSIS

CALCINOSIS CUTIS

- Amorphous or crystalline, basophilic, calcium deposits within the dermis and subcutis

NODULAR AMYLOIDOSIS

- Large and fissured amorphous pale pink nodular deposits with prominent plasm cells frequently present

COLLOID MILIUM

- Homogeneous, pale eosinophilic, fissured colloid masses filling the papillary dermis

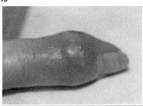

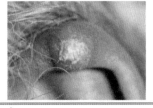

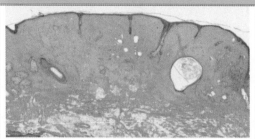

Nodular amyloidosis: large dermal deposit of amorphous pale eosinophilic material

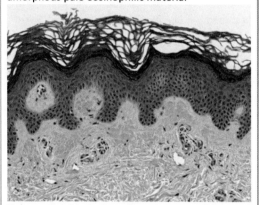

Lichen amyloidosis: hyperkeratosis, acanthosis and sparse deposits of pale pink amorphous material in the papillary dermis

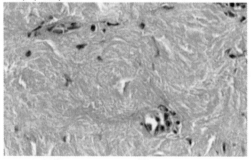

Path Presenter   Path Presenter

AMYLOIDOSIS

CLINICAL FEATURES

- Three main forms of primary localized cutaneous amyloidosis: macular amyloidosis, lichen amyloidosis and nodular amyloidosis
- Affects both genders, but macular amyloidosis is more common in females
- 4th to 6th decade of life
- Macular and lichen amyloidosis are keratin derived deposition associated with frequent trauma and sun exposure (amyloid fibril protein type AK)
- Nodular amyloidosis is a light-chain derived deposition produced by plasma cells and may or may not be associated with systemic amyloidosis (amyloid fibril type AL)
- Macular amyloidosis: red to dusky pigmented macules arranged in a reticulated pattern over the upper back, and infrequently chest and upper limbs. Pruritus is associated
- Lichen amyloidosis: multiple small red to brown keratotic papules and lichenified plaques over the anterior legs and less frequently extensor surfaces of upper extremities, back and head
- Nodular amyloidosis: solitary or multiple brown waxy nodules over the acral sites such as distal limbs, head, and neck

HISTOLOGIC FEATURES

- Amyloid deposits are composed of amorphous and pale eosinophilic material
- Macular amyloidosis: subtle deposits in the papillary dermis with pigment incontinence and occasionally melanophages
- Lichen amyloidosis: Similar to macular amyloidosis with hyperkeratosis and acanthosis
- Nodular amyloidosis: large nodular deposits in dermis and subcutaneous with admixed plasm cells frequently present

SPECIAL STAINS

- PAS Positive
- Congo red stain amyloid brick red with apple green birefringence under polarized light
- Pagoda red no 9 stain amyloid red and is more specific
- Thioflavin T shows an intense yellow-green fluorescence under fluorescent microscope
- Crystal violet: metachromatic staining

DIFFERENTIAL DIAGNOSIS

PORPHYRIA

- Amorphous hyaline deposits around the superficial dermal capillaries

LIPOID PROTEINOSIS

- Concentric hyalin deposits around capillaries, sweat gland and dermis

COLLOID MILIUM

- Homogeneous, pale eosinophilic, fissured colloid masses filling the papillary dermis

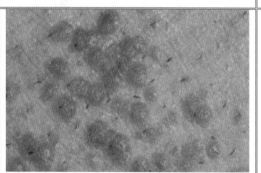

LIPOID PROTEINOSIS

CLINICAL FEATURES

- Rare autosomal recessive disorder
- Papular and nodular lesions on the face, may cause pitted scars (pigskin-leather appearance)
- Characteristic string of pearls on eyelid margin (moniliform blepharosis)
- Diffuse infiltration associated with hyperkeratosis observed in elbows, knee, hands
- Verrucous plaques can form in areas of friction
- Diffuse infiltration of the tongue and vocal cords resulting in hoarseness
- Convulsive seizures are common due to calcification of hippocampus

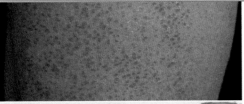

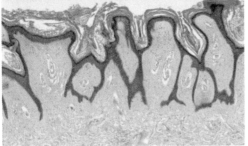

Hyperkeratosis, papillomatosis, concentric deposits around vessels and in the upper dermis

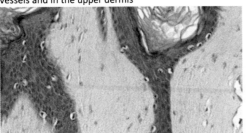

Thick bundles of hyaline deposits perpendicularly oriented to the skin surface

Path Presenter

HISTOLOGIC FEATURES

- Hyperkeratosis and occasional papillomatosis
- Eosinophilic hyaline deposits surrounding capillaries, sweat gland and also throughout papillary dermis
- The thick bundles are perpendicularly oriented to the skin surface (vertical streaking)
- Concentric deposits around vessels and adnexal (onion-skin pattern)
- Focal deposits found in the deeper dermis
- Periodic acid-Schiff-positive and diastase resistant deposits

DIFFERENTIAL DIAGNOSIS

ERYTHROPOIETIC PROTOPORPHYRIA

- Amorphous hyaline deposits around the superficial dermal capillaries. Sweat gland deposits is rare and dermal deposits not present
- Lipoid proteinosis is much deeper and more extensive than porphyria

AMYLOIDOSIS

- Pale pink amorphous deposits, Congo red stain positive

JUVENILE HYALINE FIBROMATOSIS

- Uniform, round to spindle cells without atypia
- Deposit of PAS + diastase-resistant, hyalinized, pale, amorphous material

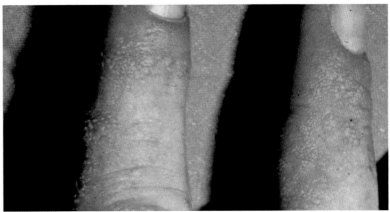

Lipoid proteinosis: papules on the fingers of the hands

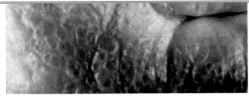

Light brown waxy papules

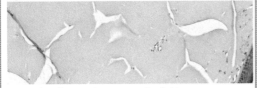

Fissured pink amorphous mass of colloid

Path Presenter

COLLOID MILIUM

CLINICAL FEATURES

- Numerous small, round, or angular, skin-colored to yellow-orange, white or light brown, waxy papules
- Face, neck, and dorsal hands
- Adult type: most common, precipitated by sun exposure
- Juvenile type: onset before puberty, clinically indistinguishable from adult type. Lesion appears before development of sun damage

HISTOLOGIC FEATURES

- Homogeneous, pale eosinophilic, fissured colloid masses filling the papillary dermis
- Adult type: Grenz zone of connective tissue separating the deposits from the overlying epidermis. Solar elastosis usually seen at the base and periphery of deposits
- Juvenile type: characteristic basal cells apoptosis (colloid bodies) in overlying epidermis
- Colloid is PAS positive and diastase resistant

OTHER HIGH YIELD POINTS

- Colloid in the adult type is of dermal origin and can stain weakly with amyloid stains

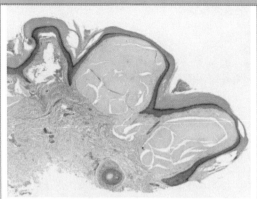

Colloid milium: Papular deposit of homogeneous, pale-pink material in the papillary dermis

- Colloid in the juvenile type is of epidermal origin, usually negative for Congo red but positive with antikeratin antibodies

DIFFERENTIAL DIAGNOSIS

NODULAR AMYLOIDOSIS

- Pale pink amorphous deposits, Congo red stain positive. May have more prominent dermal involvement compared to papular architecture of colloid milium

LIPOID PROTEINOSIS

- Concentric hyalin deposits around capillaries, sweat gland and dermis
- Perpendicularly oriented to the skin surface

PAPULAR MUCINOSIS

- Well demarcated, dome shaped papule containing a pool of mucin in the dermis

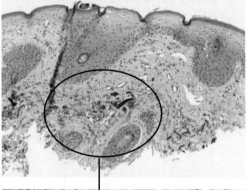

Yellow-brown, banana-shaped fibers

Ochronosis: erythema and mild blue-gray hyperpigmentation

OCHRONOSIS

CLINICAL FEATURES

- Discoloration of collagen-containing tissues due to homogentisic acid accumulation and deposition
- Exogenous or iatrogenic ochronosis: most common, induced by exogenous applied substances, such as hydroquinone and phenols
- Three clinical stages of exogenous ochronosis: erythema and mild blue-gray hyperpigmentation; macular hyperpigmentation with pinpoint "caviar-like" lesions; papulonodular hyperpigmented lesions. Localized to the area where the substance is applied
- Alkaptonuria: autosomal recessive disorder, due to lack of homogentisic acid oxidase enzyme
- Pigment deposition in alkaptonuria is disseminated and usually observed in sclera, tympanic membranes, cartilage (such as ear, nose), joints. Discoloration of skin of thenar and hypothenar eminences, axillary and inguinal areas may be seen

HISTOLOGIC FEATURES

- Ochre pigment deposition in the papillary dermis forming glassy, yellow-brown, banana-shaped fibers
- Elastic and collagen fiber disorganization and degeneration
- Pigment incontinence and melanophages and multinucleated giant cells may be seen in dermis
- Colloid milia, sarcoidal granulomas and transepidermal elimination of pigment may be observed in exogenous ochronosis

DIFFERENTIAL DIAGNOSIS

POSTINFLAMMATORY HYPERPIGMENTATION

- Melanin pigment incontinence and melanophages in dermis without ochre deposits

MELASMA

- Increase melanin in all epidermal layers and increase number of melanosomes among keratinocytes. No dermal pigment deposit

TATTOO

- Exogenous black or multicolor granular pigment material within the cytoplasm of histiocytes or free in the dermis

Path Presenter

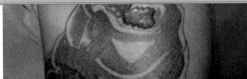

Exuberant granulomatous reaction

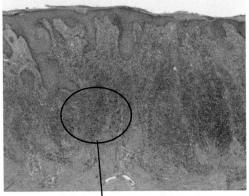

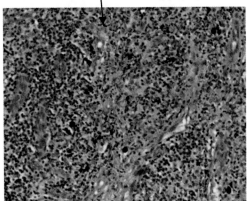

Black, irregularly shaped, granular tattoo pigment can have granulomatous inflammation

Path Presenter

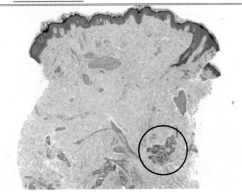

TATTOOS

CLINICAL FEATURES

- Clinical features is related to the type of inflammatory reaction present
- Granulomatous reaction presents with papules, plaques or nodules
- Pseudolymphoma-like lesions presents as erythematous or violaceous nodules
- Allergic contact dermatitis produce a vesicular or scaly rash with papules and plaques
- Hypertrophic scars and keloids may be associated

HISTOLOGIC FEATURES

- Tattoo pigments are easily visualized in tissue sections
- Exogenous black or colored, irregularly shaped, granular pigment
- After several weeks, they localize around vessels in the upper and mid-dermis in macrophages and fibroblasts
- Extracellular deposits of pigment are also found between collagen bundles; the pigment is generally refractile
- Inflammatory reactions may or may not be associated
- Granulomatous reactions may be either sarcoidal type, foreign-body type or rarely tuberculoid with caseation
- Non-granulomatous inflammation includes a perivascular lymphocytic infiltrate with pigment containing macrophages; a lichenoid reaction with band-like lymphocytic infiltrate with vacuolar change, necrotic keratinocytes and pigment incontinence
- Pseudolymphomatous lesions shows a dense nodular or diffuse, predominantly lymphocytic infiltrate, with well-formed germinal centers may be associated
- Combined reactions patterns such as lichenoid granulomatous dermatitis may be seen and is more frequent with red tattoo ink

DIFFERENTIAL DIAGNOSIS

MELANOCYTIC NEOPLASMS

- Exogenous granular pigment may be mistaken for heavily pigmented melanocytic neoplasms
- Melanocytic proliferation with variable degree of atypia
- Positive stains for melanin and melanocytic markers, such as Fontana-Masson and immunoperoxidase

SARCOIDOSIS

- Well-defined, non-caseating granulomas with few to no surrounding inflammation (naked granulomas)
- Clinical evaluation required because sarcoidal granulomas secondary to tattoo may be indistinguishable from true sarcoidosis occurring in the site of tattoo

ARGYRIA

CLINICAL FEATURES

- Prolonged exposure to silver through topical application (localized argyria) or via ingestion (systemic argyria)
- Blue-gray pigmentation to the skin, most notable in sun-exposed areas
- Mucosa and nail bed can be affected
- Develops with years of exposure
- Localized argyria: occupational exposure with silver containing substances, silver sulfadiazine creams, eye drops, dental amalgam with silver, silver earrings
- Systemic argyria: occupational exposure due to ingestion of dust during processing of silver, dietary supplements containing silver
- Silver pigment may stimulate melanogenesis in presence of light, worsening hyperpigmentation

Normal epidermis with minute black silver granules outlining membranes of sweat glands, not very well appreciated in this magnification

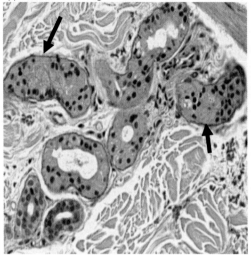

Minute black silver granules, outlining basement membrane of sweat glands

Path Presenter

- Permanent and irreversible

HISTOLOGIC FEATURES
- Normal epidermis
- Minute black silver granules in dermis, usually outlining basement membrane of sweat glands and in the lamina propria of vessels
- Granules may also be present adjacent to elastic fibers, in perifollicular sheath, and nerves

DIFFERENTIAL DIAGNOSIS

TATTOO
- Exogenous black or multicolor, irregularly shaped, granular pigment material within the cytoplasm of histiocytes or free in the dermis
- With or without chronic inflammation response

OCHRONOSIS
- Ochre pigment deposition in the papillary dermis forming glassy, yellow-brown, banana-shaped fibers

BLUE NEVUS
- Normal epidermis with dendritic melanocytes with heavy pigmentation in a sclerotic stroma in the dermis
- Absence of dark granules

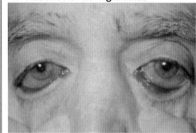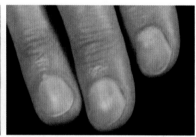

Argyria: Mucosa and nail bed are affected with blue grey pigmentation

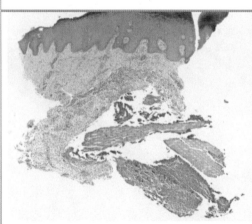

Splinter surrounded by granulomatous reaction, with brown fragments of degenerated plant material with honeycomb pattern of cell walls

Path Presenter

SPLINTER

CLINICAL FEATURES:
- Small speck of wood under the skin, usually in hands and feet
- Associated symptoms include pain, redness, swelling, warmth or pus

HISTOLOGIC FEATURES
- Brown fragment of degenerated plant material with honeycomb pattern of cell walls
- There may be abscess formation, granulomatous infiltrate, and/or inflamed granulation tissue in the adjacent dermis
- Contaminating microorganisms may be present

OTHER HIGH YELD POINTS:
- Perform stains for bacteria and fungi is judicious to exclude contaminating organisms

DIFFERENTIAL DIAGNOSIS

SUTURE
- Birefringent braided filaments surrounded by granulomatous foreign body inflammation

RUPTURED FOLLICLE CYST
- Remnants of keratin or squamous cells are often present surrounded by variable inflammation

POLY-L-LACTIC ACID
- Polarizable spiky translucent particles

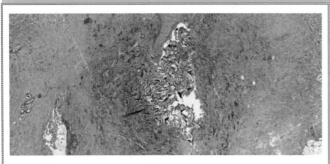

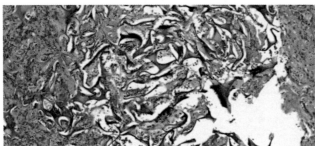

Uniformly homogenous, blue-purple, netlike pattern within fibrillar bands of pink collagen

Path Presenter

GEL FOAM

CLINICAL FEATURES:

- Gel foam is a gelatin material commonly used in dermatologic surgery to obtain hemostasis
- Usually is an incidental histopathological finding following cutaneous surgery
- Typically, no clinical lesion

HISTOLOGIC FEATURES

Gel foam appears uniformly homogenous, blue-purple, netlike pattern within fibrillar bands of pink collagen

- Deposits may be located in the dermis or percolating through the epidermis
- Granulomatous reaction surrounding the deposit and/or mixed inflammation (histiocytes, lymphocytes, eosinophils, neutrophils, and plasma cells)
- Adjacent dermal scar may or may not be identified

DIFFERENTIAL DIAGNOSIS

HYALURONIC ACID

- Absence of prior gel foam application
- Angulated basophilic dermal deposits in variable size and Shape. May be surrounded by granulomatous reaction

ALUMINIUM CHLORIDE

- Absence of prior gel foam application
- Light gray-blue granules, usually within histiocytes, underlying a scar

TRIAMCINOLONE

- Absence of prior gel foam application
- Lake of light blue amorphous material, may be surrounded by histiocytic inflammation, typically localized within hypertrophic scar or keloid

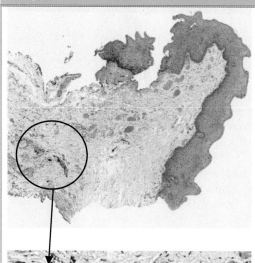

Brown black granular pigments deposited on connective tissue fibers, histiocytes and around blood vessels

Path Presenter

AMALGAM

CLINICAL FEATURES:

- Amalgam is a commonly used dental filling material containing silver, mercury and tin
- Usually occurs after accidental implantation during dental procedures
- Gray-blue asymptomatic small macules on the buccal, gingiva, and alveolar
- mucosa
- Borders may be well defined, irregular or diffuse

HISTOLOGIC FEATURES

- Brown-black granular pigments free in the dermis or deposited on connective tissue fibers, histiocytes or around blood vessels
- Mast cell infiltration is commonly seen
- Lichenoid reactions or multinucleated giant cell reaction, less frequently observed

DIFFERENTIAL DIAGNOSIS

ORAL MELANOCYTIC MACULE

- Increased melanin in basal cell layer of the epithelium with melanin incontinence in the superficial connective tissue
- Multifocal presentation may be seen in a systemic disease, such as Addison disease or Peutz-Jegher syndrome

DRUG RELATED HYPERPIGMENTATION

- Melanin pigment noted in basal cells and melanophages, and incontinent pigment is present in superficial connective tissue
- Brown-yellow granules in connective tissue
- Histologic features similar to melanotic macule

SUBMUCOSAL HEMORRHAGE

- Hemosiderin in the connective tissue from trauma
- Positive for Prussian blue

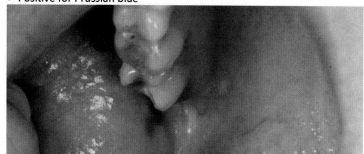

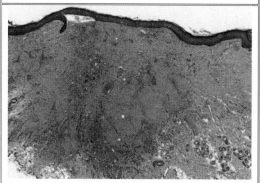

Horizontal fibrosis with collagen necrosis, and ferrugination of fibrin, dermal collagen, and striated muscle fibers

MONSEL SOLUTION

CLINICAL FEATURES:

- Ferric subsulfate solution used in dermatologic surgery to obtain hemostasis
- Monsel's solution produces artifacts that can be troublesome if rebiopsied
- Irregular brown macular area of hyperpigmentation within scar

HISTOLOGIC FEATURES

- Epidermis can be unremarkable or have reactive changes
- Epidermal effacement and horizontal fibrosis with collagen necrosis
- Ferrugination of fibrin, dermal collagen, and striated muscle fibers
- Brown-black pigment in dermis and in siderophages – large polygonal, multinucleated, and sometimes atypical histiocytes with clumps of refractile dark golden-brown fine pigment
- Adjacent dermal scar may or may not be identified

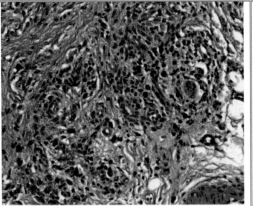

Siderophages – large polygonal, multinucleated, and sometimes atypical histiocytes with clumps of refractile dark golden- brown fine pigment

Path Presenter

SPECIAL STAINS

- Iron stain (Perl's method) is strongly positive, distinguishing the pigment from melanin

DIFFERENTIAL DIAGNOSIS

NODULAR MELANOMA

- Absence of prior biopsy or use of Monsel solution
- Preferential growth in the dermis rather than epidermis
- Melanin pigment is non refractile
- Positive for S100, Melan-A, SOX10 and other melanocytic markers

ATYPICAL FIBROXANTHOMA

- Absence of prior application of Monsel solution
- Hemosiderin deposition may be present
- Highly atypical and pleomorphic dermal proliferation of spindled to epithelioid cells
- Multinucleated giant cells may be seen

SPINDLE CELL VARIANT OF SQUAMOUS CELL CARCINOMA

- Absence of prior Monsel solution application
- Proliferation of invasive atypical spindle shaped keratinocytes often with areas of keratinization
- Absence of hemosiderin deposition
- Positive for Cytokeratins and p63

SILICONE IMPLANTS

CLINICAL FEATURES

- Silicone implants are used in soft tissue augmentation, such as breast implants and injectable cosmetic fillers
- Can cause local, distant, or immunologic reactions
- Leakage can occur after trauma to breast and may migrate to distant sites
- Breast implants: nodules in skin and soft tissue months to years following surgery. May have axillary nodules or along the lymphatic chain
- Injectable fillers: erythema, edema, or hyperpigmentation early after the implantation. Nodules may appear weeks to months after the injection

HISTOLOGIC FEATURES

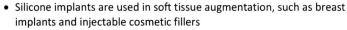

Empty variable-sizes vacuoles

- Empty variable-sizes vacuoles ("swiss cheese" appearance)-dimethicone dissolves out during processing
- Clear silicone may occasionally be seen in the vacuoles
- Vacuoles can be localized in dermis, subcutaneous tissue, or deeper soft tissues
- Granulomatous inflammation with foreign-body giant cells, lymphoplasmacytic infiltrate and variable fibrosis

DIFFERENTIAL DIAGNOSIS

PARAFFINOMA

- Similar histologic features to silicone implants but with more prominent fibrosis and sclerosis

POLY-L-LACTIC ACID

- Polarizable spiky translucent particles

HYALURONIC ACID

- Angulated basophilic dermal deposits in variable size and shape. May be surrounded by granulomatous reaction

Swiss cheese appearance

Path Presenter

Path Presenter

PARAFFINOMA

CLINICAL FEATURES

- Implantation or injection of paraffin under the skin, sometimes oils, Vitamin E, Grease gun lubricant
- Custom among Asian population to enlarge penis

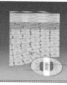
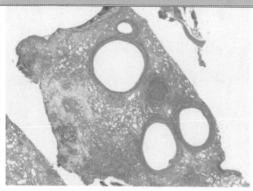

Empty vacuoles of variable sizes in a sclerotic stroma

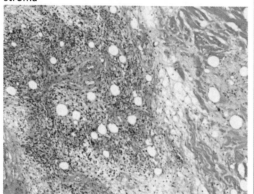

Empty vacuoles surrounded by granulomatous inflammation with foreign-body giant cells and fibrosis

- Palpable subcutaneous firm plaques and nodules
- May cause fistulas or ulcers

HISTOLOGIC FEATURES

- Empty vacuoles of variable sizes in a sclerotic stroma
- Vacuoles can be localized in dermis, subcutaneous tissue, or deeper soft tissues
- Granulomatous inflammation with foreign-body giant cells and fibrosis surrounding the inserted material

DIFFERENTIAL DIAGNOSIS

LIPOSARCOMA

- Mature adipocytes intermixed with atypical spindle cells or multipolar stromal cells with hyperchromatic nuclei
- Paratesticular soft tissue is a common location

SILICONE GRANULOMA

- Similar histologic features with less fibrosis and sclerosis

FAT NECROSIS

- Usually secondary to trauma
- Ghost outlines of necrotic adipose tissue with foamy histiocytes, chronic inflammatory cells and multinucleated giant cells

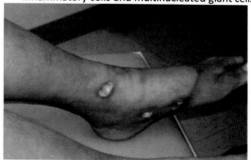

HYALURONIC ACID

CLINICAL FEATURES:

- Commonly used as injected cosmetic fillers
- Reaction to injected material may present with nodules, plaques, and discoloration overlying injected areas

HISTOLOGIC FEATURES

- Angulated acellular basophilic dermal deposits in variable size and shape
- May be surrounded by foreign body granulomatous reaction with multinucleated giant cells and dermal fibrosis

DIFERENTIAL DIAGNOSIS

CALCIUM HYDROXYLAPATITE

- Blue-gray spheres with granulomatous inflammation
- Calcium is positive with von Kossa stain

POLY-L-LACTIC ACID

- Polarizable spiky translucent particles

SILICONE GRANULOMA

- Empty variable-sizes vacuoles in dermis, subcutaneous tissue, or deeper soft tissues, surrounded by foreign body granulomatous inflammation
- Absence of basophilic material

Path Presenter

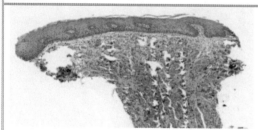

Angulated acellular basophilic dermal deposits in variable size and shape

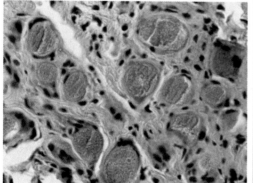

Angulated acellular basophilic dermal deposits in variable size and shape

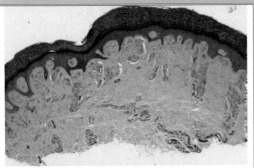
Hyaline cuffs around superficial blood vessels

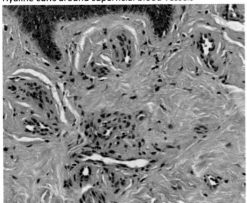
Hyaline cuffs around superficial blood vessels

Path Presenter

ERYTHROPOIETIC PROTOPORPHYRIA
CLINICAL FEATURES:

- Disorder of porphyrin metabolism associated with deficiency of ferro chelatase
- Photosensitivity with erythema, edema, and burning pain with sun exposure
- Waxy thickening of the face and knuckles
- Erosions and shallow scars on the face
- Increased protoporphyrin in blood and feces
- Normal urine porphyrins

HISTOLOGIC FEATURES

- Amorphous hyaline material around the superficial dermal capillaries, forming a cuff around these vessels
- Variable thickening of the blood vessel walls
- PAS positive, diastase resistant
- Positive for laminin, collagen IV, and immunoglobulin light chains on immunohistochemistry

DIFFERENTIAL DIAGNOSIS

LIPOID PROTEINOSIS

- The hyaline material involves the superficial and deeper vessels as well as eccrine glands

PORPHYRIA CUTANEA TARDA

- Demonstrates smaller hyaline deposits around superficial vessels associated with solar elastosis
- May have caterpillar bodies, subepidermal bullae, and festooning

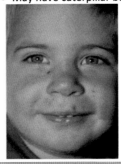
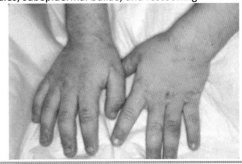

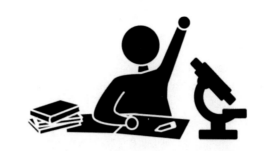

ACE MY PATH

Come Ace With Us!

REFERENCES AND
SUGGESTED READING

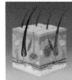

- Ronald P Rapini: Practical Dermatopathology 3rd Ed, Elsevier, 2021
- J Eduardo Calonje & Thomas Brenn & Alexander J Lazar & Steven D Billings: McKee's Pathology of the Skin, 5th Ed, Elsevier, 2020
- James W Patterson: Weedon's Skin Pathology, 5th Ed, Elsevier 2021
- Klaus Busam: Dermatopathology: A Volume in the Series: Foundations in Diagnostic Pathology 2nd Ed, Elsevier, 2015
- Steve Billings, Jenny Cotton: Inflammatory Dermatopathology: A Pathologist's Survival Guide 2nd ed Springer 2016
- Werner Kempf & Markus Hantschke: Dermatopathology 1st Ed, Springer, 2008
- Dirk M Elston MD, Tammie Ferringer MD, Christine Ko MD, Steven Peckham MD, Whitney A High MD JD MEng, David J DiCaudo MD: Dermatopathology: Expert Consult - Online and Print 3rd Ed, Elsevier, 2018
- Barnhill's Dermatopathology, Fourth Edition 4th Edition
- Raymond Barnhill, A Neil Crowson, Cynthia Magro, Michael Piepkorn, Heinz Kutzner, Garrett Desman: Barnhill's Dermatopathology, Fourth Edition 4th Ed, McGraw Hill, 2023
- Elder DE, Massi D, Scolyer RA, Willemze R WHO Classification of Skin Tumors 4th Ed, Volume 11, 2018

Made in the USA
Middletown, DE
17 March 2024

51487040R00210